The Human Disease

How We Create Pandemics, from Our Bodies to Our Beliefs

Sabrina Sholts

Foreword by Lonnie G. Bunch III

The MIT Press
Cambridge, Massachusetts
London, England

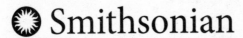 Smithsonian

The MIT Press would like to thank the anonymous peer reviewers who provided comments on drafts of this book. The generous work of academic experts is essential for establishing the authority and quality of our publications. We acknowledge with gratitude the contributions of these otherwise uncredited readers.

This book was set in ITC Stone Serif Std and ITC Stone Sans Std by New Best-set Typesetters Ltd. Printed and bound in the United States of America.

Library of Congress Cataloging-in-Publication Data

Names: Sholts, Sabrina, author.
Title: The human disease : how we create pandemics, from our bodies to our beliefs / Sabrina Sholts ; foreword by Lonnie G. Bunch III
Description: Cambridge, Massachusetts : The MIT Press, [2024] | Includes bibliographical references and index.
Identifiers: LCCN 2023018028 (print) | LCCN 2023018029 (ebook) | ISBN 9780262048859 (hardcover) | ISBN 9780262377935 (epub) | ISBN 9780262377928 (pdf)
Subjects: MESH: Pandemics | Disease Transmission, Infectious—history | Anthropogenic Effects | Social Factors
Classification: LCC RA643 (print) | LCC RA643 (ebook) | NLM WA 105 | DDC 614.4—dc23/eng/20231103
LC record available at https://lccn.loc.gov/2023018028
LC ebook record available at https://lccn.loc.gov/2023018029

10 9 8 7 6 5 4 3 2 1

For David and Issac

Contents

Foreword

In late 2019, reports out of China began to circulate about what looked like a troubling new pneumonia. By January 2020, the novel coronavirus, or COVID-19, had been identified and had spread to the United States. By February, it was clear that this pandemic was going to be a major world-wide crisis.

Of all the challenges I could have anticipated when accepting the responsibility of leading the Smithsonian, a pandemic would not have been high on my list. Perhaps I should have been more prepared for the eventuality, given Sabrina Sholts's 2018 exhibition at the National Museum of Natural History, *Outbreak: Epidemics in a Connected World*. Its prescient theme was the certainty of another pandemic and the critical role humans' behaviors would play in both its spread and response.

When the quickly evolving information about COVID-19 began to come in, I had to determine the best course of action for the Institution. As a historian, my first instinct was to look to historical precedents that the Smithsonian has had to navigate, such as the 1918 influenza pandemic and outbreaks of typhoid and scarlet fever in Washington, DC.

As much as history can be a guide, though, no analogy in the past is perfect. Science has drastically changed our understanding of communicable disease during the 176 years of the Smithsonian's existence. But as scientific knowledge has grown, so has the subsequent technological advances it has allowed, giving pathogens the means to travel around the globe with us, unwelcome partners on our vacations and business trips.

I knew if we were going to get through the pandemic and all its effects, we would need to lean on the doctors and scientists at the Smithsonian who were not only informing the medical community at large, our staff, and our public but also helping us chart a course to navigate this unprecedented crisis.

I had full confidence in our COVID-19 team's ability to lead us to the safest possible outcome, and they did. In accordance with CDC and WHO guidelines, they created protocols that mitigated risk, educated staff and visitors, and provided vaccines.

We could not simply hunker down and wait for the storm to pass, though. The Smithsonian has a responsibility to the nation and the world. To continue fulfilling our mission, a full team effort was needed. As the world shut down, we needed to become nimbler, more savvy with technology, more creative in our programming and exhibitions. Our curators, IT experts, researchers, scholars, and educators—including Sabrina and the rest of the *Outbreak* team—worked with singular purpose to use our resources to combat COVID-19 misinformation, to help keep students engaged and informed, and to give hope and solace in a time of profound hardship and sorrow.

It was truly a Smithsonian-wide effort like none I had ever seen—not just at our museums, research facilities, and education centers in the DC region, but across the country and world. The experience proved that the Smithsonian is unique in its ability to provide a comprehensive view of contemporary issues by using history to contextualize current events and using scientific discovery to foster understanding about the natural world.

The Human Disease is fully in keeping with that tradition, a holistic look at pandemics through the broad sweep of history. It is told from a scholar's perspective and with scientific precision, all illustrated through deft storytelling. But at its heart is the profound insight that each of us holds the key to resilience despite our most daunting shared challenges. I hope the main takeaway for everyone who reads Sabrina's terrific book is that even though we have not experienced our last pandemic, we can help each other survive by leading with our humanity.

Lonnie G. Bunch III
Secretary of the Smithsonian Institution

Prologue: An Empty Museum

Over the course of my career as a biological anthropologist, I've doubled back to my lab or office for many reasons: to change a sample, check an instrument, retrieve a hard drive, grab a book, and so on. It's a fairly common happening for any scientist, especially a forgetful one, regardless of your specific field or place of work. But for one at a natural history museum, it's a reentry into a wondrous place. Navigating the quirks of a century-old building, I might see the fossilized remains of a dinosaur if I glanced left or those of an ancient whale if I looked up. Truthfully, I usually don't even notice. Too often I'm hurrying past them without pause, my eyes and thoughts on something modern and probably mundane. After all, it's not like I won't be back again tomorrow, right?

On March 16, 2020, it was different. When I returned to my office in the Smithsonian's National Museum of Natural History (NMNH) in Washington, DC, beckoned by an unemptied trash can in my office, I took none of my surroundings for granted. I had come back to retrieve a banana peel, haunted by the cascading consequences of fruit decay that I envisioned in my absence. Seriously, I really did. And with every step through the museum, I took a mental snapshot for my memory bank. I had no idea when I'd see any of it again.

Only days before, on March 11, the World Health Organization (WHO) declared that the worldwide spread of a novel coronavirus, named SARS-CoV-2, was a pandemic. It was a pronouncement that many people, including me, thought was already weeks overdue. Then, that evening, US president Donald Trump abruptly declared a travel ban on visitors to the United States from Europe. I was in London at the time, and flew back to Washington amid a transatlantic wave of confused and panicked travelers the next day. By the time that I landed at Dulles International Airport, the Smithsonian had announced the temporary closing of all of its museums to the public. Restricted access for employees was imminent and indefinite.

Like so many of the impacts of COVID-19, the disease caused by SARS-CoV-2, the shuttering of the Smithsonian in March 2020 was unprecedented. The impacts of the 1918 influenza pandemic, which caused an estimated fifty to hundred million deaths in less than two years, didn't even come close. First off, there were only three Smithsonian museums at that time, compared to nineteen museums today. Furthermore, even though the NMNH opened with great fanfare as the United States National Museum (USNM) in 1910, it was already closed to the public by 1918 due to the US entry into World War I. At the request of US president Woodrow Wilson and through the courtesy of the Smithsonian's Board of Regents, the building was placed at the disposal of the recently established Bureau of War Risk Insurance of the Department of the Treasury. Their need for space was met by the USNM, then Washington's second-largest building, where "stuffed animals and innumerable cases of historical exhibits were moved to make room for the patriots engaged in administration of the war risk insurance act."[1] From October 1917 to April 1919, thousands of federal clerks and makeshift desks were packed into repurposed exhibit halls, laboratories, and storage spaces, while the museum's scientific and administrative staff tried to continue their normal activities and duties on the floors above.[2]

The 1918 influenza pandemic goes unmentioned in the Smithsonian's annual reports from these years, despite many references to the impacts of World War I. But some information survives in correspondence from the Bureau of Public Health Service.[3] Even though the infectious agent of influenza was a mystery to health officials—scientists didn't confirm a virus as the cause until more than a decade later—they understood the flu as a crowd disease that spread between people via air and contaminated surfaces. To help protect the health of US government employees, numerous precautionary measures were recommended to the Smithsonian in October 1918: "flushing out" the USNM building with fresh air before employees arrived for work and during mandatory fifteen-minute recesses outdoors; maximum ventilation within reasonable comfort at all times; careful cleaning of the transmitters of all telephones with disinfectant solution twice a

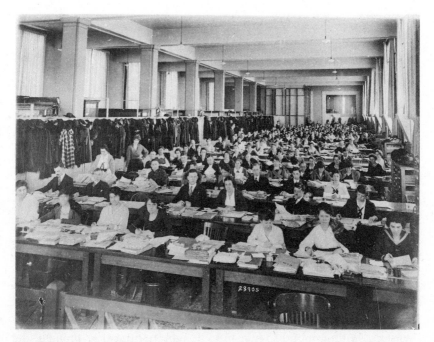

Figure 0.1
The Smithsonian during the 1918 influenza pandemic. Clerks of the Bureau of War Risk Insurance work at makeshift desks packed into areas not meant for offices, such as one of the display spaces of the US National Museum (now the National Museum of Natural History building) in 1918. *Source:* Smithsonian Institution Archives. Image # MAH-23905.

day; and the wearing of gauze masks covering the nose and mouth during business hours by all employees who worked indoors and whose duties necessitated coming in contact with a large number of people.

These directives came during an autumn surge in Washington, as District officials responded to the community spread of the deadly disease by canceling all public gatherings, closing churches and schools, and placing shops on a staggered schedule of operating hours.[4] Even the Smithsonian's National Zoo closed some of its animal houses to prevent influenza from spreading through the weekend crowds.[5]

On the afternoon of March 16, 2020, I was only beginning to realize the repetitions of history around me. As I crossed the Constitution Avenue lobby of the NMNH, a neoclassical behemoth of pale granite that flanks the National Mall for three city blocks, the emptiness was profound. The

Treasury clerks of 1918 were gone from the building, but so were the masses of visitors that have filled its galleries ever since, even those visitors who, in the preceding years, had come to our museum specifically for a lesson on pandemic risks.

*   *   *

Pandemics have been central to my work as a museum curator for about as long as I've held the position. I was hired as a research anthropologist and curator of biology anthropology at the NMNH in February 2014, when by coincidence, a terrible disease epidemic was unfolding in West Africa. Although Ebola virus disease (EVD) had been known and studied by scientists for decades, this situation was different. All the known EVD outbreaks since 1976 had been in central and eastern African countries. Yet in the forested areas of southeastern Guinea, a country of more than eleven million people on the Atlantic coast, an EVD outbreak had claimed dozens of lives by March.

From Washington, I followed the news of the growing crisis with apprehension. Within months, human-to-human transmission brought the deadly virus into the capital cities of Guinea and its neighboring countries, Liberia and Sierra Leone. A traveler from Liberia also carried the causal pathogen (commonly known as Ebola virus) to the capital city of Lagos in Nigeria, the largest metropolitan area in Africa. This terrifying development was another first: EVD had never before reached densely populated urban centers, where many health care facilities were soon overwhelmed with desperately ill patients. By August, with a rising death toll in the thousands, the WHO declared a Public Health Emergency of International Concern, recognizing that the disease could spread to other countries through regional and global travel networks. And it did. Before the end of the year, the virus was transported by road and air to seven more countries in Africa and Europe as well as the United States.

In the United States, there was a nationwide panic. In October, a traveler from West Africa died from EVD in a hospital in Texas, also infecting two nurses who cared for him. The nurses recovered, as did physician Craig Spencer, who was diagnosed with EVD in New York City after returning from treating EVD patients in Guinea. Although these were limited and largely nonfatal incidents, many people in the United States saw the disease as a grave and immediate threat. In a Gallup opinion poll in November

2014, the US public ranked EVD as the third most urgent health problem in the country, above diabetes, obesity, flu, and even cancer.[6] Misperceptions about how the disease spread, such as believing that someone can transmit EVD through casual contact without showing symptoms, had a lot to do with it. These false beliefs about the disease likely stemmed from a mistrust of institutions, according to a study of 179 public opinion polls about EVD, which reported that only 7 percent of people in the United States had "a great deal" of trust in US public health officials to share complete and accurate information about Ebola virus.[7] And the US media, by sensationalizing the EVD cases and criticizing the public health response to them, certainly didn't reassure anyone of their safety.

The bigger problem, in my view, was that lots of people were worried about the Ebola epidemic for the wrong reasons. In the United States, the odds of being infected with the virus, and much less dying from it, were vanishingly small. But the causes of its emergence and spread in West Africa should have been alarming to everyone. They were promises of more threats to come, and more communities at risk, no matter who you were or where you lived.

These misplaced concerns weren't only the result of fears, assumptions, and bad information. Unfortunately, there also wasn't a whole lot of *good* information that the public could easily access and understand, at least not in a way that folded the Ebola crisis into a larger story about our pandemic-prone species. Fortunately, I was given the chance to do something about it.

It came during the "Ebola Autumn" of 2014, as White House Ebola response coordinator Ron Klain later called it. That's when the NMNH decided to help the public understand the Ebola epidemic and the threats of others in the future. The idea came from infectious disease physician Daniel Lucey in August, the day before he flew to Sierra Leone to care for EVD patients there. Dan had been on the front lines of practically every major infectious disease epidemic since severe acute respiratory syndrome (SARS) in 2003. And along the way, he and his colleagues recognized an increasingly common origin: wild and domesticated animals. These diseases—SARS and EVD as well as many others that sounded alarms with growing frequency—were caused by pathogens from nonhuman animals (called zoonotic pathogens) that "spilled over" to humans through various interactions. These interactions were the kind of human activities and behaviors that change ecological relationships and encounters between people and

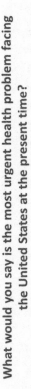

What would you say is the most urgent health problem facing the United States at the present time?

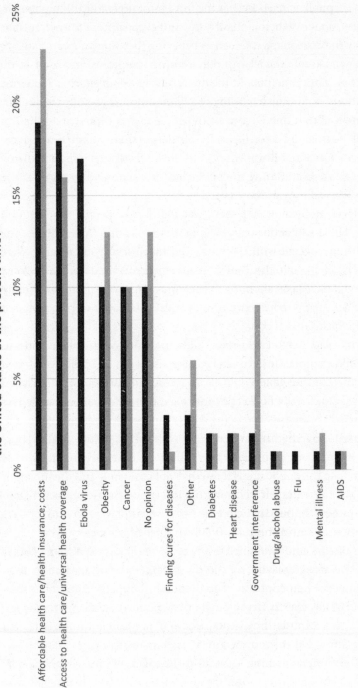

Figure 0.2
Ebola fears top US health concerns in 2014. EVD was ranked in the top three health problems facing the United States by a poll of people in United States in November 2014, in the month following four cases of EVD reported in the country. *Source:* Gallup, Inc. https://news .gallup.com/poll/179429/ebola-ranks-among-americans-top-three-healthcare-concerns.aspx.

our fellow organisms, such as industrialized food production, deforestation, and animal trade. It's a complicated story, but a seriously important one. And not enough people were hearing it.

Dan proposed that the NMNH create a major public exhibition in which the Ebola epidemic, and human health in general, was connected to animal and environmental health in an all-encompassing concept, "One Health." The museum agreed that One Health was a message that we were uniquely qualified to deliver given our mission to understand the natural world and the place of humans within it. And thus a large team and network of collaborators including Dan, with me as the lead curator, formed in 2015 to develop an exhibit that eventually became *Outbreak: Epidemics in a Connected World*. The exhibit opened in May 2018 with plans for a three-year run and high hopes about pandemic prevention. But in March 2020, like most everything in the world, the show came to a grinding halt.

When I walked out of the NMNH on March 16, 2020, uncertain of when or under what circumstances that I'd return, the last view that I tried to memorize was the *Outbreak* exhibit. For years, while it was being built and almost two years after it opened, I passed it daily as I walked up the marble staircase to my office on the floor above. On days when I really felt like *Outbreak* was doing some good and making a difference, I'd take a moment to look down on the gallery and all the visitors within it. But in that last long look, I could only hope that was true. Millions of people had visited the exhibit by that point. The COVID-19 pandemic would be a test of what, if anything, they had learned.

*   *   *

The next few months felt a waking dream, where things are both familiar and strange at the same time. All the ways that *Outbreak* explained how pandemics can disrupt and devastate people's lives—not only with respect to illness and death, but in their social, cultural, and economic consequences—were playing out in reality. Our carefully selected images and finely crafted descriptions of pandemics in the past, from face masks to overfull infirmaries to "an aura of fear" as portrayed by a survivor of the 1918 influenza, kept flashing through my mind like déjà vu. And the pandemic warnings and concerns that I'd heard *for years* from so many of our collaborators, on issues from One Health to international cooperation to health equity, were repeated by these people when I saw them again—not face-to-face, but on television.

As the COVID-19 pandemic continued to spread and worsen through 2020 and beyond, I understood why *Outbreak* had elicited so much help and enthusiasm from the professional community: it already saw another pandemic around the corner and wanted the public to be ready. Yet nobody could have predicted how catastrophic the crisis would become. Furthermore, the attacks on scientists, doctors, and public health officials trying to save lives, particularly in the United States, were like nothing that I ever would have imagined. Several of my colleagues received death threats.

Being a scientist myself, I did what I could to help. We couldn't access our labs and collections at the NMNH, which meant, ironically, that my colleagues and I couldn't move forward with our research on the evolutionary history of zoonotic pathogens such as influenza viruses and coronaviruses, which we planned to study using historic specimens of birds and bats at the museum. In my fruit-free office, the only thing happening was . . . dust. But our public education efforts for *Outbreak* continued despite the Smithsonian's physical closure, as we organized and offered more than a dozen free webinars on COVID-19, vaccines, and a variety of related topics.[8] These conversations gave me valuable insights into the status of both scientific and public knowledge about the evolving pandemic situation. They were the kind of interactions that happened every day and all the time in the exhibit gallery, where volunteers and guest experts were always on hand to explain topics and answer questions for our visitors. Without those in-person encounters, virtual engagement was the next best thing.

All over the world, scientists and science communicators were doing the same thing. And in one respect, some of them kept *Outbreak* going even while the NMNH was closed. That's because when we opened the exhibit in Washington in 2018, we also launched a free do-it-yourself tool kit called Outbreak DIY. Consisting of digital resources derived from or used for *Outbreak*, including information panels, videos, games, 3D models, and promotional materials as well as a how-to guide written by the *Outbreak* team, Outbreak DIY could be used by people anywhere for local One Health education. People didn't have to make other exhibits, but many of them did, in all kinds of ways and places that met their audiences where they were: libraries, parks, gardens, airports, beaches, hospitals, community health centers, markets, malls, conference venues, and yes, museums. Hundreds of versions of Outbreak DIY popped up in over fifty countries on almost every continent. We offered ten translations for the materials, including Arabic, Hindi, and Swahili, but some people did their own, such as in Burmese, Hebrew, and Korean. In addition, lots of Outbreak DIY users chose to create their own panels using our templates in order to focus their exhibits on the stories, issues, and people most relevant to their communities. And given that Outbreak DIY was distributed as digital files and adaptable to outdoor settings, the tool kit was practically pandemic proof. Thus even when COVID-19 was at its worst, which happened in countless ways at different times and places, Outbreak DIY continued to spread. To be honest, it was the only kind of spread that gave me hope.

Throughout all of this public education, the oft-used mantra of pandemics was loud, clear, and constant. *We're all in this together.* To some ears, it rang hollow. After all, for many people and places, such as those with front line exposure to disease risks or with back-of-the-line access to effective vaccines, COVID-19 was anything but fair. But in the sense of needing to work together across disciplines and borders to prevent pandemics, it was true. And the expression means something even more to me. Simply put, the problems that cause and come with pandemics are shared by everyone, no matter how or where we live. That's because we—people—are the most formidable problem of all.

*   *   *

As human beings, we tend to ascribe human characteristics to things that are nothing like us. We perceive faces in clouds, anger in storms, and terrible intentions in pathogens. Called anthropomorphism, this human universal makes the unknown seem more familiar and predictable. I believe this habit is misleading and sometimes unhelpful, though, when talking about pandemics because, let's face it, pathogens have no plan. They don't scheme and strategize, nor do they like and want. In fact, a virus is nothing more than a piece of genetic code in protein packaging, totally unable to function outside a host (that is, the organism in which it replicates). Viruses can't even move on their own, even though they're frequently described as "jumping" or "hitching a ride" to their hosts, as if—like humans—they had propulsive legs and prehensile hands. In cartoons they may borrow our behaviors, but in reality they have none of them.

The downside of projecting our own powers onto pathogens, by anthro-
pomorphizing them, is that we misdirect attention from our true oppo-
nent: ourselves. That's right, *Homo sapiens*. Although humans can wrongly
place our species at the center of every story and scenario in the universe
(another ism called anthrocentrism), we *absolutely* have a starring role
when the tale turns to pandemics. And by discounting all the ways that
humans cause and contribute to the cross-continental spread of infectious
disease, we deny ourselves enormous control over how these events unfold.
Because pandemics don't just happen. Humans make them happen. And
we will continue to make them happen. Yet how often they occur, how far
they go, how long they last, and how bad they get . . . much of this is in
our uniquely human hands. As unsettling a prospect as this may seem, it
should give us optimism: if we're the problem, then we're also the solution.
The more that we understand how humans cause pandemics, the better
equipped we are to do something about them.

In a nutshell, that's what this book is about: pandemics as a feature of
modern humanity. And so chapter by chapter, we're going to look at some
of the most common human traits, tendencies, and activities that double
as pandemic liabilities. My goal is to help you understand how a pandemic
is, by definition, a human disease.

One of the biggest concerns when it comes to the emergence of new
pathogens in the first place relates to our evolutionary and ecological relationships with other animals. The former extends into our deep history as
a species, but the latter reflects more recent turns, particularly toward agriculture and domestication. That's chapter 1.

Then there are the risks that are baked into our biology—the focus of
chapter 2. Talking and touching, for instance, increase opportunities for the
spread of many pathogens, helped by some human-specific brain and body
functions. But the everyday conditions in which many people live and
work, within dense and interconnected urban settings as no other species
does, can create the ideal conditions for rapid disease transmission among
and between communities. We examine these factors in chapter 3. In addition, as we see in chapter 4, humans also create social and cultural environments that compel us to gather—not just to talk and touch, but to eat, love,
and pray—in ways that make us feel human beyond the sum of our parts.
And in an epoch defined by human domination over the planet, our travel
and trade stretches across oceans, bringing pathogens and the animals who

carry them into new environments and naive populations. The so-called Anthropocene provides a framework for chapter 5.

Unfortunately, no matter where they are, people can increase transmission risks through misperceptions and social constructions of difference, magnifying the harm and spread of infectious diseases through the human-specific phenomena of xenophobia, racism, and stigmatization. At the same time, these processes can fuel mistrust and resistance to the very public health measures designed to flatten an epidemic curve. We take a closer look these issues in chapters 6–9.

Finally, chapter 10 focuses on misinformation, which often accompanies a new virus, and in the information age, spreads and mutates as quickly as one. This unique human talent is uniquely destructive to disease prevention and control efforts, and creates the greatest obstacles for science communication during a pandemic. The *Outbreak* exhibition, and now this book, are part of the epic battle against it.

This book is neither a history of plagues nor an encyclopedia of them. The early chapters address particular diseases and outbreaks more briefly than you'll find in some of the later chapters because they are integrated with information about microbes, evolution, and epidemiology for the readers who are new to these topics. The varying formats are intentional. Yet every chapter is filled with examples and accounts of past epidemics and pandemics in order to illustrate the human factors that long preceded the latest disease crisis. Each epidemic and pandemic deserves its own book, and many of them already have quite a few. As a devoted booklover, I give references and call out titles for the resources that I particularly recommend, and those whose authors provide more detail and depth that I can cover.

Stories are powerful tools for communicating information, despite the difficulties in condensing the trauma and suffering of epidemics into narrative form. Another difficulty is deciding which ones to write about, as the stories are countless. With the stories I tell in the following pages I've made my best effort to engage with the readers learning about these tragedies as well as to honor the people who lived them. These stories don't appear chronologically, and that's also by intention. As an anthropologist, I'm cautious about linear or directional representations of humanity through time. Therefore some epidemics, such as EVD in West Africa, are told across multiple chapters in different parts. Elsewhere, in back-to-back chapters, I write about two US epidemics a century apart: the bubonic plague and acquired immunodeficiency syndrome (AIDS). Both of these epidemics were part of global pandemics, and so they're just a small geographic slice of a much larger whole. I write more frequently about the United States than any other country, not to privilege or center one national experience over others, but simply because it's the one that I know best. Even so, I've tried to bring as much geographic and sociocultural diversity to this book as the subject of pandemics deserves.

Lastly, a few words about *we* and *us*. My goal in this book is for every reader to see themselves in it because it's about humanity writ large—and so the *we* and *us* are people in general. Not every person does every single thing or thinks in every which way that I describe. But many do. Likewise, not every community or country bears the same level of responsibility for the global patterns and processes that I discuss, such as the ones related to human-caused environmental change. The entire world, however, is still affected. I hope that across the chapters of this book, our shared challenges are felt that way. One thing that we have in common is that, well, we're all in this together. But there's a lot more than that. The challenges that I describe in this book are part of being human. In better understanding ourselves, through the prism of pandemics, I hope that we can better understand each other, too.

1 *Homo sapiens:* The Evolutionary Upstart

When news broke that a novel coronavirus had emerged in China, relatively few people in the world knew what those words meant. Most people had probably never heard of any sort of virus doing any such thing. Yet with an alarming capacity to surprise and spread, the never-before-seen pathogen was a wake-up call for the twenty-first century.

After setting off alarms with an outbreak of unusual pneumonia, the infections skyrocketed in a mystifying spectrum of manifestations, ranging from no symptoms to mild flu-like illness to acute respiratory distress. Doctors didn't recognize the pathogen, and neither did their patients' immune systems. Some people couldn't breathe on their own and required mechanical ventilation in intensive care units. Stories about mysterious and sudden deaths in hospitals began to circulate online and across the globe.

The novel coronavirus appeared to spread primarily via respiratory droplets between people. But a nonhuman animal origin was suspected, as several of the early patients had connections to a market where live animals were handled, butchered, and sold. It thus seemed most probable that cross-species transmission of the virus had occurred there. And eventually, scientists found similar viruses in several different animal species, with the closest match in a horseshoe bat, its likely source in nature.

Unsuspecting travelers, infected with the virus, carried it onto airplanes and across borders. Within weeks of the initial outbreak, dozens of countries around the world confirmed their first cases. Powerful and unprecedented, this new pathogen devastated economies, immobilized international trade and travel, and wreaked havoc on some public health systems.

By then, the disease had a name: severe acute respiratory syndrome. SARS for short. That's right, I'm not talking about SARS-CoV-2 here but rather its older cousin, SARS-CoV-1.

*   *   *

SARS shook the world. Or at the very least it shook the WHO, which used these words to open its official account of the epidemic, *SARS: How a Global Epidemic Was Stopped*, with a record scratch.[1] Following initial reports of the disease in Guangdong Province in late 2002, the WHO coordinated the international response to SARS, which resulted in nearly eight hundred deaths and over eight thousand cases in twenty-nine countries and territories, mostly within an unnerving period of seven months. SARS was the first emerging and readily transmissible disease of the twenty-first century, caused by the first human coronavirus ever known to manifest in severe illness. And after the virus was contained and disappeared, the WHO's lesson #1 was chilling: *We were lucky this time.*

I don't entirely agree. Some successful elements of the SARS response, like strong leadership and international coordination, had little to do with good fortune. Expertise and competence helped save the day. Also, the SARS virus (called severe acute respiratory syndrome coronavirus, or SARS-CoV-1) was anything but lucky for the people who became ill from it, most of whom were health care workers or patients in hospitals. With a fatality rate above 50 percent for patients aged fifty-five years and older, the virus was downright terrifying. But granted, things could have been a lot worse.

For example, the virus could have infected so many people and spread for so long that it became endemic (meaning constantly present) in certain parts of the world. And yet thankfully, some characteristics of SARS-CoV-1 made containment feasible. For starters, there was little or no asymptomatic transmission of the virus, meaning that people weren't really contagious until they began to show symptoms. Even then, SARS patients usually didn't transmit the virus until several days after the symptoms started, and they were most contagious when their symptoms turned severe, by the tenth day or so of illness. In addition, the incubation period (that is, the length of time between the initial infection until the appearance of symptoms) could last for a week or longer. These characteristics made it easier to trace contacts and isolate patients before they were able to infect anybody else, thus ending the chain of transmission.

The world faced a far greater challenge with COVID-19. The causal virus (dubbed severe acute respiratory syndrome coronavirus-2, or SARS-CoV-2) is so closely related to the SARS virus to be named after it, but it emerged with critical differences. Most significantly, asymptomatic transmission of SARS-CoV-2 is common. Plus infected people can be most contagious for days before showing symptoms or early in their illness, and therefore can transmit the virus without even knowing that they have it. These features gave SARS-CoV-2 some of its pandemic potential. But more than anything else, humans turned that potential into reality.

Disease emergence is a game of chance, and humans are constantly playing it. The name of the game? Evolution. As the process by which populations experience genetic changes over time, evolution is the machinery of natural history, whose workings give rise to new species, and cause them to vary across time and space. Humans wouldn't exist without evolution, and we continue to evolve today through mechanisms of *microevolution* (a term for evolutionary change within a species or group of organisms). For instance, as a human population adapts to the challenges of a new environment, beneficial traits may be passed down from parents to their children as heritable information in their DNA. This kind of adaptive evolution is driven by a mechanism known as *natural selection*, which naturalist Charles Darwin (who coined the term) also described as "survival of the fittest," meaning that individuals who are better suited to survive in a particular environment are more likely to reproduce and contribute genes to the next generation. Another evolutionary mechanism is genetic drift, where population changes from generation to generation occur through random events, such as when certain people survive a disaster that kills off everyone else. Natural selection and genetic drift, however, can only change the frequencies of genetic elements that already exist in the pool. Which is to say, they can't introduce entirely new traits into a population. The evolutionary mechanisms that *can* do this, and frequently do, are migration and mutation. The former is when people from genetically different populations meet and mate, resulting in exchanges of genes (called gene flow) that increase diversity in subsequent generations, while the latter is when the DNA sequence of a gene is altered by errors in its replication or repair.

In viruses, the evolutionary process is turbocharged. When viruses replicate, they do so in a rapid exponential fashion that generates millions of new virus particles and many genetic mutations, potentially leading to the "survival" of viruses that can better infect, replicate, and cause disease in a host. Mutation is one of the principal mechanisms by which genetic changes occur in viruses, such as when SARS-CoV-2 went from a single, wild type virus in 2020 to a series of alphanumeric variants and subvariants as the pandemic wore on. One reason that SARS-CoV-2 evolved so quickly is that it's an RNA virus (like influenza viruses, Ebola viruses, and many other notorious pathogens), meaning that its genetic material is RNA. Since the virus's hosts don't have enzymes that can correct for errors in RNA replication, its mutation rate is enormous. Recombination, the exchange of genetic material between different organisms, is another mechanism that generates diversity in viruses: multiple viruses can give rise to a new hybrid by co-infecting a single cell and exchanging genetic material.

This is why disease emergence is a gamble: the more opportunities for replication, mutation, and recombination, the more likely that a new virus with pandemic potential will emerge. My colleague Dennis Carroll, former director of the Pandemic Influenza and Other Emerging Threats Unit at the US Agency for International Development, likens the game to a slot machine. In his analogy, the evolution of a highly pathogenic virus that can easily infect and spread among humans is like hitting a triple-cherry jackpot: despite the slim chances, if we keep feeding quarters into the machine, eventually we're going to get three cherries in a row. Or three mutations. Which is all it would take for a highly pathogenic avian flu virus, specifically one known as H7N9, to become easily transmissible between people.[2]

Those who were shaken by SARS, such as the global health community, recognized that SARS-CoV-1 was possibly a few mutations away from a pandemic, and that every replication was another pull of the lever. The unshaken ones might not even remember or know anything about SARS—making COVID-19 a complete surprise for most people. And when SARS-CoV-2 kept spreading, with constant infections and mutations in people and other animals, more and more variants of the virus emerged as the COVID-19 pandemic wore on; with SARS, the situation was brought under control before this happened. Understanding how humans *create* the opportunities for new pathogens to suddenly appear among us, and how they can cause harm, is the enlightenment that all of us need. And it requires a thoughtful consideration of the unique place of humans within the natural world.

In this chapter, we're going to examine the broader context of disease emergence in order to clarify the position of humans therein. Microbes have been around for much longer than humans, as have most of the other species that can carry and transmit them to us. The evolutionary and ecological relationships through which these microbes mutate and spread can be friendly arrangements for some animals, but disastrous when we disrupt them. With an appreciation for the deeper history and present-day diversity of pathogenic threats, we can make smarter bets on a healthier and safer future.

Microbes and Friends

Any organism that can only be seen with a microscope is generally considered a microorganism or microbe. Thus in a historical sequence of scientific landmarks, the microscope came first. But like many human discoveries, microbes existed for ages before we knew about them. Actually, that's an understatement. They were the earliest organisms (that is, living creatures) on Earth, represented by traces of microbial life in rocks that are more than 3.5 billion years old. Knowing how they, and we, figure into our planetary past is critical for understanding human-pathogen relationships today.

If the history of Earth happened in a single day, with 4.5 billion years crammed into 24 hours, then the first few hours were pretty much unlivable.[3] At midnight, the planet was molten, sterile, and oxygen free, while under constant bombardment by asteroids and comets. This hot and hellish eon is known as the Hadean, named after the underworld of ancient Greek religion.

But by 4:00 a.m., as the planet cooled, and continents and oceans formed, the conditions became less hostile and more stable. In these pre-dawn hours, the earliest organisms developed as single-celled microbes, probably near hydrothermal vents (basically, underwater hot springs) at cracks in the ocean floor. This 2.5-billion-year eon, named the Archean from the Greek word for "beginning," thus gave rise to cellular life.

Bacteria and *Archaea* ruled the rest of the morning. These two domains of life are both prokaryotes, meaning that they're single-celled microbes that lack a nucleus and other membrane-bound internal structures, but differ in some genetic, metabolic, and structural aspects. Following their divergence from the last universal common ancestor, an inferred evolutionary link between the abiotic and biotic phases of Earth's history, some bacteria evolved into the first photosynthetic organisms.[4] This means that they could convert sunlight into energy and generate oxygen gas as a by-product. Appearing around 5:30 a.m., these cynobacteria led to the greatest change in the history of our biosphere. Oxygen continued to be released

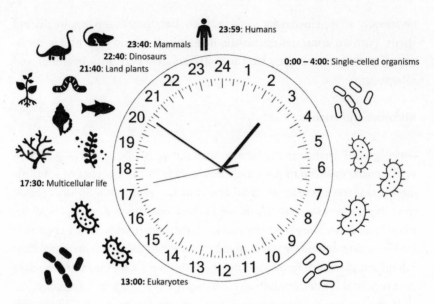

Figure 1.1
A condensed chronology of life on Earth. If the history of Earth were crammed into
24 hours, microbes would appear by 4:00 a.m. and humans at the stroke of midnight.

over millions of years and became abundant in the atmosphere by about
2.4 billion years ago, allowing for complex life-forms to evolve. By then, it
was nearly lunchtime.

From around 1:00 p.m. on, the rest of the day was dominated by the
evolution of *Eukarya*, the third domain of life that includes humans. The
first eukaryotes were single-celled like bacteria and archaea, but their cells
contained a nucleus and organelles. Multicellular organisms appeared by
around 5:00 p.m., but the first animals, such as sponges, didn't show up
in the oceans until 8:00 p.m. or so. There was an explosion of biodiversity
around 9:00 p.m., from which almost all modern animal forms began to
appear. Dinosaurs made a late-night cameo for about an hour.

Our earliest humanlike ancestors arrived only in the last couple minutes
of this eventful day, by around 5.8 million years ago. But modern *Homo
sapiens* were the ultimate latecomers. We crashed the party as the clock
struck midnight, about 300,000 years ago at least, almost a full day after
microbes arrived and hours after everyone else got acquainted.

This snapshot of biological history covers the origins of most microbes,
including bacteria, archaea, and eukaryotes (such as helminths, fungi,

protists, protozoa, and algae). But did you notice a missing guest? That's right . . . viruses. And that's because, at present, viral origins are a bit of a mystery.

Viruses aren't organisms, even though they're often classified as microbes, including in this book. They have a special place in biology, but none within the tree of life. The reason is that they're not alive. Essentially, a virus is a nucleic acid genome (that is, all the genetic information of a virus or organism, consisting of nucleotide sequences of DNA or RNA) wrapped in a protein coat. That's all, folks. Hence unlike humans, a virus has no means of metabolism or self-replication on its own. Instead, a virus has to infect a living cell and hijack its energy and molecular machinery in order to make copies of itself. That's why virologists Marc van Regenmortel and Brian Mahy say that viruses, at best, lead "a kind of borrowed life."[5]

Given that viruses depend on living cells in order to multiply, one might assume that viruses evolved from or after cellular organisms. This may be true, but the timing and nature of such an event is far from certain. One possibility (known as the reduction hypothesis) is that viruses were once complex intracellular parasites that lost their ability for independent metabolism and retained genes only for the functions that viruses have today.[6] In a different scenario, sometimes called the escape hypothesis, viruses evolved from genes that escaped from inside early cells and infected others. Notably, retroviruses such the human immunodeficiency virus (or HIV, the causal pathogen of AIDS) replicate through similar mechanisms by entering a cell and inserting their DNA within the genome of the host.[7] In fact, up to 8 percent of the human genome is composed of genetic sequences of retroviral origin, the relics of ancient infections that were experienced by our evolutionary ancestors over the last 100 million years.[8]

Yet another hypothesis of viral origins suggests that they preceded cells in the history of life on Earth. According to the primordial virus world hypothesis, viruses are direct descendants of primitive molecules that existed in the precellular stage of evolution, presumably in the early morning of our 24-hour chronology of planetary existence. If this is correct, as virologist Susan Payne points out, then our evolutionary history has been impacted by viruses since the earliest beginnings of cellular life.[9]

Even without knowing exactly when they arose or how, it's safe to say that viruses have existed on this planet for a long time. The fact that they infect all kinds of organisms, from every type of ecosystem and kingdom of life, points to an extreme antiquity.[10] Plus they exist and infect organisms in a huge array of forms, which we've only learned about since the twentieth century. Until then, we only knew the diversity of diseases that viruses and other microbes can cause.

To be clear, none of this means that individual microbes around *today* are billions of years old. Microbes mutate and multiply constantly, as often as they're killed or destroyed, and the new ones—like SARS-CoV-1 and SARS-CoV-2—are the biggest concern for people. But our slim summary of biological history has a simple takeaway: we are living in a microbial world. And figuring that out is one of the smarter things that we've done as a species.

*   *   *

The first person to describe microbes, after viewing them at hundreds of times their actual size, was Dutch tradesman-turned-microscopist Antoni van Leeuwenhoek in 1684. Peering through his handcrafted lenses, van Leeuwenhoek saw magnified scenes of bacteria and protists (which he named "animalcules") that lived in varied environments, ranging from pond water to his own mouth. He didn't know what they did, but he marveled at their multitudes. "The number of animals in the scurf of the teeth are so many," he wrote about his discovery of bacteria in dental plaque, "that I believe they exceed the number of men in a kingdom."[11]

Talk about an understatement. Today we know that microbes are everywhere on the planet, even in the most extreme environments, and that they account for more than 15 percent of Earth's total biomass.[12] We also know that most of the genetic diversity of Earth resides in viral genomes, which are ten times more abundant than the number of cells in all organisms.

But even within a single human body, millions of microbes can occupy a site no larger than a freckle. Every mammal plays host to enormous and essential communities of microbes called the microbiome, a diverse and dynamic part of your biology from birth until death. Thriving in the mouth, gut, and other body parts, these collectives of microbial colonists serve a variety of metabolic, protective, and regulatory functions throughout life. We describe them as commensal (which translates to "sharing a table" in Latin; more about this in chapter 4) because it's a win-win relationship in which all sides are served. And given that some resident microbial species

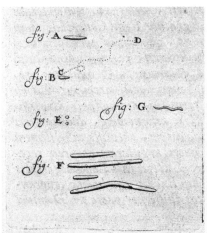
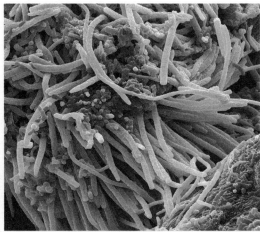

Figure 1.2
Left: Drawings of bacteria in the seventeenth century. The first observations of microbes by Antoni van Leeuwenhoek included his own sketches of bacteria in dental plaque. *Source:* Wellcome Collection. Arcana naturae detecta / Ab Antoni van Leeuwenhoek. **Right: Microscopic views of bacteria in the twenty-first century.** Today bacteria can be recorded in magnified images produced by high-powered electron microscopy. *Source:* Steve Gschmeissner / Science Photo Library.

have coevolved with their host species over millions of years, it's a partnership that can withstand the test of time.

The microbiome is thus an essential component of humanity. Usually its constituents and indeed most microbes on the planet can be harmless, if not helpful, to the health of host organisms. That's why recent alterations to the human microbiome due to changes in diet and antibiotic use have been linked to the increased prevalence of health problems like obesity and asthma.[13]

Microbes, however, get the most attention when they cause disease, which is when they're usually called pathogens. Some scientists think that we should stop using the term *pathogen* altogether because disease is just one of many possible outcomes from microbe-host interactions.[14] None of them are inherently "good" or "bad." In fact, microbes can be *both* commensal and pathogenic depending on the circumstances. For instance, the bacteria *Staphylococcus aureus* and *Escherichia coli* are commensals in many people, but also opportunistic pathogens under the right conditions. And as we'll discuss further, a microbe can be a pathogen for a human but cause no harm to a different host species. Although I've chosen to refer to disease-causing microbes as pathogens in this book, the objections to the word are duly noted.

Van Leeuwenhoek didn't make the causal link between microbes and diseases, although he experimented plenty with the wee beasties that he found and even figured out that wine vinegar could kill them. Back then, medicine was dominated by the miasma theory of contagion, which blamed infectious diseases on foul-smelling vapors from decomposing matter. Astonishingly, scientists didn't recognize the pathogenic potential of bacteria for nearly two more centuries.

Two scientists are best known for advancing the germ theory of disease, wherein microbes replaced miasmas in explaining how sickness could occur and spread. French chemist Louis Pasteur made countless bacteriologic breakthroughs during the second half of the nineteenth century, proving the role of microbes in fermentation, putrefaction, and the spoiling of food as well in causing illness. At the same time, German physician Robert Koch was equally prolific, formulating criteria to confirm a specific microbe as the agent of a specific disease. For instance, using his postulates, Koch announced that *Mycobacterium tuberculosis* was the bacterial agent of tuberculosis in 1882. As his evidence, guinea pigs (*Cavia porcellus*) infected with *M. tuberculosis* not only succumbed to the disease but also grew *M. tuberculosis* in their lungs, which Koch used to infect and transmit the disease to healthy individuals of the same species.[15]

Pasteur and Koch also developed tests, treatments, and vaccines for well-known diseases among humans and nonhuman animals, both bacterial and viral. Viruses weren't visually identified until the 1930s, after the invention of the electron microscope, because they're ten to a hundred times smaller than bacteria. But their rapid rates of replication and mutation were advantageous to experimentation, allowing early scientists to guide and indirectly observe their evolution across different organisms and species. Pasteur thus developed a method to attenuate (that is, weaken) pathogens by transferring infected material from a sick animal to a healthy one, again and again. Called serial passage, the pathogen adapted to new hosts and became less virulent to others, causing mild infection without severe disease. With experiments on dogs, monkeys, and rabbits, Pasteur weakened the rabies virus by serial passage and exposure to dry air, resulting in the first human vaccine produced in a laboratory. In 1885, the critical test of his vaccine, a nine-year-old boy bitten by a rabid dog, was celebrated as a lifesaving success.[16]

The prominence of animals in the development of germ theory shows that many of the diseases of greatest concern to nineteenth-century scientists were zoonotic, meaning that they originate in animals and spread between them. Furthermore, these investigations illustrated the diversity of host-microbe interactions among species. Pasteur's study of fowl cholera, for example, highlighted the importance of healthy carriers in the transmission of disease. Caused by the *Pasteurella multocida* bacterium (which Pasteur identified and named), fowl cholera infects a variety of animal species worldwide, with severe symptoms and death in some of them. Pasteur found that chickens and rabbits were equally susceptible to *P. multocida* infection, but guinea pigs showed a particular resistance, with no observable impacts on their health or appetite.[17] Yet chickens or rabbits living in contact with an infected guinea pig would suddenly become sick through cross-species transmission—also known as spillover—of the pathogen.

As early as the 1870s, it therefore became clear that one animal species could serve as a reservoir for infection in another species, including humans.[18] Humans themselves can be a *reservoir*, a common epidemiological term for a habitat or host in which an infectious agent normally lives, grows, and multiplies. This means that some people can be healthy and highly contagious at the same time, with no signs of infection except for the outbreaks that erupt in their wake. We'll meet one such individual in the next chapter. But first, there are other risky meetings to consider.

Disruptions and Disease

Generally speaking, a pathogen is classified as *emerging* when it newly appears in a population, or rapidly increases in incidence or geographic range. There are numerous ways this can happen among humans, and many of them involve interactions with other animals. That's because the majority of emerging pathogens are zoonotic, with more than 70 percent of them originating in wildlife. A lot of these pathogens have multiple animal hosts, both as reservoirs that enable their persistence within a community and as incidental hosts who aren't required to maintain them. Sorting out what's what is urgent business, especially as zoonotic pathogens have been emerging with increasing frequency since the twentieth century.[19]

Emerging pathogens are responsible for some of the most alarming disease events in recent decades, and represent a growing and significant threat to global health. If we consider the following examples of zoonotic pathogens that have emerged or reemerged from wildlife in recent decades, it's easier to see how humans play a notable and unique role in driving them through ecological changes as well as disruptions.

*   *   *

After a new coronavirus was discovered in SARS patients in early 2003, the pathogen still needed to be confirmed as the cause of the disease. When crab-eating macaques (*Macaca fascicularis*) were infected experimentally with the virus and showed similar symptoms as humans, Koch's postulates were fulfilled.[20] But animals provided a lot more information about disease than its etiology. They indicated where it came from and how it spread to humans too.

At first the medical community was stunned by the emergence of a new coronavirus with such serious effects on healthy adults.[21] Since the 1960s, human coronaviruses (named for their solar corona-like appearance in an electron microscope) had been known to produce only mild symptoms such as the common cold.[22] Veterinarians were less surprised, though. As early as the 1930s, they had recognized severe respiratory diseases and other illnesses caused by coronaviruses in a variety of animal species.[23] Also, they were familiar with the emergence of new coronaviruses from unknown reservoirs, often with fatal symptoms in immunologically naive animal populations.[24]

Because some of the first SARS patients in Guangdong were restaurant workers who handled wild mammals as exotic food, these animals were an early target for investigations into the source of the virus. In a live animal market, researchers found that at least three different animal species—masked palm civets (*Paguma larvata*), Chinese ferret badgers (*Melogale moschata*), and a common raccoon dog (*Nyctereutes procyonoides*)—were infected with a closely related virus that showed 99.8 percent similarity to SARS-CoV-1.[25] Some workers at the market also showed evidence of previous infection, especially those who dealt with animals. Among the people tested, antibodies for SARS-CoV-1 were detected in 40 percent of wild animal traders and 33 percent of animal slaughterers, compared to 5 percent of

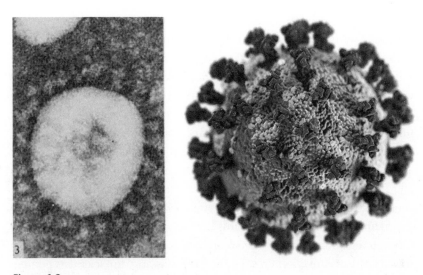

Figure 1.3
Left: The earliest imaging of a human coronavirus. Microscopy images of human coronaviruses were first published in a virology journal in 1967. *Source:* J. D. Almeida and D. A. Tyrrell, "The Morphology of Three Previously Uncharacterized Human Respiratory Viruses That Grow in Organ Culture," *Journal of General Virology* 1, no. 2 (1967): 175–178. **Right: A modern rendering of a human coronavirus.** Coronavirus images were everywhere during the COVID-19 pandemic, such as the illustration of SARS-CoV-2 created by the US Centers for Disease Control and Prevention (CDC) in 2020. *Source:* Alissa Eckert, MSMI, and Dan Higgins, MAMS/CDC.

vegetable traders. The conclusion? Between the market workers and menagerie of animals sold there, a lot of spillover was going on. And SARS was the unfortunate outcome.

The exotic animals sold at the market were hunted and raised on farms in order to meet the demands of a southern Chinese culinary tradition that considers them delicacies. The catlike civets, which have been farmed in China since the 1980s, accounted for the most infections of SARS-related viruses among all the market animals tested. Researchers found no evidence of widespread infections among farmed civets, however, suggesting that civets were most likely infected at live animal markets, where the overcrowding and commingling of various species were the perfect conditions for cross-species transmission.[26]

Civets became the mascot of SARS in China. Soon after market civets were identified as a likely source of human infections, the Guangdong government launched a campaign to cull all civets in the province to reduce the risk of transmission to people. More than ten thousand civets and other mammals were killed in early 2004—a move criticized by the WHO at the time. The culling not only prevented more extensive sampling from civets for SARS research, some opponents argued, but also had the potential to lead to a false sense of security. "For all we know," warned WHO official Julie Hall, "they could be an intermediary carrier."[27]

Well as it turned out, they were. In 2005, two teams of scientists announced evidence of SARS-CoV-like viruses in bats in southern China and Hong Kong, particularly among small, insect-eating species of horseshoe bats (*Rhinolophus* spp.).[28] Both teams declared that horseshoe bats were the natural reservoir of coronaviruses closely related to those responsible for the SARS outbreak and civets were most likely incidental hosts caught in the crossfire of contagion. In support of this scenario, the scientists pointed to experimental evidence of civets that showed clinical signs of SARS-CoV-1 infection, which wouldn't be expected in a natural reservoir host that had coevolved for a long time with the virus.[29] Civets were even suggested to be an amplifier host for SARS-CoV-1 that provided an effective environment for efficient interspecies transmissions.[30]

If bats are the origin of SARS, then they had to transmit their SARS-like viruses to civets or other animals in one way or another. Unfortunately, we don't know exactly how it happened. Both groups of scientists noted that spillover could have occurred in the wild, but more likely took place in live animal markets in southern China, where bats are sometimes sold for food and used in traditional medicine.[31] Given that many of the market vendors sold multiple animal species, caged close together, the opportunities for spillover were abundant. Wild and domesticated animals were suddenly face-to-face, shedding and sharing microbes through excretions and emissions, and forced into interactions that probably wouldn't happen in natural settings.

Bats made sense as the natural reservoir of SARS-CoV-1 for other reasons too. They account for about 20 percent of mammalian diversity worldwide, consisting of more than fourteen hundred species, and their genetic diversity creates diverse habitats for many viruses. They live longer than most other small mammals, and often in large, densely packed colonies, which gives them countless chances to acquire and transmit viruses. They're also the only mammal that's capable of sustained, powered flight, which allows them to travel long distances and carry viruses across their diverse, wide-spread homes. Some of their metabolic adaptations for flight may actually help them tolerate viral infections, as bats generally don't show disease symptoms from many of the viruses they carry. But this impressive resistance may reflect their coevolution with viruses over a longer period than many other mammals given that bats have been adapting to viruses for more than fifty million years.[32]

Today, bats are known as the reservoir host for numerous diseases prioritized by the WHO (due to their epidemic and pandemic potential), such as Nipah virus disease, EVD, Marburg virus disease, SARS, and Middle East respiratory syndrome (MERS).[33] Since the emergence of SARS-CoV-1 in 2002, coronaviruses have been detected in 16 percent of bat species, resulting in more than four thousand genetic sequences of bat coronaviruses on six continents.[34] Some of this diversity was highlighted in 2013, when one study reported that at least seven different SARS-CoV-like strains were circulating within a single colony of Chinese horseshoe bats (*Rhinolophus sinicus*), including some viruses with the ability to infect human cells through direct bat-to-human transmission.[35]

Coronaviruses are scary for numerous reasons, such as their ability to rapidly mutate and recombine, as when multiple viruses infect a single host cell and produce a different one. Their threats to human health have become increasingly obvious with the additional emergences of coronaviruses that cause MERS in 2012 and COVID-19 in 2019. We now know about three of them that infect and cause severe illness in humans through person-to-person transmission. And as long as we keep dropping quarters in the slot machine, the better the odds that more will be coming.

*   *   *

The same year that SARS swept around the globe, a much smaller and more localized outbreak offered similar warnings about mixing animals and their microbes. It wasn't just about animal trade but also species translocation. Moreover, the problem wasn't exotic foods but rather exotic pets.

Mpox was never detected in the Western Hemisphere before 2003. Most of the human cases had been documented in the Democratic Republic of Congo (DRC), where it was first recognized as a human disease called monkeypox in 1970, although it's endemic in both Central and West Africa.[36] Caused by the monkeypox virus (or MPXV for short), a close relative to the variola virus that causes smallpox and produces similar symptoms, this potentially fatal disease got its name by sickening a research colony of crab-eating macaques (*Macaca fascicularis*) in 1958. And herein lies the most important difference between mpox and smallpox: mpox is zoonotic. In fact, MPXV infects a broad range of mammalian taxa, whereas smallpox was an exclusive disease of humans. Thus unlike smallpox in 1979, mpox can't be eradicated. And unfortunately, its wildlife reservoirs are yet to be determined, although several species of African rodents are suspected.[37] Monkeys are not part of the puzzle, to be clear; the name of the virus is a misnomer that's led to confusion as well as racist and stigmatizing language, and even fed into conspiracies (as we'll see in chapter 10). For this reason, the WHO began using mpox as a new name for monkeypox in late 2022.

MPXV can spread from infected animals to people through physical interactions, such as bites or scratches, direct handling, or the use of contaminated animal products. In humans, the symptoms of mpox are milder than those of smallpox, often beginning with fever and progressing to a rash within a few days. Sometimes there are no symptoms at all. Yet in some cases, patients have shown characteristic pustules prior to flu-like symptoms and developed skin lesions at different stages of the disease.[38] Human-to-human transmission of the virus occurs primarily through close proximity or direct physical contact with these skin lesions, virus-laden respiratory droplets and possibly airborne particles, and to a lesser extent, contaminated materials and objects.

In 2022, mpox achieved global infamy with an unprecedented explosion of concurrent cases in more than a hundred countries around the world. Within the span of a few months, over sixty-five thousand people were confirmed with MPXV infections, almost entirely in places that hadn't reported mpox cases in the past. At that point, the people most affected by the disease were young and middle-aged men who have sex with men, mostly through close sexual contact with an infected individual. Although relatively few people died from the infection (as the pandemic entered 2023, less than a hundred mpox-related fatalities had been reported), the variable symptoms went far beyond a skin and respiratory disease.[39] Clearly the virus had mutated through countless replications, across years of undetected spread, but more research was needed to understand which behaviors and routes of transmission were most dangerous. In the 2003 outbreak in the United States, for instance, researchers found that mpox patients were more likely to experience severe illness and hospitalization if they were scratched or bitten by animals infected with MPXV, compared to patients with noninvasive exposures (such as touching an infected animal or cleaning the cage of one).[40]

The first case of mpox in the 2003 outbreak was in the US state of Wisconsin, where a three-year-old girl was hospitalized with a fever and skin infection following a bite from a black-tailed prairie dog (*Cynomys ludovicianos*). Her family had recently purchased the small rodent from an exotic animal distributor at a local flea market where animals were bought and traded.[41] The girl's parents also soon became ill with a febrile rash, as did the distributor after being scratched by another prairie dog in his stock. In the preceding weeks, the Wisconsin-based distributor had purchased thirty-nine prairie dogs from a supplier in the neighboring state of Illinois and sold a number of them to two pet stores. Some of the prairie dogs developed symptoms of illness after arriving at the stores, and some of them died shortly thereafter.

By the time that several of the early patients had laboratory-confirmed diagnoses of mpox, the outbreak had spread across the midwestern United States. Within the time span of five weeks, there were seventy-two human cases of monkeypox in six US states. Many patients were veterinary staff who treated ill prairie dogs, while other patients included pet store employees or visitors as well as members or visitors of households with prairie dogs.[42] The majority of infections resulted from handling, feeding, or being scratched or bitten by a prairie dog, although some infections may have been due to human-to-human transmission or environmental exposure via contaminated feces or urine. Fortunately nobody died, as the human cases were milder than those generally seen in the Congo Basin, where a distinct clade of mpox (known as clade I) has a case fatality rate of around 10 percent and significant potential for human-to-human transmission.[43] That's because the MPXV that appeared in the United States was from a West African clade (known as clade II), which is less virulent and less transmissible between people.

More specifically, it was from Ghana. That's where a shipment of 800 small mammals was prepared and exported to Texas one month before the outbreak. The shipment contained 762 African rodents, including rope squirrels (*Funiscuirus* spp.), African dormice (*Graphiurus lorraineus*), and

Gambian giant pouched rats (*Cricetomys* spp.), some of which later tested positive for monkeypox.[44] Quite a few of these animals ended up with the Illinois-based distributor, who kept them in captivity with about 200 prairie dogs. From there 39 prairie dogs went to Wisconsin, along with a Gambian giant pouched rat.[45] The giant rodent (which is no hyperbole, being up to one meter long including the tail) was ill and later died, probably having infected prairie dogs with whom it should never have crossed paths in the first place.

It's reasonable to wonder if the containment of the 2003 monkeypox outbreak wasn't another "lucky" outcome that could have been much worse. Even though none of the human cases were fatal, the potential ecological consequences of species translocation are serious. An invasive population of Gambian giant pouched rats has already been introduced in Florida, after several of them were released into the wild by a local exotic breeder between 1999 and 2001, suggesting the possibility of an African reservoir species for mpox to become established in the Western Hemisphere.[46] But prairie dogs represent another opportunity for a pathogen to cross oceans and become endemic in North America. It's a scenario with historical precedent.

The bubonic plague, the feared killer of perhaps one-third of Europeans in the fourteenth century, didn't reach the United States until 1900. It arrived by sea, when ships carrying plague-infested rats made landfall in San Francisco during the third plague pandemic. The rodent stowaways disembarked with the other passengers, carrying the plague bacterium (*Yersinia pestis*) into the Bay Area. There, as early as 1903, plague started to spread through local rodent populations of California ground squirrels (*Otospermophilus beecheyi*) and their fleas, which are the primary vector (an agent that transmits pathogens between hosts) for the disease. We'll discuss the details of how and why this happened in chapter 6, but for the moment it's enough to know that plague is now endemic in the western United States. The sylvatic (or enzootic) plague, as it's known when the pathogen cycles in natural populations of mammalian hosts and flea vectors, has been reported in at least seventy-six species of mammals across the region.[47] The black-tailed prairie dog, a ground squirrel whose natural habitat is the Great Plains of North America, is one of them.

Only a handful of people in the United States are infected with *Y. pestis* each year, unlike in other parts of the world where plague is endemic; globally, over two hundred rodent species carry the bacterium, and some eighty flea species transmit it, on every continent except Australia and Antarctica. But in endemic regions of Madagascar, where *Y. pestis* was most likely first introduced via infected rats on steamships from India in 1898, plague still infects hundreds of people on a seasonal basis.[48] Among the many factors involved in the outbreaks, deforestation appears to be one of them by encroaching on natural habitats and thrusting humans into sylvatic cycles that were previously isolated from our species.[49]

Thankfully we now have antibiotics to treat infections of *Y. pestis*, as long as patients can access them and the bacteria don't develop resistance to them. If untreated, these infections can progress to a deadly pneumonic form that spreads directly from person to person via respiratory droplets. When this happens in densely populated urban settings, such as in Madagascar in 2017, thousands of people can quickly become infected and gravely ill. Thus even old pathogens can create new problems when they reemerge, especially if we don't detect them right away. Put another way, as my colleague Dan Lucey says, "What's next is already here. We just haven't recognized it yet."

*　　*　　*

While Madagascar experienced an urban outbreak of pneumonic plague, with almost twenty-five hundred probable cases and over two hundred deaths in four months, another disease was reemerging in the Americas. And in Brazil in particular, deforestation was again a factor in bringing humans in contact with the vectors and reservoirs of an ancient scourge.

Yellow fever is a zoonotic viral disease transmitted by mosquito bites, which can manifest in a variety of symptoms within days of infection, from fever and aches to liver damage (causing jaundice; hence the "yellow fever" name) to fatal organ failure. The yellow fever virus is endemic to tropical and subtropical regions of Africa and Central and South America, possibly having arrived in the Americas on slave-trading ships from West Africa as early as the sixteenth century. Its primary urban vector, the *Aedes aegypti* mosquito, made the Atlantic crossing with the virus. In the Americas, however, the yellow fever virus encountered favorable ecological conditions that allowed for a sustainable and seasonal sylvatic cycle.[50] In Brazil, where the earliest yellow fever outbreak was recorded in 1685, this cycle involves forest mosquitoes (such as *Haemagogus* spp.) feeding on the infected blood of primate reservoirs like howler monkeys (*Alouatta* spp.) who live in the same forest habitats.

In late 2016, the most significant epidemic of sylvatic yellow fever in seventy years began in the rural state of Minas Gerais in Brazil. From there it followed an alarming spread into urban states and cities that had been free of the disease for many decades. Over the next three rainy seasons, 2,237 cases of and 759 deaths from yellow fever were recorded, and the patient demographics were telling. As noted by microbiologist Poliana de Oliveira Figueiredo and colleagues, the majority of cases were males of working age in rural areas, probably due to their work activities and proximity to forest sites.[51] This male bias was part of an increasing trend since 2001, following a pattern of infections among loggers, hunters, farmers, and other Amazonian dwellers likely to be bitten by virus-carrying forest mosquitoes. Farmers and rural workers were also the first groups to be infected during the epidemic overall and at the start of each wave.[52]

Unlike in previous outbreaks, though, the forest mosquitoes carried the virus further southeast along forest corridors inhabited by monkeys and toward large urban centers.[53] Severe drought may have forced mosquitoes and monkeys to congregate closer to rural-urban boundaries for food and water, while increasing the rates of mosquito bites.[54] But deforestation also helped the virus spread near and into urban environments by reducing buffer zones as well as creating more opportunities for human exposure to fragmented forest areas where sylvatic cycles occur.[55] Insufficient vaccination coverage was another factor in the epidemic, despite the availability of an effective vaccine for yellow fever, thereby leaving many people vulnerable to the disease.

Because there's no specific treatment for yellow fever, vaccination is the best tool for preventing severe illness and death from infection. Unfortunately, efforts to vaccinate the public during the epidemic were slowed by false rumors about the vaccine, which made some people more hesitant to get it.[56] Furthermore, misinformation led to hostility toward and shocking violence against wild monkeys. As fears about the virus grew, authorities in several areas of southeastern Brazil found monkeys poisoned, beaten, burned, and shot to death.[57] Presumably the assailants thought that these killings would stop the spread of the virus, not realizing that their actions would actually make it worse. To be sure, more monkeys than humans died of yellow fever in epizootics (animal disease outbreaks equivalent to human epidemics), which made them valuable sentinels for the disease. "They're putting human beings at greater risk by killing the messenger," lamented

Brazilian public health official Renato Alves at the time. "Monkeys are a crucial alert mechanism that we monitor to deploy vaccines and prevention efforts in the right places."[58]

Nonhuman primates are far from alone in acting as message bearers for disease threats, as epizootics are common warnings among many species. Nonhuman primates are a particularly important source of information, however, having been involved in about 20 percent of major human diseases, even though they represent only 0.5 percent of all vertebrate species.[59] This pathogen sharing is likely due to our evolutionary and physical closeness, primate to primate. Our species, *Homo sapiens*, doesn't descend from our living primate relatives, but we do share not-too-distant ancestors, most recently with chimpanzees around six to eight million years ago (or about 11:58 p.m., if we think back to our twenty-four-hour compression of Earth history). Given these lower cross-species barriers for transmission, many pathogens that affect nonhuman primates also affect us, and vice versa.

Without question, the best-known example of a pathogen that originated in nonhuman primates and was sustained in humans is HIV, which has caused at least forty million deaths to date. Around the world, almost forty million people are living with HIV today, with more than one million new cases each year. There are two types of HIV, which both evolved from simian immunodeficiency viruses (SIVs) carried by nonhuman primates in Africa. The pandemic viruses are HIV-1, and mostly Group M (a subdivision of HIV-1, which is further divided into subtypes A, B, C, and so on), derived from a strain of SIV carried by chimpanzees (*Pan troglodytes*). SIV in chimpanzees takes longer to weaken their immune system than HIV in humans, but eventually the virus can cause them to get sick and die. The spillover that led to HIV-1 seems to have occurred around the turn of the twentieth century in Central Africa, possibly when a hunter made contact with SIV-infected blood while butchering a chimp.[60] Perhaps for most of a century, HIV-1 circulated and diversified among people, spreading undetected into urban centers and across oceans until it was finally recognized in 1981. The less famous HIV-2 is closely related to SIV in sooty mangabeys (*Cercocebus atys*), which are thought to have first transmitted the virus to humans in Guinea-Bissau during the first half of the twentieth century.[61] The two types of HIV share many similarities, but HIV-2 is less transmissible and less likely to progress to AIDS. Also, since its emergence

HIV-2 has been confined mostly to West Africa, whereas HIV-1 infections occur worldwide.[62]

Another zoonotic pathogen that affects our primate cousins, and can be transmitted to and between humans through blood and other infected fluids, is Ebola virus. There have been dozens of human outbreaks of EVD since 1976, when the virus was first identified. In 2014, however, an Ebola epidemic in West Africa led to more cases and deaths than all the previous ones combined in another disease emergence linked to deforestation and urbanization (which we'll get into more in chapters 3–4). But the Ebola virus is even deadlier for other great apes, and may be responsible for killing one-third of the world's gorillas (*Gorilla* spp.) and chimpanzees since the 1990s.[63] And like the yellow fever virus in New World monkeys, Ebola virus has caused massive die-offs of African apes that preceded human Ebola outbreaks in the same areas. These epizootics could have served as lifesaving warnings, if people saw them as such. Wildlife veterinarian William Karesh summed up the situation with a simple yet consequential statement to the *Washington Post* in 2003. "Human or livestock or wildlife health can't be discussed in isolation anymore," he said. "There is just one health. And the solutions require everyone working together on all the different levels."[64]

What's Now, What's Next

Since its debut into the public lexicon twenty years ago, "one health" has become a lot more than a slogan. One Health is now a professional framework and established field of practice, with academic degrees, journals, research centers, and professional communities that focus on the fact that human, animal, and environmental health are inextricably connected. Around the world, public and global health organizations have adopted One Health as an approach to anticipating and preventing infectious disease threats through cross-disciplinary and international collaboration, such as the WHO, US Centers for Disease Control and Prevention (CDC), and World Bank. There's even a One Health Day on November 3 every year to bring attention to the need for One Health partnerships and their achievements.

And of course, One Health was the main message of the *Outbreak* exhibit. That's because it was the best way that we could easily summarize the challenge of disease emergence *and* offer a solution to it. By understanding how and where pathogens might emerge or reemerge, spreading across species and bypassing borders as a result of human activities, we can take actions to stop the next pandemic before it starts. Reduce the spillover, reduce the spread.

Staying informed about current outbreaks is one way to be prepared. The largest publicly available system for the global reporting of infectious disease outbreaks, created by the International Society for Infectious Diseases, is the Program for Monitoring Emerging Diseases (ProMED).[65] Using a One Health approach, ProMED was launched in 1994 as an internet service to identify unusual health events related to emerging and reemerging infectious diseases and toxins affecting humans, animals, and plants. Today it has subscribers in almost every country in the world, adding to a global network of users who might share and respond to posts at any moment, twenty-four hours a day, seven days a week. In February 2003, ProMED published the earliest public description of SARS, at a time when the Chinese government was actively suppressing news of the outbreak.[66] Over the next two decades, ProMED was the first to report on the early spread of EVD, MERS, COVID-19, and many other disease outbreaks and biothreats.

Another action that we can all support, if not all participate directly in, is the global surveillance of zoonotic pathogens that can spill over into the human population. This is the monitoring of outbreaks that *could* happen, if we're not careful. One of the most ambitious efforts to operationalize this strategy was the PREDICT project, which was funded by the US Agency for International Development from 2009 to 2019. With the Smithsonian as one of its implementing partners, the PREDICT consortium worked in over thirty countries to detect emerging disease threats at their source and build local capacities to keep them in check. By sampling more than 164,000 nonhuman animals and people, keeping a focus on the ecological interfaces of human-livestock-wildlife interaction, the PREDICT project identified nearly a thousand novel viruses.[67] Its findings included more than five hundred coronaviruses in bats in China and the detection of Ebola virus in a bat in Liberia that was the same type responsible for the 2014 Ebola epidemic in West Africa, thereby providing the first evidence for a reservoir of the disease in the region. The project also incorporated social scientists into its teams, and they identified high-risk behaviors and educational tools for human behavior changes related to zoonotic pathogen transmission.

Lastly, as a museum curator I feel compelled to emphasize the importance of collections-based research in generating and disseminating information about zoonotic pathogens and pandemic risks. Certainly, exhibitions and public programs are effective ways to raise awareness as well as catalyze conversations about issues of infectious disease emergence and the role of humans within it. That's the dissemination part. But for generating new data on microbes and the animal hosts, historical specimens and samples offer unique opportunities to recover lost microbial diversity and elucidate the evolutionary history of pathogens circulating among us today. For example, rodent specimens from Central Africa have produced viral evidence of mpox in rope squirrels dated as early as 1899, more than half a century prior to the first described case of the disease, as well as in some species not previously identified as hosts.[68] Furthermore, estimations of the timing of the chimpanzee-human spillover event that led to the HIV pandemic were only possible through the nearly complete recovery of an HIV-1 genome from a preserved tissue sample from 1966.[69]

Microbes are everywhere around and in us. They outnumber and sometimes undermine us. Yet there's only so much that they can do without us. In this chapter, we looked at some activities that bring us closer to animals as well as facilitate the emergence and reemergence of zoonotic pathogens, which will probably cause the next pandemic—but only to the extent that we let that happen. In the next chapter, we're going to explore how we physically transmit diseases among ourselves in ways that only a species like us can do.

2 The Human Body: A Perfect Host

The human body is distinctive and remarkable in many respects that we often take for granted. For better or worse, it allows us to do things that no other species on Earth can do. Your ability to hold this book and turn its pages, comprehend this sentence and read it aloud, and communicate this experience to another person—such as by voicing your opinions or writing a review—is made possible by a number of highly specialized, and specifically human, features.

Today we use some of these features in ways that our human ancestors didn't. In fact, evolutionary biology is full of traits that came to serve different functions than those for which they were originally selected—sometimes called exaptations.[1] One classic example of an exapted trait is feathers, which may have started out as thermal insulation for some dinosaurs. (The warming effect of feathers, which trap air close to the body and limit the amount of heat that can escape, should be verifiable by anyone who's ever been zipped into a down jacket or sleeping bag.) But some feathers evolved to allow for other functions, eventually making it possible for birds to fly.

Over on the hominid branch of the tree of life, our vocal tract consists of structures that most likely evolved for purposes of breathing and eating. They still provide these abilities, but later became instrumental (and instruments) for speech.[2] Using the same respiratory system of tubes and tissues, the modern human can do it all: respiration, mastication, and conversation. Contagion too.

An unfortunate complication of some of our special faculties is that we've become uniquely equipped to transmit pathogens, which enter and exit our bodies through numerous routes and portals therein. They may sound bloodless in epidemiological terminology (in my mind, routes and portals are infrastructure, not anatomy), but these structures and functions are the necessities of our lives. Biologically speaking, they're the physical means by which we breathe, excrete, procreate, and interact with the world. Thus without any intention or hint of awareness, we can spread pathogens simply by being human.

But the good news is that we're in control. We can reduce our vulnerabilities to these risks by understanding how they're embedded in our bodies and intertwined with how we use them. Although it may seem like pathogens are out to get us, the fact is that we spread them much more effectively than they can spread themselves. And so in this chapter, we're going to drill down on two aspects of our biology and behavior that can do the most damage: the ones that let us touch and talk. They're the fundamentals of the human body that help and essentially make us. They can also work against us when it comes to pandemics, yet only if we let them.

Handy Anatomy

"There is no act of life so dangerous to others," fumed physician Robert Eccles in 1909, "as carelessness concerning the condition of our hands."

He really meant it. In a seven-page rant titled "Dirty Hands," published in the *Dietetic and Hygienic Gazette* of New York City, Eccles blamed filthy fingers for the deadliest crimes of the age. Causing more deaths than "bullets, poisons, railway accidents, and earthquakes combined," the human hand was a weapon of mass destruction that extinguished innocent lives by the hour, according to this Brooklyn-based doctor. And Eccles was fighting back. With ample ammunition from bacteriology, a field in its heyday by the close of the nineteenth century, he had scientific proof that uncleanliness could transform hands into petri dishes of pathogens. "Until the HABIT is established of purifying the hands, both timely and properly, no lessening of this human misery seems possible under existing conditions," Eccles declared.[3]

The main target of the doctor's ire was a private cook named Mary Mallon, the notorious Typhoid Mary of medical lore, who was serving a sentence of forced isolation on North Brother Island in New York City's East River. Mallon was arrested as a public health threat in 1907 after being identified as the source of seven household outbreaks of typhoid fever since

1900.[4] Epidemiological evidence suggested that she infected her clients by preparing their meals with unclean hands—a charge that Mallon rejected. She didn't deny her poor hand hygiene but also failed to see how she could have infected anyone. Typhoid fever has many symptoms, such as a prolonged high fever, headache, and malaise, and Mallon had none of them.

Typhoid fever is caused by the bacterium *Salmonella typhi*, which was well-described and identifiable with diagnostic tests by the 1890s. Untreated typhoid fever can be fatal in up to 30 percent of the cases, and before the advent of antibiotics, it caused thousands of deaths in the United States each year.[5] Only humans are infected by and transmit the pathogen, usually through food and water contaminated with *Salmonella*-filled urine or feces. This is likely how Mallon spread the disease given that laboratory analyses of her feces showed pathogens aplenty. Apparently none of her trips from the bathroom to the kitchen (also known as fecal-oral transmission) involved soap.

Mallon refused to believe that she was an asymptomatic carrier of typhoid fever, even after her release in 1910. She continued to cook, but didn't adopt the handwashing habit that Eccles preached. Thus he was probably pleased by the further punishment that she faced for her dirty hands when health authorities tracked her down again. After more people had fallen ill and died from her contaminated cuisine, she was arrested and isolated for a second time in 1915, with a sentence that lasted the rest of her life.[6]

The story of Mallon holds many lessons, and the danger of unclean hands is one of them (with more to be discussed in chapter 9). But still today, disease risks frequently involve pathogens and routes of transmission that we fail to recognize. I recall when virologist Matt Frieman made this point effectively at a workshop sponsored by the National Academy of Sciences in 2017. The scientists in attendance were invited to present and discuss their research with a group of filmmakers, and Matt's topic was perfect for a Hollywood movie: deadly viruses that have recently emerged in humans. When Matt finished his presentation, one filmmaker asked him how much we needed to worry about these pathogens at present. You could hear the alarm in her voice. And without missing a beat, Matt replied, "Right now, *our* most immediate threat is a norovirus outbreak from that jar of cookies by the bathrooms."

He was right. In our meeting venue, arranged by one of the premier scientific organizations in the United States, there was an inviting jar of chocolate chip cookies on a small table . . . directly on the path to and from the toilets. Like *Salmonella typhi*, norovirus is an intestinal pathogen that's commonly spread through contaminated food, water, and surfaces. It's one of the world's leading causes of gastroenteritis (also known as stomach flu) and extremely contagious, partly because a small dose can cause infection. Incredibly, a sick person can shed billions of tiny particles of norovirus in their stool and vomit, but infect another person with as few as eighteen of them.[7] Yet norovirus is also highly transmissible because it's picked up and left all over the place by our grabby hands.

For an example, look to the utterly miserable weekend of an Oregon girls soccer team. While sharing hotel rooms at an out-of-state tournament, eight of the team's players fell ill with acute gastroenteritis. The first girl to become sick (called the index patient) had used a bathroom where a grocery bag of snacks was being stored. She didn't actually touch the bag or its contents but instead contaminated their surfaces by vomiting, excreting diarrhea, and flushing the toilet—all of which can aerosolize noroviruses, thereby making them airborne. The index patient went home the next morning, but the food in the grocery bag (consisting of cookies, chips, and fresh grapes) was passed around at the team's lunch that afternoon. Within forty-eight hours, seven other girls became sick too.

Sickness is often a helpful signal of infection risks for the patient as well as the rest of us. But like *Salmonella typhi*, norovirus can be contagious without any symptoms at all. People can shed the virus in their feces before they start to feel sick or for weeks after they begin to feel better. Handwashing is therefore the simplest and most effective way to prevent transmission. Placing treats far away from the restrooms is another one.

*   *   *

Our hands wouldn't work so well as disease vectors if we didn't use them so much. And we wouldn't use them so much if there wasn't so much that they can do. So before we get further into a discussion of how we give a helping hand to pathogens in their transmission, let's consider what makes our hands so helpful in the first place. A round of applause, if you will.

If you place one hand flat on a surface, palm down, you might be able to make out the contours of fourteen short bones (called phalanges) in your thumb and fingers, in addition to five longer ones in your palm (called metacarpals) that articulate with your wrist. There are also eight small bones in the wrist (called carpals), which are mostly hidden from external view. Some of them are surprisingly charismatic in shape, resembling miniature forms of common objects that range from a boot to a boat—as every student of human osteology knows by heart. But there's nothing cute about what they do. These twenty-seven bones give each hand its rigid, knuckled structure, while joined and surrounded with muscles, tendons, ligaments, blood vessels, and nerves that connect with other elements of the body and carry out directions from the brain. Together they're critical components of the anatomical architecture that allows your hand to move.

At each of your fingertips there's an ever-growing, translucent plate of fibrous protein called keratin, otherwise known as a nail. Although they're nice for decoration, your nails protect and enhance your sensitivity to touch too. If you flip your hand over, you can better understand how. The nails provide a hard backing for fibrofatty cushions of flesh at each of your fingertips, five apical pads in addition to several palm pads on the underside of each hand. Extremely creased and furrowed, these pulpy apical pads of nerve endings have some of the highest concentrations of mechanoreceptors and thermoreceptors in all the skin, making them highly sensitive to sensory stimuli. Try them out with a tap or two—but be careful! Fingertip injuries are potentially debilitating and common, particularly in curious young children who use their hands to explore their environment without realizing the physical dangers involved.[8] Even beyond childhood, through touch sensations and tactile perceptions of temperature, texture, and vibration transmitted to the brain, fingers are essential to how most people contact and interact with the external world throughout life.

For a primate, our hands have some minor distinctions that make a big difference. The human hand can be distinguished from other living apes by a high thumb-to-digit ratio, meaning that we have a relatively long thumb when measured against the fingers on the same hand.[9] (Among primates, however, we overlap with some monkeys in this index.) One major advantage of these hand proportions is that our thumb can be placed squarely in pad-to-pad contact with, or positioned diametrically opposite to, any or all of our fingers. Thumb opposition isn't unique to humans, and in fact an opposable thumb facilitates the enhanced grasping abilities of many primates.[10] But what sets our thumb apart is its power. Modern humans have a unique combination and greater number of forearm muscles versus other primates, as well as a notable musculature in the thumb.[11] Altogether, these features allow humans to firmly and precisely grip objects for certain types of manipulation that other animals, even our living primate relatives, can't achieve.

Imagine pinching a piece of paper between your thumb and index finger, for example. Maybe you already are, as you turn this page. We use this type of forceful, pad-to-pad precision gripping without thinking about it, and literally in a snap. Yet it was a breakthrough in human evolution. Other primates exhibit some kinds of precision grips in the handling and use of objects, but not with the kind of efficient opposition that our hand anatomy allows. In a single hand, humans can easily hold and manipulate objects, even small and delicate ones, while adjusting our fingers to their shape and reorienting them with displacements of our fingertip pads.[12] Our relatively long, powerful thumb and other anatomical attributes, including our flat nails (which nearly all primates possess), make this possible. Just picture trying—and failing—to dog-ear this page with pointy, curved claws.

With a unique combination of traits, the human hand shaped our history. No question, stone tools couldn't have become a keystone of human technology and subsistence without hands that could do the job, along with a nervous system that could regulate and coordinate the necessary signals. Anybody who's ever attempted to make a spear tip or arrowhead from a rock (as many archaeologists do, through a process called knapping) knows that it requires strong grips, constant rotation and repositioning, and forceful, careful strikes with another hard object. And even with a fair amount of know-how, it can be a bloody business.

But our manual dexterity isn't determined by our hand anatomy alone. There are neurological components to our hand movements, which involve the brain, spinal cord, and a complex system of nerves. Neurological factors may partly explain why primate species with similar hands can differ quite a bit in their mechanical abilities.[13] For example, the brown capuchin (*Cebus apella*) and common squirrel monkey (*Saimiri sciureus*) both have pseudo-opposable thumbs, but only the capuchin displays relatively independent finger movements and precision gripping in picking up small objects and manipulating tools.[14] Functional differences in their neuroanatomy may be the cause.

Of course, the most common object that people touch nowadays is a screen. And the *tap-tap-tap* movements of our fingers is a unique human ability, as no other primate can move their fingers as rapidly and independently

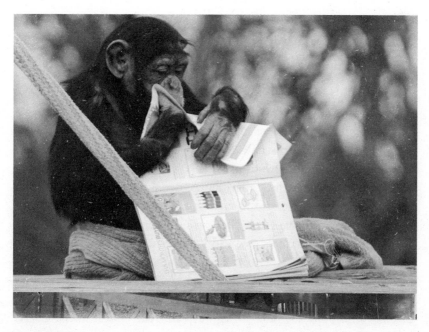

Figure 2.1
Ape hand movements. While a human can turn the page of a book using forceful thumb-finger opposition, other apes can't form this pad-to-pad "precision grip" due to the relative shortness of the thumb compared to the other fingers, as seen in the left hand of this chimpanzee. Instead, this chimpanzee is gripping the pages of a magazine by holding them between the knuckles of their right hand. *Source:* Mertie/flickr.

as we do.[15] Here again, we can thank the extraordinary human brain given that normal finger tapping requires the functional integrity of the corticospinal tract, cerebellar motor circuitry, and kinesthetic pathways.[16] Moreover, repetitive rapid finger tapping is a common test of fine motor control of the upper extremities as well as a standard means of assessing the potential effects of neurodegenerative disease and traumatic brain injury.

Our use of information technology, like smartphones and computers, is often described as having the world at our fingertips. But as we'll see, this metaphor makes sense when it comes to microbes too.

*   *   *

The vast majority of microbes on and in the human body are persistent but harmless colonists, as we discussed in chapter 1. The hand is no exception.

Many of the microbes at our fingertips are commensal, and some provide important benefits for human health. For instance, one of the key functions of the skin microbiota, which are mostly bacteria (accounting for over 80 percent of the microbes at most sites), is acid resistance.[17] By regulating the acidity of the skin, these microbes help to maintain a powerful permeability barrier that prevents water and electrolyte loss from the body—a requirement for life in terrestrial animals like us.[18]

Our skin barrier also prevents infectious diseases and allergies by blocking external substances such as pathogens, allergens, and chemicals from invading the body.[19] At least that's how it's supposed to work. But even though many of the microbes that come in contact with or reside on the skin are normally unable to establish an infection, any break in the skin from a cut, scrape, burn, or bite can be the entry point of an invading pathogen, such as Ebola virus from the infected blood of a mammalian host or Zika virus from the infected saliva of a mosquito vector.

But these aren't the most frequent ways that our hands participate in the spread of infectious diseases. Rather, our hands are critical in the *indirect* transmission of pathogens between people via contaminated objects and surfaces, as Mallon did throughout her career. Called fomites, these risks are everywhere: phones, faucets, doorknobs, elevator buttons, dishtowels, utensils, food, you name it. We touch these things and the microbes on them literally all the time.

It will surprise no parents that children can touch objects and surfaces more than six hundred times *per hour* during outdoor play.[20] At the same time, these little explorers might touch their mouths or someone else's about twenty times an hour. Yet adults do this quite a bit too. Regardless of age or sex, we touch our faces up eight hundred times a day.[21] Often it's an automatic and unconscious movement, and so if you think you're an exception, it could be that you simply don't remember. For instance, when prompted to recall nonverbal behaviors during interpersonal interactions, the subjects of a study showed the lowest accuracy in estimating how many self-touches they made.[22]

Hand contact with the mouth, nose, and eyes (sometimes called the facial T-Zone by infectious disease researchers) is the riskiest kind of face touching. That's because the mucous membranes that line these structures can serve as staging grounds for microbial pathogenesis, the process by which microbes cause disease. People have been observed touching their T-Zone around eight times an hour in public places, and the number nearly doubles for kids.[23] In medical offices, some health care workers make T-Zone touches with the same frequency as people do in public, although clinicians do so slightly less often.[24] But believe it or not, medical students can be even worse. In one study, they were observed touching their face twenty-three times per hour while listening to a lecture—after completing coursework in infection control and transmission precautions, no less! And almost half of those touches involved contact with a mucous membrane.[25]

Hand contacts with fomites and mucous membranes are a potentially dangerous combination. People who are infected with pathogens can expel them from their bodies (in a process known as shedding) in saliva, mucus, blood, urine, and feces as well as in respiratory secretions in the form of droplets and aerosols. These pathogens can be deposited on or transferred to fomites in a variety of ways, from an explosive sneeze or casual touch. Then the pathogens can survive and remain infectious on fomites for varying lengths of time, from a few hours in some cases to several months in others depending on variables related to the pathogen, the fomite, and their environmental conditions.[26] Many people were made aware of these possibilities during the COVID-19 pandemic, when the earliest recommendations from health officials included washing your hands, cleaning surfaces, and *not* touching your face.

Some pathogens are more likely than others to spread via fomite and hand-to-hand contact, even if SARS-CoV-2 doesn't appear to be one of them. This is the case for some enteric pathogens like *Salmonella typhi*, norovirus, and poliovirus, which usually follow a route of fecal-oral transmission. Others such as *Vibrio cholerae* (bacteria that cause cholera) and *Escherichia coli* (normally commensal bacteria that can cause a variety of infections depending on the strain) are more likely to spread through fecal contamination of food and water. But fomite-mediated transmission is also a concern for some respiratory pathogens like rhinovirus, which is the predominant cause of the common cold. One study found that around 14 percent of the rhinovirus on an individual's fingers was transferred to another individual via a doorknob or faucet, and half as much via hand-to-hand contact.[27] Furthermore, another study found that after an overnight stay in a hotel, adults with natural rhinovirus colds contaminated about 35 percent of the 150 environmental sites tested, such as pens, light switches, remote controls, and telephones.[28] As well, in one-third of the trials, the study's subjects indirectly transferred the virus to other people's fingertips up to eighteen hours after contaminating these surfaces. If this isn't an argument for hand hygiene, then I don't know what is. And it's an argument that long preceded Mallon.

In 1847, when Hungarian physician Ignaz Semmelweis devised the interventions that would earn him the title of "the father of hand hygiene," the discipline of medicine was on the verge of a revolution. Surgeons had just started using general anesthesia when operating on patients, who were able to experience painless operations as never before. Anesthesia was also first used for childbirth in 1845, at a time when maternal death was far too common; in general, for every thousand babies born during the nineteenth century, as many as ten mothers died. One of the major causes of maternal mortality was childbirth-related septicemia, known as puerperal fever or childbed fever (and later found to be caused by *Streptococcus pyogenes* bacteria). Between 1841 and 1847, puerperal fever was responsible for up to 16 percent of maternal deaths at the Vienna hospital where Semmelweis worked.[29] Mothers died far more frequently, however, in one of the hospital's obstetric wards than in the other one. And Semmelweis seized the opportunity to understand why and how.

He examined the mortality statistics at the hospital over decades, finding that the mortality rates of the two wards diverged after 1841.[30] At that time, one of the wards became staffed only with midwives. In the other one, deliveries were performed by medical students and doctors, who also conducted autopsies in a nearby room. After one of the hospital's pathologists died following a scalpel slip during an autopsy, from which he succumbed to a condition similar to puerperal fever, Semmelweis made the cadaver connection.

Concluding that the medical students and obstetricians were causing puerperal fever in their pregnant patients by infecting them with cadaverous particles on their hands, Semmelweis instituted some harsh protocols. Everyone had to scrub their hands with a chlorinated lime solution after leaving the autopsy room and before contact with a patient. Why chlorinated lime? Because Semmelweis didn't think that soap and water were strong enough to remove the culprits of contagion from postautopsy hands, and chlorinated lime solution was the strongest product used by the housekeeping staff at the hospital.[31]

The new system worked, complaints notwithstanding. Maternal mortality rates in the two wards soon evened out, with a dramatic drop in deaths from puerperal fever in the obstetricians' ward from 18.3 percent in 1847 to 2.2 percent in 1848.[32] Even though Semmelweis was unappreciated for his achievements during his lifetime, his experiment remains powerful proof that hand hygiene is one of the simplest and most effective human behaviors that can prevent the spread of disease.[33] And certainly by the early twentieth century, his crusade against dirty hands counted more than a few allies.

Diseased Discourse

After examining how the human hand can function as a vehicle for spreading germs, we're now going to move headward and look deep within. The human vocal anatomy, which allows for the production of sound via altered breathing, is the factor in focus here. That's because of its critical role as a highly effective and specifically human mechanism for disease transmission: speech.

While Mallon was unwittingly spreading typhoid fever among the upper classes of New York society, an outbreak of a different sort was under investigation on the other side of the Atlantic. After a wave of influenza hit the House of Commons of the UK Parliament in 1903, British bacteriologist Mervyn Henry Gordon was appointed to conduct an inquiry into the air quality and ventilation of the Debating Chamber. It happened to be a place where some members of Parliament (MPs) spent time during their convalescence, and there were complaints that the closed atmosphere created "a feeling of heaviness."[34]

Intimate and adversarial by design, the Debating Chamber was a venue of spirited discourse—the noisy kind. Seated opposite each other at a distance of two swords, hundreds of MPs gathered tightly in the Debating Chamber in order to discuss legislative matters, or in Gordon's polite wording, "loudly articulate." And thus the level of salivary pollution that resulted from all the raised voices was a main target of his experiments in 1904 and 1905.

The respiratory transmission of influenza was already known to scientists by the twentieth century, even if its causal pathogen was not yet (correctly) identified. In 1899, German bacteriologist Carl Flügge and his collaborators first advanced the theory of droplet transmission as the primary route through which respiratory diseases spread. Their work showed that microbes (specifically, *Serratia marcescens* bacteria) could travel at least one meter in distance via respiratory droplets emitted while sneezing, coughing, and speaking.[35] Using the same approach, Gordon wanted to see how far microbes might travel across the Debating Chamber from the utterances of a single MP during an act of oration. And so with his mouth and throat filled with *S. marcescens*, Gordon stood at the dispatch box where the MPs spoke. From there, he recited an hour of dramatist William Shakespeare's writings to an audience of agar plates.[36]

The results were stunning. Gordon's speaking experiments produced colonies of *S. Marcescens* throughout the Debating Chamber, mostly in plates nearest to the speaker, but also in those more than twenty-one meters away. Moreover, ventilation seemed to only increase the spread. In his report to Parliament, Gordon concluded that the chief source of air contamination of the Debating Chamber during debates was the mouths and upper respiratory passages of the MPs themselves. His recommendations, however, mainly concerned structural changes to improve the temperature, humidity, and flow of air throughout the complex. He did not suggest that the legislators lower their voices or lessen their speech.

By the time that influenza emerged as a global pandemic in 1918, Gordon's findings about the transmission risks of speaking were well supported. Following a similar protocol (without the Shakespeare), US researchers found that five minutes of loud speech could propel respiratory droplets of *S. marcescens* over a distance of more than one meter and five minutes of conversational speech had a slightly shorter range.[37] They identified a "4-foot danger zone" around an influenza patient while speaking, but only in the absence of a mask. Not just any kind of mask, however. From additional experiments, they concluded that a three-layer buttercloth mask was efficient in blocking infectious droplets while speaking or coughing, whereas ones made of gauze were worthless as barriers.

The study made headlines in the United States. During the second wave of the pandemic in fall 1918, mask mandates and other public health measures were in effect around the country. And like elsewhere in the world, people had to adjust to temporary closures and restrictions in other aspects of life, including religious institutions, schools, and recreation facilities. But the UK Parliament didn't close, and the only mention of the influenza pandemic in the records of the House of Commons was a discussion about pensions.[38] Perhaps Gordon's recommendations were implemented and wildly successful. In any case, the MPs didn't stop talking.

*   *   *

All animals communicate, but none are known to have a system of communication that comes close to human language in expressiveness and sophistication.[39] Wild parrots can mimic our words when in captivity, although they make chirps and screeches in the wild. Baby bats can babble much like human infants and develop an extensive system of high-frequency squeaks in maturity.[40] Many animals use sounds not only for communication but also hunting and navigation. Yet one distinguishing feature of humans is that we communicate about, well, everything. Not just things in the here and now, but those far away and in the future as well as things that already happened or might someday occur.

Our speech is a unique feature of our species, the result of vocal and cognitive capabilities that allow us to make sounds with vast acoustic and symbolic complexity. In doing so, though, we can emit more than just sounds. Respiratory pathogens, like influenza viruses and coronaviruses, are associated with some of the biggest pandemics in human history because these pathogens can spread so easily via our respiratory anatomy. As easy as breathing. And coughing. Plus sneezing. But also, and especially, by talking.

Human speech can release dramatically greater numbers of virus-laden particles than coughing does, and even speaking quietly yields significantly more of them than breathing normally and wordlessly.[41] Furthermore, human speaking while breathing is about 90 percent exhalation, with quick intake breaths about 10 percent of the time, whereas intake and outtake breaths in other animals are about the same duration.[42] Most of us probably don't realize how much air we breathe out in a casual chat—and everything that we share besides words.

Our prospects for contagious conversations are highly alarming given that generally speaking, people speak all the time. One study found that adults use an average of about sixteen thousand words per day.[43] It's difficult to date the origins of this behavior because physical evidence in the fossil record is scarce. Anatomically, modern humans have been around for several hundred thousand years, and a vocal tract capable of producing the sounds of human language has existed for even longer. Our capacity for speech clearly differentiates humans from other primates, suggesting that some of these mechanisms diverged from our prelinguistic ancestors.[44] Our brains, however, only reached their modern form perhaps about a hundred thousand years ago, so it's possible that we didn't acquire language until then.[45] Human vocal anatomy wouldn't have been nearly so useful for language without a brain that can direct and control all the mechanics of speech, as cognitive scientist Philip Lieberman notes.[46]

In the human body, speaking involves a lot more than simply opening your mouth. Our vocal sounds are emitted through a process of altered breathing, and the entire respiratory system is involved. The lungs are the primary organs of the respiratory system of humans and most other animals, and the largest organs of our lower respiratory tract (also known as the lower airway). They're central to a general mechanism that produces nearly all voiced sounds of vertebrates, and the buildup of air within them creates a pressure that provides the primary energy source of human speech. The trachea (or windpipe) carries inhaled air into the lungs through tubular branches called bronchi, which divide into increasingly smaller branches of air tubes called bronchioles. These branching structures resemble an upside-down tree, and so we call them the tracheobronchial tree. And at the end of the bronchioles are small ducts connected to clusters of microscopic air sacs called alveoli. Tiny but mighty, the alveoli are where the lungs and blood exchange oxygen and carbon dioxide during the process of breathing in and out—otherwise known as respiration. When the alveoli become infected with a pathogen, the unfortunate owner can experience pneumonia, a severe and sometimes deadly illness associated with diseases like plague, SARS, and COVID-19.

The bronchi are connected via the trachea to the larynx, an organ composed of muscle and cartilage in the upper respiratory tract (also known as the upper airway) at the top of the neck. The larynx is commonly referred to as the voice box because it holds the vocal cords in humans and other mammals. And in humans, this is where things get a little . . . different. Adult humans are unusual in having a larynx that rests low in the throat, permanently descended, unlike in many other mammals.[47] This is a derived feature of our species relative to other primates, as opposed to an ancestral one, meaning that it evolved in humans to be quite distinctive.[48] The horseshoe-shaped hyoid bone, which anchors the muscles of the larynx (as well as the tongue, epiglottis, and pharynx), also sits in a much lower position in humans than found in other apes, roughly at the level of the jaw and third cervical vertebra.

Like any wind instrument, the shape and proportions of our airways affect the kind of sounds we make. Vocal sounds are produced by air passing from our lungs through the two flexible bands of our vocal folds (also known as cords) in the larynx, causing them to vibrate and create sound waves in the throat, nose, and mouth. The volume and pitch of these sounds are dependent on the rate and volume of exhaled air moving through them. But once a sound wave leaves the larynx, its quality changes considerably as it passes through an L-shaped configuration known as the supralaryngeal vocal tract.

Picture two tubes that form a right angle at your tonsils, one running up your throat and the other running out of your mouth. The vertical tube (through the throat) and horizontal tube (through the mouth) are equally long in humans, due to our short and retracted faces. In other mammals, whose noses and mouths protrude as snouts and muzzles, the horizontal tube is at least twice as long as the vertical tube. But even though we don't howl and bark, the human configuration provides many advantages for varied vocals. That's because the equal lengths of our L-shaped vocal tract can produce vowels with frequencies that are more distinguishable and require less effort, while our lips, tongue, and jaw modify its shape to make an impressive range of sounds as we talk.[49]

With all of these unusual human features of vocal anatomy, we could easily overlook the critical role of a superpowered brain in allowing us to communicate as we do. As a motor control behavior, speaking involves the supremely complex and rapid orchestration of more than a hundred muscles of the respiratory system, not even counting the other elements involved in hearing and understanding the words spoken by others. The complex sequences of motor commands for speech are regulated by neural circuits, which carry out specific functions as populations of nerve cells in the brain (also called neurons) that communicate via synapses. The human brain consists of an estimated eighty-six billion neurons, at least half of which are in the cerebellum where motor control functions are coordinated. But recent advances in brain-imaging methods have shown that language production and comprehension involve numerous regions of every major lobe of the brain, rather than being localized or isolated in a particular area as long believed.[50]

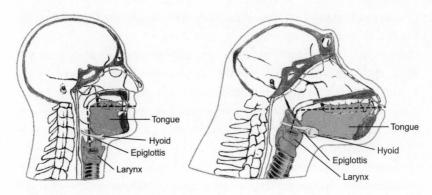

Figure 2.2
Primate vocal anatomy. Humans are unique among primates for our ability to communicate through speech, which is made possible in part by the distinctive anatomy of our vocal tract. Compared to a chimpanzee (*right*), a modern human (*left*) has a larynx and hyoid that are positioned low in the throat, with horizontal tubes and vertical tubes of nearly equal length. *Source:* Modified from D. Gokhman, M. Nissim-Rafinia, L. Agranat-Tamir, G. Housman, R. García-Pérez, E. Lizano, O. Cheronet, et al., "Differential DNA Methylation of Vocal and Facial Anatomy Genes in Modern Humans," *Nature Communications* 11, no. 1 (2020): 1189.

Yet there's a genetic basis for language related to cognitive and motor capacities that shouldn't be overlooked either. To date, the best-known gene involved in human speech is the Forkhead box protein P2 (FOXP2) gene, which encodes a transcription factor that regulates the extent to which other genes are expressed as proteins—including many genes linked to brain development and function. Lots of vertebrates have some version of the FOXP2 gene, which may help birds to sing and bats to echolocate, but the human version is slightly different than even those found in nonhuman primates.[51] (Interestingly, the human variant has been found in Neanderthal and Denisovan DNA too, which raises questions about the speech abilities of these extinct evolutionary relatives.) The importance of the FOXP2 gene in speech is most apparent when someone inherits a damaged copy of it, which happened to more than a dozen people across three generations of one extended family. Those family members who had a mutated version of the FOXP2 gene were affected by an array of speech and facial movement issues that made them agrammatical and sometimes intelligible.[52]

Many people have difficulties with speaking in some respect, and some don't speak at all. And while speech is a feature of our species, lacking or losing the ability to speak does not make anyone less human. In the United States alone, approximately 7.5 million people have trouble using their voices, sometimes due to an injury or disorder affecting the vocal anatomy.[53] These conditions might influence their emissions of respiratory pathogens given that speech plays a significant role in airborne transmission, but their risks of infection are the same as anybody else's.

*   *   *

Respiratory infections start with interactions between pathogens and mucosal surfaces of the respiratory tract, usually through inhalation or direct hand contact. These infections are generally described as affecting either the upper or lower respiratory tract, a fuzzy division that's often drawn beneath the voice box. Airways of the upper respiratory tract are found in the mouth, nose, and throat, and their job is to move (or conduct) air between the external environment and lungs. They also work hard to eliminate pathogens and keep them from getting into the lower airways of the lungs. Lined with an epithelial barrier of sticky mucus and hairlike cilia, the upper airways can catch and kill pathogens that enter their zone. This process of mucociliary clearance pushes the germs to the pharynx, where they're expelled from the airways through swallowing, coughing, and sneezing.[54] Some pathogens don't even make it to this stage, as when they get entangled in our nose hair and forced out with a loud *achoo*! But even if they do survive all of these defenses, they still have to contend with antimicrobial proteins, phagocytic cells, and other components of a healthy immune system.[55] And to progress into the lower airways, they need to pass through a gauntlet of smaller and smaller structures: the branches of the tracheobronchial tree.[56]

Inhalation is one way for a pathogen to reach the most distant tips of the branches, deep in the lungs, depending on the size of the liquid droplets that carry them. The smallest droplets, called aerosols, are particularly tiny and numerous when a person speaks, allowing them to be suspended in air and breathed in by someone who's not even within hearing distance. Inhaled droplets are deposited in the upper regions of the respiratory tract, from which they might be promptly kicked out. But inhaled aerosols can penetrate into the depths of the lungs, where they can establish an infection in the alveoli.[57]

The pathogens that manage to adhere, invade, and replicate in our tissues can be trouble. The most frequent infections of the upper respiratory tract are the result of viruses, such as those responsible for the common cold, and they usually cause disease by growing at their mucosal entry sites. That means most of them will replicate only in the upper respiratory airways. Some of them, however, can continue to infect deeper tissues and other body parts, with specific genes in individual strains that determine where and how they spread.[58] The same goes for other types of pathogens, such as *Mycobacterium tuberculosis* (the bacterial agent of tuberculosis), which can settle and grow in the lungs, but then travel through the bloodstream to infect the kidney, spine, and brain.

The severity of respiratory infections can be vastly different for a number of reasons. Those in the upper respiratory tract tend to be far less deadly than the ones in the lower respiratory tract, possibly because the lower airways have the critical job of gaseous exchange with the blood, whereby oxygen is absorbed and carbon dioxide is released. Upper respiratory tract infections (such as those caused by rhinoviruses, common coronaviruses, and some influenza viruses) typically manifest in manageable symptoms such as a fever, sore throat, and runny nose. Yet lower respiratory tract infections (such as those caused by *Streptococcus pneumoniae*, *Mycobacterium tuberculosis*, and SARS-CoV-1) are more likely to give you a wet cough, chest pain, abnormal breathing, and host of other problems.

Pathogens don't take turns, though. We can be infected with multiple pathogens, both viruses and bacteria, at the same time. And in many cases, they cooperate. During the 1918 influenza pandemic, for instance, the majority of the fifty to hundred million deaths likely resulted directly from secondary infections of bacteria that commonly colonize the upper respiratory tract.[59] They were able to spread into the lower respiratory tract and cause fatal pneumonia because the influenza virus broke down the mucociliary barrier that should have gotten rid of them.

Influenza virus is a good example of a respiratory pathogen for which speech is a significant source of transmission, and SARS-CoV-2 is another one. The reason is that the COVID-19 coronavirus is likely to first infect the airways of the upper respiratory tract after being inhaled through respiratory droplets and aerosols. Some patients experience mild to moderate symptoms of respiratory disease as a result of infection (and for others, the infection can be severe and highly variable), but many people have no symptoms whatsoever. And as long as there's an active infection in the upper respiratory tract, there are opportunities for aerosolizing the virus by speaking. Indeed, high viral loads of SARS-CoV-2 have been detected in oral fluids of COVID-19 patients, including asymptomatic ones.[60] Given that normal speech generates droplets that can remain suspended in the air for tens of minutes or longer, the infection risks are even greater in confined environments.[61]

Many studies have shown that microscopic particles emitted during normal speech and breathing are large enough to carry a variety of respiratory pathogens, such as measles virus, influenza virus, *M. tuberculosis*, and SARS-CoV-2, potentially at the same time. The processes by which these respiratory particles are aerosolized in significant quantities is an area of active research. It's been hypothesized that these small particles are generated from the mucosal lining of the respiratory tract by a "fluid-film burst" mechanism caused by the opening and closing of the lower bronchioles during breathing. But a similar mechanism seems to occur in the larynx as the vocal folds repeatedly open and closed during vocalization.[62]

A study by chemical engineer Sima Asadi and colleagues produced another important finding: the louder we speak, the more we emit particles. However, in a another Asadi-led study, surgical and KN95 masks reduced outward particle emission rates by 90 percent during speaking, even though people spoke more loudly while wearing them.[63] It didn't measure or show anything about viruses directly, so the results are silent about the influence of speaking and masking on airborne disease transmission. But in yet another study, Asadi and her coauthors suggested that language might modulate the airborne spread of respiratory pathogens, given that some vowel sounds (like the long e of *please* in English) released more aerosol particles than others (like the short i of *bitte* in German).[64] In other words, it's not what you say but how you say it.

Internal Struggles

The routes of disease transmission under examination in this chapter are by no means the only ones in which humans engage. Sexual transmission, for instance, is a major factor in the spread of many pathogens around the world, including the current HIV pandemic (which is the focus of chapter 7). Yet in all honesty, I can't make a strong argument that human sexual behavior is so different from other species. Certainly not compared to the things we do with our hands and voices, everywhere and all the time.

Despite the narrow focus of this chapter, the challenges outlined here are enormous. But again, they're largely within our control. Historical events show how long that we've known about these problems of disease transmission as well as how long their solutions have been understood. And one unifying element of this discussion of touching and talking has been the role of the human brain. We shouldn't overlook the fact that humans have the brainpower to use their bodies to increase infectious disease risks, and we have just as much cognitive capacity to decrease them.

Semmelweis left a legacy of hand hygiene that continues into the twenty-first century, showing that a good scrub could stop hospital-associated fomite transmission. Today, his interventions are comparable in efficacy to the alcohol-based hand rubs recommended by the WHO for hand hygiene in health care settings.[65] Elsewhere, most people became more accustomed to hand rub formulations during the COVID-19 pandemic, when dispensers and packets of hand sanitizer were hard to avoid. Others became friendlier with soap and water than ever before. Ironically, handwashing has been part of human history for thousands of years, as shown by washing equipment placed in ancient Egyptian tombs and warnings about dirty hands written on Mesopotamian tablets long before people knew what pathogens were.

Truly, with the fate of the world in our human hands, you would think that the least we can do is keep them clean. Unfortunately, we still have a long way to go. "About 20 percent of humans worldwide wash their hands with soap after toileting," notes Miryam Wahrman in *The Hand Book: Surviving in a Germ-Filled World*. "That leaves 80 percent who do not."[66] Some of us don't wash our hands by choice, either by lack of awareness or motivation, although Mallon was perhaps the last person to be publicly vilified for it. For many people, however, it's simply not possible. The United Nations International Children's Emergency Fund (UNICEF) estimates that currently 40 percent of the world's population, or three billion people, don't have a handwashing facility with water and soap at home. Three-quarters of them live in the world's poorest countries and are among the most vulnerable populations. With its Hand Hygiene for All campaign to provide resources, supplies, and education for hand hygiene, UNICEF estimates that it is possible to prevent around 165,000 deaths from diarrheal diseases each year as well as a range of other diseases, including common colds, flu, and pneumonia.[67] When it comes to hand hygiene, as a global society, we're not lacking in knowledge or resources but rather in urgency and resolve in matters of health equity.

We face a different challenge with the transmission of pathogens through speech because at least one remedy for this problem has taken on symbolic significance beyond its intended functions. Mask wearing has a briefer human history than handwashing, as the earliest use of protective masks during an epidemic was little more than a century ago. European surgeons began to wear masks while treating patients by the end of the nineteenth century, but Malayan physician Wu Lien-Teh popularized them while working to control an outbreak of pneumonic plague in Manchuria in 1910–1911. In fact, his gauze mask design is considered the forerunner of the N95 respirator mask. Mask wearing was central to his antiplague measures (which we'll discuss further in chapter 4) and became a pillar of public health practices in East Asia from then until today. But in the United States, mask wearing during the 1918 influenza pandemic was erased from social memory by the time that COVID-19 emerged in 2019. And when it was reintroduced, many rejected the practice, as did a small subset of the population in 1918, despite abundant scientific evidence to support it (another topic of further exploration in chapter 8).

In all fairness, the science on mask wearing was difficult to follow during the COVID-19 pandemic, and masking policies and recommendations didn't always reflect the latest scientific evidence. But as researchers began to look at the impact of mask interventions in various parts of the world, it became clear that they helped to prevent SARS-CoV-2 infections. In rural Bangladesh, for example, a study of more than 340,000 adults in 600 villages observed a thirty percent increase in mask wearing among adults who were encouraged to do so, which led to a nine percent reduction in COVID-19 cases—and in communities where the researchers promoted surgical mask use, the COVID-19 cases were reduced by eleven percent.[68] Given that it was a voluntary mask-wearing program, the researchers emphasized, it is likely that even greater reductions would have occurred if more people had masked up.[69] Indeed, the effectiveness of mask requirements was evident in a study in Germany, where it was estimated that after 20 days of mandatory mask wearing in a region, new infections fell by around forty-seven percent.[70] This estimation was based on results from the city of Jena, which saw almost zero new infections after face masks became mandatory between April 1 and April 10, 2020.

To reduce infectious disease risks, masks are especially important in closed and crowded settings, as research on aerosol transmission and epidemiological evidence shows. But in the same way that we're always talking and touching, these are the kinds of conditions in which many people around the world reside and work. The types of urbanized environments in which more than half the planet lives, where the spread of crowd diseases like those we've highlighted in this chapter, are a feature of how humans live today. In the next chapter, we'll examine how this happened, what it means, and what we can do about it.

3 Permanent Residents: Setting the Stage

Modern society is the perfect storm of conditions for the sustained transmission of pathogens between people. What could be better for spreading infectious disease than large populations of potential hosts living practically and sometimes literally on top of each other? The answer: when those populations are inextricably connected through travel, trade, and technology. This panoply of pandemic risks is the nature of human existence today.

Yet it wasn't always so. In fact, it was almost always *not* so. From traces of prehistory over hundreds of thousands of years, we know that early humans lived quite differently than most people do today, as small groups that foraged for food and frequently moved across wide swaths of land. Without a steady supply of susceptible hosts to maintain their transmission, acute viral infections like influenza, measles, EVD, and COVID-19 couldn't go far. But as our prehistoric predecessors began to settle down and grow food—constructing permanent settlements, domesticating animals, and adopting agriculture—they altered the dynamics of infectious diseases for hundreds of generations to come. And as we evolved as the engineers of ecosystems, we became the architects of unanticipated adversity.

Our urbanized world, created by the unmatched skill of our species to modify environments to accommodate our needs, is full of opportunities for the rapid and widespread sharing of germs. All the makings of a pandemic are already in place. Fortunately, we have some powerful protections against pandemic threats due to remarkable scientific advances. Humans today benefit enormously from ever-expanding knowledge and tools to identify pathogens as well as mitigate their impacts with vaccines, therapeutics, and public hygiene.

All over the world, there are recent examples of outbreaks that occur in the absence of these resources, underlining their critical importance for human health—such as more than a million cases of cholera among families affected by war in Yemen or thousands of deaths from measles among unvaccinated children in the DRC. And of course in early 2020, people everywhere experienced the devastating consequences of a new disease for which vaccines and specific treatments did not yet exist with the global spread of COVID-19. But we need only look a few centuries into the past in order to see these vulnerabilities laid completely bare, before the rise of modern medicine. Amid the contagious conditions that developed with the astronomical growth of cities, we can recognize some of the epidemic and pandemic risks that we've carried into the modern age.

*   *   *

When poet John Donne composed his famous lines, "No man is an island, entire of itself; every man is a piece of the continent, a part of the main," he was recovering from illness. Winter 1623 had taken a dark turn when he became sick. Fifty-one years old and serving as the dean of Saint Paul's Cathedral, a towering sanctum above the city of London, he could hear the somber ringing of the cathedral bells from his residence in the deanery: "Any man's death diminishes me, because I am involved in mankind, and therefore never send to know for whom the bell tolls; it tolls for thee."[1]

The cause of Donne's illness isn't entirely clear from his writings. In a manner of self-diagnosis, he blamed "pestilent vapours" that were at the time believed to carry disease—a discredited idea now referred to as miasma theory, which we discussed in chapter 1. (Remember, nobody knew that microbes existed in 1623, let alone that such invisible creatures had pathogenic powers.) To be fair, London's air was fouled in those days. Smoke and soot thickened the skies and blackened the buildings, causing such damage to Saint Paul's Cathedral that even King James I was concerned.[2] Diarist John Evelyn wrote about how Londoners were "never free from *Coughs* and importunate *Rheumatisms*, spitting of *Impostumated* and corrupt matter" due to impure vapors and the diseases they delivered.[3]

Frankly, the air stunk. In addition to visible fumes from heavy coal and lime burning across the capital, an array of rank odors wafted through its narrow and congested streets from piles and splatterings of waste. The stench of rotting refuse and excrement mixed with the masses of people and other animals who lived there, particularly in tightly packed places with minimal sanitation.[4] It surely made a person feel sick, causing plenty of problems that resembled an infectious disease.

But the air wasn't directly responsible for Donne's sickness. Today the cause is explained by germ theory, which didn't supplant miasma theory until the discoveries led by Pasteur and Koch in the late nineteenth century. His signs and symptoms, such as fever and rash, support recent theories that he suffered from louse-borne or epidemic typhus.[5] These modern names for an ancient disease refer to how it spreads.[6] The vector of the disease is the body louse (*Pediculus humanus humanus*), a remarkably well-adapted human parasite: it lives and reproduces in clothes. For this reason, it's also known today as the clothing louse, although bedding is another common habitat. Emerging from an egg laid and hatched in the folds of fabric, the tiny insect immediately moves onto the skin for the first of many blood meals, leaving behind small marks that can cause intense itching. Yet this miniscule bloodsucker can also leave its host with something even smaller and indeed microscopic: the rod-shaped bacterium *Rickettsia prowazekii*.

As the etiologic agent of epidemic typhus, *R. prowazekii* has played a deadly part in the human story for millennia. Although this bacillus has a wildlife reservoir in the southern flying squirrel (*Glaucomys volans*) of North America, it spreads mainly via louse-borne transmission between people all over the world. In any case, it's a zoonotic pathogen, passed between species. The body louse catches this bug itself by sucking the blood of an infected host.

The *R. prowazekii* bacteria invade and replicate in the cells of the body louse, which excretes the bacteria by the millions while feeding. If an unsuspecting person scratches, rubs, or inhales the louse's bacteria-laden feces (or crushed remains) into an itchy bite wound or perhaps a mucous membrane—say, by touching the eye with unclean fingers—then *bingo*. It's another human infection of *R. prowazekii* for the history books. The bacteria can then infect the endothelial cells that line blood vessels, causing restricted blood flow along with damaging effects on organs and tissues in the human body. This is how the disease can become fatal if untreated. Although Donne survived epidemic typhus, countless numbers of his contemporaries did not, including his brother.[7]

With a good idea of what caused Donne's illness, we can surmise how he may have been infected. Cold and crowded living conditions with poor sanitation and hygiene are conducive to body lice infestations. Through unwashed clothes and blankets, particularly in circumstances of squalor and confinement, epidemic typhus can thus spread quickly between people. Commonly associated with the dismal settings of soldiers, prisoners, and refugees, this vector-borne disease has also been called camp fever, jail fever, and war fever, respectively.[8] Still today, outbreaks of epidemic typhus occur among people who are displaced, unhoused, and/or living in the wake of conflict, famine, and natural disasters.[9] But when he got sick with epidemic typhus, Donne wasn't quartered in a camp or confined to a prison. In my opinion, the most interesting aspect of his disease experience is where it happened: in the heart of a booming, bustling city.

On a basic level, cities are permanent settlements of a large number of people, most of whom don't grow food for a living.[10] From an archaeological perspective, cities tend to be political, economic, and religious centers, with a wide range of specialized production and services.[11] Historically, they're crossroads that exist for and by exchange.[12] In Donne's time, London was all of these things and more. With a constant inflow of migrants from outlying regions, its population rose to hundreds of thousands of people during the seventeenth century. "This Head grows three times as fast as the Body unto which it belongs. . . . [O]ur *Parishes* are now grown madly disproportionable," wrote demographer John Graunt about London in 1662.[13] Already one of the largest cities in Europe, London flourished as a massive hub of international commerce with a busy river and thronging markets. Even Saint Paul's churchyard swarmed with merchants and dealmakers—a congregation of social classes that formed the harbinger of the shopping mall at the core of the urban ecosystem.[14]

For centuries London's leading commodity was cloth, but pathogens were arguably its most significant trade. Epidemic typhus was raging in London when Donne was ill, as it was wont to do given that clothes and beds were extensively reused and infrequently deloused. This is probably how Donne became infected, a hard-to-avoid consequence for even the most privileged Londoners, with lice endemic to the city and human hosts abound.

But for the urban poor, things were even worse. Large and rapid population increases led to overcrowding in impoverished areas, where houses were partitioned, rooms were shared, and even space in a bed could be rented—resulting in numerous people, sometimes strangers, soiling the same sheets.[15] Typhus went hand in hand with plague, which ravaged London's pestered parishes along with smallpox, measles, dysentery, typhoid fever, and tuberculosis, as many cramped accommodations lacked plumbing and proper ventilation too. In addition, body lice may have transmitted the causal bacterium of plague between people, although its best-known vector is the Oriental rat flea (*Xenopsylla cheopis*), a go-between for humans and the black rat (*Rattus rattus*), a common urban reservoir of plague.[16] Also known as house or roof rats, these rodents could move through porous walls and carry infected fleas between households, especially where houses were subdivided as tenements and joined as blocks. Sometimes called ship rats, they were transported into London by trade ships, whose excesses of food in stores, granaries, and rubbish heaps supported the rodents along with their fleas as huge populations and ever-present health threats. High mortality rates among Londoners reflected a lack of effective treatments for the resulting diseases as well as their limited understanding of the role of humans in their transmission.

No man is an island. In his contemplation of funeral tolling in London, which must have seemed incessant in the midst of so much death, Donne had more insight into the cause of his illness than he realized. His theological view of humankind as interdependent was, in fact, an epidemiological reality. This has never been more accurate than today. Whereas about 1 billion humans were sharing the planet 200 years ago, there are around eight billion of us at present. Currently over half the world's human population resides in urban areas, and 1 in 5 people live in a city with at least 1 million other coinhabitants.[17] These trends are increasing dramatically, as more cities turn into megacities of 10 million people or more. Our constant interactions in large, dense, and highly connected conglomerations have become a part of a fundamental element of the human experience. And at the same time, they've become a powerful driver of epidemic and pandemic diseases.

How did people come to live in highly populated and urbanized settings, and what are the implications of these changes for the emergence and spread of infectious diseases? How were things different in the past? When did they change? The forces that gave rise to pandemics actually began long before humans started to make the materials of the modern city, before environments were built to last. Before the crowds arrived.

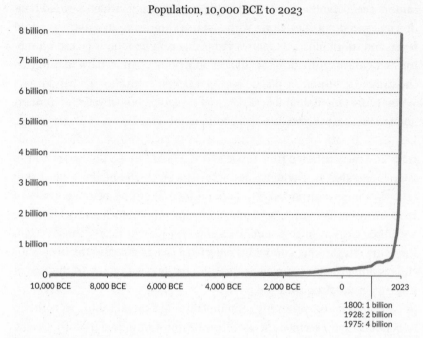

Figure 3.1
Human population growth over the last 12,000 years. The majority of the world's human population growth has occurred in the last two centuries, increasing from around 1 billion to nearly 8 billion people. *Source:* Data published in Global Burden of Disease Collaborative Network, *Global Burden of Disease Study 2019 Results* (Seattle: Institute for Health Metrics and Evaluation, 2021), via Our World in Data.

Spreading Out

Not long ago, geologically speaking, humans were few and far between. Only a little further back in time, there were none at all. And until relatively recently, everyone was African. Our species, *Homo sapiens*, evolved during a slice of time that geologists define as the Pleistocene epoch between around 2.58 million and 11,700 years ago. To date, the earliest fossils that have been identified as *Homo sapiens* are about 315,000 years old—an astonishing discovery in Morocco that pushed back the timing of modern human origins in Africa by more than 100,000 years.[18] Many scientists have long held that *Homo sapiens* evolved in a particular African region, as a "cradle of humanity," but it now seems possible that the evolutionary processes behind the emergence of *Homo sapiens* may have involved the whole African continent. New finds such as the Moroccan fossils have raised tantalizing possibilities of connections and contacts among a larger, interbreeding population of ancient humans, making for a pan-African origin of our species.[19]

Early humans spread not only across Africa but also out of it. First reaching Eurasia by about 210,000 years ago and finally the Americas by at least 16,000 years ago, the global dispersal of *Homo sapiens* was a prelude to our planetary domination today—a topic of further discussion in chapter 5.[20] Thanks to a special combination of advantages, including bipedal locomotion, tool manufacture, and extraordinary cognitive capacity, our Pleistocene ancestors were able to move and adapt to environments just about anywhere.

Mobility was a big part of survival for most early humans, who procured much of their diet from hunting, gathering, fishing, collecting, and scavenging the local fare—a broad range of subsistence activities known as foraging. Some of these movements and behaviors have subtle signals in bones, stones, and genomes recovered from the archaeological record, while others literally left tracks, such as fossilized footprints of small groups of foragers on the trails of their prey.[21] Although people didn't invent writing systems until much later in history (around 5,400 years ago), we have additional insights into early human lifeways and ecosystems through pictorial scenes and animal representations in cave paintings as early as 45,000 years before the present time.[22]

Early human experiences with pathogens and illnesses are difficult to reconstruct, but scientists can make some inferences about the infectious disease profiles of early human foragers from archaeological, skeletal, and molecular information. For starters, there's no evidence to suggest that our earliest ancestors were unhealthy in general. On the contrary, they appear to have eaten quite well by modern nutritional standards, particularly in ways that would have supported a strong immune system.[23] Of course, that doesn't mean good health was a piece of cake, so to speak. Foraging would have required significant energy investments, and seasonal shortages could have easily occurred. But what ancient African diets lacked in predictability, they made up for in breadth and balance. For instance, consider the 315,000-year-old fossils of *Homo sapiens* found in Morocco. More specifically, they were found in a cave. And even more specifically, they were found in a cave with the likely leftovers from many meals, such as broken bones and shells, representing an impressive menu of gazelles, wildebeests, buffalo, porcupines, hares, tortoises, mollusks, snakes, and ostrich eggs.[24]

Additionally, at other sites in South Africa and elsewhere, human remains up to 130,000 years old have produced microscopic evidence of an omnivorous appetite. From dental calculus (that is, calcified plaque on the teeth) and stone tools, the remnants of starch grains and phytoliths indicate that our ancient ancestors ate a wide variety of plants too.[25] These findings add to an enormous body of scientific support for diverse diets of high-protein and high-fiber foods during the Pleistocene, inspiring the Paleo diet as a modern weight-loss fad. Yet according to one of my NMNH colleagues, paleoanthropologist Briana Pobiner, "The real 'Paleo diet' is eating whatever you can get."

Pleistocene foragers likely had more exposure to wildlife than many of their nonforaging successors and thus ample opportunities for spillover. The potential pathogens would have varied from one habitat to another, posing new threats where humans moved into new environments.[26] This hasn't changed. Today more than 70 percent of emerging or reemerging zoonoses have a wildlife origin, such as coronaviruses that cause SARS, MERS, and COVID-19, as we learned in chapter 1. And they've been on the rise in recent decades, largely because of changing human-animal interactions related to urbanization, industrialized food production, and other ecologically disruptive enterprises.[27] Recent research shows that bats, nonhuman primates, and rodents harbor especially high proportions of zoonotic viruses worldwide, but other kinds of animals, such as carnivores and even-toed ungulates in Africa, deserve increased surveillance.[28]

Given that even-toed ungulates like gazelles account for the majority of leftovers in the aforementioned Moroccan cave, our earliest human ancestors may have risked spillover from at least some of the animals they killed and consumed. Nowadays wildlife hunting and butchering are well-known to increase risks for blood-borne zoonotic infections, with potentially far-reaching impacts. For example, these behaviors have been implicated in the origin of the pandemic spread of HIV from Central Africa during the twentieth century. So does this mean that Pleistocene foragers faced the same epidemic and pandemic concerns as we do now?

Probably not. Like a fire running out of fuel, outbreaks can burn out when susceptible hosts—the organisms necessary for a pathogen's replication and spread—are in short supply. This can happen in cases of acute viral infections with epidemic and pandemic potential, such as EVD, measles, and influenza, which tend to be self-limiting in small, isolated communities.[29] Our early ancestors probably lived in ways that weren't conducive to the rapid and widespread transmission of such diseases, scattered across broad expanses of land in small, mobile groups.[30] Archaeological evidence suggests that residential groups of no more than thirty to forty individuals were common among foragers of the Pleistocene, possibly with seasonal or periodic aggregations into larger groupings.[31] Like modern foragers of the tropics and subtropics, early *Homo sapiens* may have lived in temporary camps as groups of them moved from place to place, making short-term constructions from expedient and perishable materials, or taking advantage of natural shelters in rock features.[32] There are good reasons that caves are frequent sites of early human discoveries in light of their benefits for protection during life and preservation after death.

Genetic and paleoenvironmental data also suggest that early human populations throughout Africa were small and strongly subdivided, connected by sporadic interbreeding amid strong climatic fluctuations and across shifting ecological boundaries over time.[33] Combined with fossil and archaeological evidence, these findings point to the likelihood that some populations were semi-isolated for millennia by distance or habitat. Here again, it seems unlikely that enough people were living in sufficiently close and frequent contact for the human-to-human transmission of diseases over large spatial extents. Recent genomic research, however, indicates that seasonal concentrations of early *Homo sapiens* populations in riverine, lacustrine, and coastal environments of Africa were able to maintain the transmission of malaria from *Plasmodium* parasites (*P. vivax* and *P. falciparum*) via *Anopheles* mosquitoes.[34] Additional studies show that *Helicobacter pylori* (a common cause of digestive illnesses) and *M. tuberculosis* strains may have accompanied early human movements within and out of the African continent during the Late Pleistocene. Thus even in small and low-density populations, early humans may have sustained such pathogens as low-virulence, chronic infections, in contrast to many of the epidemic diseases that were yet to come.

Coming Together

Here's where the human story takes a dramatic downward turn with respect to health. It all started with the end of the Pleistocene, which marked the beginning of one of the most transformative periods in the history of *Homo sapiens*. This was when, simply put, human populations started to settle down, grow plants, and raise animals as a way of life.[35] After hundreds of thousands of years of foraging, the transition to farming was revolutionary for human society. For this reason, the onset of the subsequent Holocene epoch (about 11,700 years ago until present) is also known as the Agricultural Revolution.

Agriculture developed independently at different times and places in the world, but likely first in a crescent-shaped region of the Near East called (surprise, surprise) the Fertile Crescent. Throughout this region, archaeological, biological, and genetic evidence shows the initial phases of domestication in both plants and animals, from small-scale trial cultivation by foragers about 23,000 years ago to signs of species management by around 12,000 years ago.[36] These experiments and investments eventually paid off in extra food and more stable social groups for the ecological engineers of the Early Holocene. Over the course of the next several millennia, agriculture spread, and year-round settlements grew in size and dependence on domestic crops and livestock. With the emergence of cities in the Near East as early as 7,000 years ago, human populations became increasingly urbanized and connected throughout Eurasia and beyond, where large sedentary communities expanded into centers of construction, consumption, and trade. And as these processes intensified, we can identify significant changes in human activities and lifestyles that raised epidemic and pandemic risks.

Let's start with the agricultural diet. Nutrition is a major factor in host responses to infection, as the immune system requires a constant supply of essential nutrients in order to fend off invading pathogens. Nutritional deficiency is therefore often associated with impaired immunologic function and infectious disease susceptibility. With shifts from foraging to farming during the Holocene, as people became more reliant on a narrower and less nutritious range of foods, human infections seem to have increased. The proof is written in bone: skeletal indicators of systemic infections, metabolic diseases, and developmental stresses are more frequent in agricultural populations than in non- or preagricultural ones.[37] And then there's the teeth. By eating more domesticated cereals and soft, carbohydrate-rich foods, agriculturists had bigger issues with periodontal disease, cavities, and plaque than foragers—the kind of problems that illustrate the importance of brushing and flossing today. Ancient oral microbiomes (the communities of microbes that colonize the mouth) reconstructed from dental calculus also show a disease-associated shift in pathogenic bacteria with the transition to farming during the Early Holocene.[38]

Sedentism, or putting down roots, involves a number of risk factors for infectious diseases. The practice of staying in one place for a long time wasn't exclusive to agriculturalists, as some foragers were (and still are) sedentary to different degrees. One big difference, however, came with surplus and refuse. A commitment to agriculture meant living with both, at least most of the time. Stored food and water can attract wildlife reservoirs and insect vectors of infectious disease, creating more opportunities for various zoonoses to infiltrate a community. For example, the yellow fever mosquito (*Aedes egypti*), which also transmits the pathogens that cause dengue, chikungunya, and Zika virus disease, breeds only in stagnant water within human-created containers. Like the body louse, it's a human-adapted insect. In addition, stores of grains can be a source of food for rodents and parasites, and hence become contaminated with their feces. We saw some effects of such excesses taken to the extreme in our visit to seventeenth-century London, with rats in the rafters, garbage in the streets, and pathogens galore. Accumulations of fecal waste posed similar risks for sedentary societies, increasing in step with swelling settlements of people and domesticated animals. Finally, when infections occurred, built shelters may have presented their occupants with greater dangers from the air within than from the elements outside. Permanent housing provides enclosed air circulation that facilitates the indoor transmission of airborne diseases, a common concern with influenza and COVID-19 infections today. Sedentism thus put more susceptible hosts within reach—or cough—of each other than ever before.

Domestication, the evolutionary process of artificial (as opposed to natural) selection by which we created new species for human use, fundamentally transformed our interactions with other animals. In so doing, we increased our exposure to new microbes from our furry and feathered friends. Whether for work, food, or companionship, domesticated animals can transmit zoonotic pathogens to humans through direct and frequent

contact with them. These animals are particularly effective as interme-
diate hosts of pathogens that originate in wildlife, often serving as con-
duits or even amplifiers for new and highly pathogenic viruses in people.
Domestic pigs (*Sus scrofa*), which farmers raised in the Fertile Crescent as
early as 9,000 years ago, provide an excellent example of a potential epidemic threat. In 1998–1999, the first human outbreak of the Nipah virus in
Malaysia and Singapore was traced to pig farms and ultimately bats known
as flying foxes (*Pteropus hypomelanus* and *Petropus vampyrus*), which had
contaminated pig feed with their virus-laden droppings from fruit trees
overhanging the pigsties.[39] Domestic pigs also act as a mixing vessel for
influenza viruses that originate in wild waterfowl and can result in human
flu pandemics, which happened with the H1N1 pandemic of 2009–2010.[40]
As illustrated in both cases, however, the *intensification* of farming throughout the Holocene is the most serious disease risk associated with livestock,
creating and confining large, high-density populations of potential hosts
as well as disturbing and destroying the natural habitats of wildlife along
with the microbes they carry.

Population growth is a dominant trend across the Holocene, and one
of the biggest factors in the spread of epidemic diseases. As humans mul-
tiplied and large aggregates of susceptible hosts formed, the urbanization
of the ancient world became increasingly conducive to highly transmissible human diseases. Measles (caused by *Measles morbillivirus*) is one of the
most contagious of them all, with highly efficient airborne spread. Its basic
reproduction number (R0) is 12–18, meaning that on average, between 12
and 18 susceptible hosts will be infected by one contagious person in the
absence of any deliberate interventions, such as mask wearing. (The 2009
H1N1 influenza virus, in contrast, had a R0 of less than 2.)

Yet as already we know, measles doesn't persist in small, isolated populations. In fact, the minimum size of a closed population in which it can
persist indefinitely is about 250,000 to 500,000 individuals. You might then
guess that the measles virus emerged around the time that human communities began to approach this critical size. If you did, you would be correct.
Recent genomic analyses suggest that the measles virus arose as early as
about 2,600 years ago, when cities such as Luoyang in China and Babylon
in Mesopotamia already had populations of 100,000 to 200,000 people.[41]
Because the virus has an infectious period of only about eight days and
must be transmitted between people sharing air, the population densities

of these urban centers could have provided the necessary conditions for its spread. And as cities grew in density and number, so did the pathogens of crowd diseases that afflicted their many inhabitants.

Making Connections

Transportation routes, as pathways of connectivity between urban centers, were critical for the long-distance, multiregional trade of goods during the Holocene. Urban populations demanded imports, but they got more than they expected through the transmission of pathogens. These connections enabled the worldwide transmission of infectious diseases, species to species and shore to shore, which are evident in cross-continental waves of plague over the last several thousand years. Genomic analyses of *Y. pestis* obtained from Late Neolithic/Bronze Age human skeletons show that less virulent strains of plague bacteria were spreading with human migrations across Eurasia thousands of years before any historical recordings of pandemics of the disease, during a period between around 5,000 and 2,500 years ago.[42] Moving with westward expansions that likely originated in the Eurasian Steppe, *Y. pestis* first arrived in Britain at least 4,000 years ago, in a form that may have not been transmissible via fleas.[43] However, strains of *Y. pestis* with the potential for flea-borne infections—and for bubonic disease—also arose at this time (if not earlier), as revealed by 3,800 year old *Y. pestis* genomes recovered from human skeletons in modern-day Russia.[44]

With the development of globe-spanning trade routes linking Asia and Europe, plague spread just about everywhere in three centuries-long pandemics. The first plague pandemic began with the Justinianic plague in ca. 541–544, which killed many inhabitants of the Byzantine Empire, particularly in its capital city of Constantinople, by then the world's largest city with a population of perhaps half a million people. The initial outbreak was reported in the Mediterranean port city of Pelusium in Roman Egypt on the eastern edge of the Nile Delta. From there, grain ships may have imported *Y. pestis* carried by stowaway rats and fleas, which thrived on the large granaries maintained by the Roman government. The geographic origin of the lineage of *Y. pestis* that led to the Justinianic plague is uncertain at present, although an introduction from Central Asia through overland or oceanic trade routes seems most probable.[45] As more outbreaks spanned the Mediterranean region and beyond, the pandemic continued until ca. 750.

The second plague pandemic was much longer and far more devastating to humanity, beginning with an initial wave known as the Black Death (ca. 1346–1353) and spreading across Europe for the next five centuries. The Black Death alone may have wiped out over half the human population of western Eurasia over its eight-year course, caused by a strain of *Y. pestis* that's been traced to fourteenth-century cemeteries near modern-day Kyrgyzstan.[46] These cemeteries contained many burial sites dated between 1338 and 1339, with some inscriptions referring to an unspecified pestilence as the cause of death. Genomes of *Y. pestis* from several individuals are indicative of a plague epidemic that preceded the Black Death in Europe by seven or eight years.

Nestled in a valley surrounded by the Tian Shan Mountains of Central Asia, these plague-stricken communities appear to have been ethnically diverse, and highly reliant on trade and connections with several regions across Eurasia, with people living in settlements in close proximity to trans-Asian trade networks. Most likely these people were infected with *Y. pestis* from flea-ridden marmots in the region (which still carry a descendant strain of the plague pathogen today), but through trade activities, more people and animals throughout Europe eventually met with the disease as well. Maritime trade routes may have been a significant source of transmission in Europe, bringing ships with plague-infected rats and fleas to urbanized ports and commercial hubs, where grain warehouses and dense populations allowed the spread to continue.[47]

The third plague pandemic began in the Yunnan region of China in 1855 and reached all human-inhabited continents by 1900. This was another feat of maritime transportation, owed partly to an unprecedented expansion of international trade following the invention of the steamship.[48] Plague was also a companion of colonialism, resulting in major outbreaks in Hong Kong, Bombay (present-day Mumbai), and other places under British rule at the end of the nineteenth century. (Out of at least twelve million deaths caused by the third plague pandemic, at least ten million of them were in India alone.) Mostly by sea, people spread the pathogen from Hong Kong to India, and then to Africa, South America, Europe, Australia, North America, and the Middle East. The pandemic started to dissipate by the 1920s and was declared over by the WHO in 1960, but *Y. pestis* was by no means gone. As we learned in chapter 1, the pathogen is still carried and transmitted by rodent reservoirs around world—an epidemiological legacy of the human activities that provided a never-ending supply of hosts.

Getting Bigger

Many cities were demographically flattened by the plague pandemics, especially during the Black Death, which laid waste to countless urban and rural communities throughout Europe. Before Donne's time, the Black Death killed about half of all Londoners in 1349.[49] The second plague pandemic continued throughout his life and well beyond; decades after Donne's death, London lost another 15 percent of its population, perhaps more than 100,000 lives in total, to the Great Plague of 1665. Still, even in periods in pestilence, Donne and his contemporaries had no idea how crowded their city would become. Between 1714 and 1840, London's population grew from around 630,000 to 2 million people, overtaking Beijing as the largest city in the world.[50] This dramatic climb was part of a major expansion in urbanization during the Industrial Revolution, a transition to mechanized production processes in Great Britain, resulting in unprecedented population increases and growth rates.

But London wouldn't hold its number one status for long. Even though the population of London has swelled to almost 9 million people today, at present it falls short of the 10-million-people marker of a megacity. New York City and Tokyo were the first cities to reach this threshold in the 1950s, and since then an increasing proportion of the world's biggest cities have been concentrated in Asia. This trend may hold over the short term, but already the population center of the world is gravitating toward a different continent. With undeniable narrative symmetry, to better anticipate our future, we should look to where we started. Because population-wise, Africa is exploding in the twenty-first century.

These were the observations of my colleague Dennis Carroll at a global health conference in 2019. The world in which we live now will be extremely different in 2100, Dennis predicted, partly because half the most populous countries will be in sub-Saharan Africa. So will the world's top megacities—Lagos in Nigeria, Kinshasa in the DRC, and Dar es Salaam in Tanzania—with an estimated 70–80 million inhabitants each.[51] By the end of the century, more than 8 out of every 10 people in the world will live in

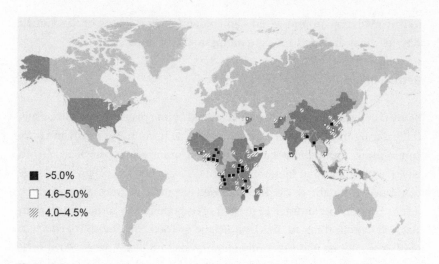

Figure 3.2
The fastest-growing cities in the world: Cities with the highest average annual growth rates between 2020-2025. While recent decades have seen rapid urbanization in Asia, in the 2020s, the fastest-growing cities are in Africa. *Note:* 2018 projections, out of all cities with 300,000 inhabitants or more. *Sources:* Statista, https://www.statista.com/chart/24298/fastest-growing-cities; data from UN Department of Economic and Social Affairs, UN World Urbanization Prospects, at https://population.un.org/wup/?_gl=1*10h60a8*_ga*MjAwNzM5ODQ4Ni4xNjg3NDA3OTE2*_ga_TK9BQL5X7Z*MTY4Nzk3MjQ0OC4zLjAuMTY4Nzk3MjQ1Mi4wLjAuMA. Reproduced under a CC BY-ND license.

Asia or Africa, although Asia will see a significant fall from almost 60 percent of the global population today to around 45 percent in 2100.[52] In Africa, on the other hand, we'll see a rise from 18 to 38 percent of the global population.

These changes in population size and distribution are intertwined with other trends, or megatrends, that will be centered in Africa. All over the world and most especially there, we'll see them converge with increases in health burdens from noninfectious diseases, infrastructure needs such as better water and air quality, habitat changes associated with agriculture and livestock production, global temperatures resulting from human carbon pollution, and transformative technologies that will connect just about everyone on the planet. Some of the most dangerous effects will be the emergence and spread of more infectious diseases. And in some places, we've already seen this happen, as with EVD in West Africa in 2014.

Since 1976, when scientists discovered Zaire ebolavirus, the most common causal pathogen of EVD, in a community near the Ebola River in the modern-day DRC, there have been dozens of periodic outbreaks and hundreds of human deaths within a number of African countries.[53] But people aren't the only casualties of Ebola viruses, which can be deadly to nonhuman primates as well. Chimpanzees and gorillas experience severe illness and mass mortality from EVD, indicating that they're not reservoir hosts of the virus, even though they can transmit it to humans. Bats make sense as its natural origin—a probability supported by the 2019 discovery of RNA fragments of Zaire ebolavirus in a bat captured near the Liberia-Guinea border in West Africa.[54] It was a major announcement around the world and a long-missing piece in the ecological puzzle of a terrifying epidemic threat.

The first Ebola outbreak in West Africa was the deadliest in the history of the disease. In blunt terms, it was a disaster of preventable proportions. In early 2014, a few cases of EVD were reported in Meliandou, a village of only thirty-one households in a forested area of southeastern Guinea.[55] The presumed source was human contact with wild animals, more likely bats than nonhuman primates, both of which are hunted and eaten by people locally.[56] The most common story about the epidemic's origins have centered on a two-year-old boy who was seen playing near a tree occupied by bats, which may have been displaced by recent deforestation from mining and logging operations around the area. The boy's role as an index patient for the epidemic has been disputed, however, based on claims that an adult EVD patient brought the virus into the village.[57] In any case, the child died two days after falling ill with EVD symptoms like fever and vomiting, while the disease spread—quickly and fatally—to members of his family and the people who took care of them in the nearby town of Guéckédou. Cases skyrocketed as those infected with the virus carried it into major urban centers, including the capital cities of Guinea, Liberia, and Sierra Leone, as well as other countries and continents via air travel. In a matter of months, the scale and geographic range of the transmission was beyond any previous EVD outbreak, reaching the United States in fall 2014. By the end of the Ebola epidemic in 2016, it had caused more than 28,600 cases and over 11,300 deaths, far exceeding the total counts of all previous outbreaks combined.[58]

The West African Ebola epidemic was a catastrophic consequence of recent changes in land use, population growth, urbanization, and transportation in the region. Rather than the outbreak in Meliandou burning out, these familiar factors fanned the flames. Industrial activities had transformed the rich ecosystems of the region, decimating once-abundant forests, and forcing wild animals like bats into new habitats and interactions with humans. Population densities had risen dramatically over the preceding four decades of Ebola outbreaks in Africa, more than tripling on average across Guinea, Liberia, and Sierra Leone.[59] Within the same span of time, the proportion of these populations that became urbanized increased by as much 223 percent. And in addition to the large, crowded centers that had grown with rural-to-urban migration since 1976, people had become more connected than ever before. By 2014, previously remote villages were linked to larger towns and high-density centers by major road networks, allowing EVD-infected individuals to move rapidly to populous places and spread the virus widely. Local hospitals were limited and overwhelmed, necessitating the construction of temporary Ebola treatment units that also became filled beyond capacity. It was the first time that the disease had taken hold of crowded metropolitan areas, and urban Ebola was a cautionary tale for dangers ahead.

In the same way that One Health looks at the dynamic interface of human, animal, and environmental health, the complexities of global health require a more holistic perspective on our rapidly multiplying, disruptive, and interconnected species. We need to mobilize global efforts, as Dennis argued and I agree, that forge alliances between government, academy, business, and communities, and understand how economics, population dynamics, geopolitics, and urban planning influence as well as intersect with infectious disease. These epidemic and pandemic factors that developed through human history remain with us even more powerfully today and for the long haul. In recognizing and understanding them, the abrupt and rapid spread of infectious disease should be less surprising and mystifying.

But demographics and infrastructure weren't the only drivers of the 2014 emergence of EVD in West Africa. There were cultural behaviors that also contributed to the spread of EVD in 2014, and behavioral changes were essential to ending it. In the next chapter, we'll look at how this happened, and consider the cultural context of habits, traditions, and rituals by which humans often unwittingly, and all too frequently, spread disease.

4   Cultural Transmission: Sharing Is Caring

Of all the factors that contribute to the spread of pathogens, human behavior can be the biggest head-scratcher. Defined as how humans act, react, and interact, human behavior is one of the major obstacles to predicting or mitigating disease threats. That's because there are layers on layers of decisions that affect a person's behaviors in every context, when sick or well, whether consciously made or not. Even the most mundane meal can be a fusion of necessity, preference, tradition, and convenience, influencing not only what one eats but also how, where, when, and with whom. Feelings and knowledge about infectious disease risks might add another layer to the decision-making, but not necessarily the one that matters the most.

Many of our behaviors are based on things that we've learned from others. Nobody is born with any information or ideas about how to interact with or conduct themselves in the world, although everybody inherits genes for biological structures and functions through which behavior is expressed. And nobody, as we learned in the last chapter, is an island. Much of our behavioral information is acquired as we grow older, passed on to us by those who raise and teach us what to do, and strengthened or modified by social lessons—from those with whom we live, work, keep company, and share experiences—throughout life.

This phenomenon is by no means unique to our species. Across the animal kingdom, there are fascinating examples of behavior shaped and reproduced through social learning.[1] Adult meerkats (*Suricata suricatta*) teach their young how to handle dangerous prey in a manner of spoon-fed scorpions by first removing the sting from scorpions before feeding them to pups, and then gradually introducing the pups to live pincers and monitoring their handling behavior.[2] Juvenile white-crowned sparrows (*Zonotrichia leucophrys*) learn songs by imitating adults in their population, mastering the distinct features and shared vocabulary of the local dialect to communicate with their neighbors.[3] Chimpanzees even copy behavior from their group members without any clear adaptive benefit whatsoever, such as sticking a blade of grass in their ears for the purpose of . . . style?[4]

We do this a lot too. Humans transmit all kinds of instructions and rules to each other through social learning by explaining, demonstrating, guiding, modeling, and reinforcing. When locked into our brains, this information governs our customs, practices, traditions, habits, and skills, and differentiates our social behaviors as groups and communities. Some anthropologists, including yours truly, might sum up this sort of information in a single word: *culture*.[5] Put simply by neuroscientist Robert Sapolsky, culture is how we do and think about things.[6]

As a species, our cultural differences vastly outweigh our biological variation. There are countless ways to eat; there's only one way to swallow. From rites and rituals to values and beliefs, culture can affirm our bonds with certain people and mark our differences from other ones, such as in the languages we speak, clothes we wear, and holidays we celebrate. It can reflect what's normal, familiar, or important to us, with multiple meanings and purposes through which we communicate emotions and affirm a shared understanding of the world. For this reason, our socially learned cultural behaviors can be the hardest ones to give up or change when faced with pandemic threats, even when, and sometimes especially when, these behaviors facilitate the transmission of pathogens.

Cultural behaviors got a lot of attention during the Ebola epidemic in West Africa from 2014 to 2016 as they influenced how EVD spread and was ultimately contained in the most affected communities of Guinea, Liberia, and Sierra Leone. In his book *Fevers, Feuds, and Diamonds*, medical anthropologist and physician Paul Farmer framed the West African epidemic within a regional history of extractive colonialism, armed conflict, and social injustice that created a public health and clinical desert in which the catastrophe was almost inevitable. Yet he also recognized the influences of cultural beliefs and behaviors on the transmission of the virus as well as in how people reacted to its harms: "Anthropology, for its part, taught me to distrust confident claims about local culture as *the* chief determinant of recurrent suffering and early death, even as it taught me that culture and context are everywhere important in facing unequally distributed misfortune; whatever the fates deal out, culture invariably shapes social responses to it."[7]

Farmer's statement could be applied to virtually any epidemic or pandemic in the past or present, when people have been called on to suspend or modify their habits and customs for public health reasons. This is why culture warrants discussion in a book about the human features and factors of pandemics. And thus in this chapter, we're going to consider how culture intersects with infectious diseases in both unusual circumstances and everyday experiences: the specific cases of caring for the dead and sharing food. Understanding why some behaviors, and behavior *changes*, are instrumental to infection control is a critical lesson in facing and fighting disease.

Death Rites

At the NMNH, a place where deceased organisms take up a lot more space than living ones, there's a special spot for an individual whose remains are especially famous for where and how they were buried. Known as Shanidar 3, the fossilized skeleton is one of a number of Neanderthals (*Homo neanderthalensis*) who dwelled in the Shanidar Cave in northern Iraq around 65,000 to 35,000 years ago. When the site was first discovered in the 1950s, nobody knew that these evolutionary cousins of *Homo sapiens* made graves for their dead. But at least some of the Shanidar skeletons show evidence of this kind of behavior, including possibly Shanidar 3. Now laid to rest on an acid-free bed, within a climate-controlled case under an airtight lid, the skeleton is treated and displayed with the utmost care, like the Hope Diamond of the Hall of Human Origins.[8] And rightly so, given how much the Shanidar remains changed our understanding of Neanderthal culture.

Mortuary practices such as interment (that is, burial) are exceptionally meaningful acts. In greater service to the living than the deceased, they serve as an emotional outlet for grief and mourning, physical means to commemorate and stay connected to those who died, and collective affirmation of social and religious beliefs among the mourners. Deliberate burials of Neanderthal and human remains in residential localities start to appear in the archaeological record after about 120,000 years ago, using familiar and accessible places that indicate extended caring for individuals across the life-death divide. As such, argues anthropologist Mary Stiner, burials provide the strongest case for symbolism among the Neanderthals and early modern humans alike.[9]

The earliest-known human burial in Africa so far, dated to around 78,000 years ago in a cave site on the coast of Kenya, is a striking example. The deceased was a young child placed in a burial pit in a tightly flexed position, lying on the right side of the body with knees drawn to the chest (often called a fetal position). The rotation of the collarbone and the first and second ribs suggests that the upper body was wrapped or shrouded in some kind of material, such as large leaves or animals skins—an act that would make little sense for a body regarded as merely a lifeless corpse, the research team noted. Additionally, in another detail described by the researchers as a tender touch, the positioning of the head was consistent with a pillow of biodegradable material being placed underneath it for support, as the dearly departed was tucked in one last time.[10]

Since the extinction of Neanderthals about 40,000 years ago, we're the only species who behaves like this. Most animals appear to show little interest in the remains of their dead, although there are exceptions. Some colony-living animals, such as social insects and brown rats (*Rattus norvegicus*) have special procedures to dispose of bodies, yet they do so to reduce the risks of disease or predator attacks in order to maintain the health of the colony.[11] Similarly, certain birds like wild American crows (*Corvus brachyrhynchos*) will gather around the corpse of the same species so that they can learn and communicate about the dangers of the area.[12]

To be sure, there are a few animals who convey concern when confronted with the death of a group member, namely chimpanzees and bonobos (*Pan paniscus*), African elephants, and toothed whales and dolphins. Numerous whale and dolphin species, for instance, support or carry dead calves at the surface of the water in a mournful reflection of the social bonds of group-living species for whom raising offspring is critical for survival.[13] None of these animals, however, bury their own.

Today burial is an exclusively human treatment of our deceased loved ones, and it's hardly the only one. Across many millennia, our mortuary practices have become as diverse as human culture itself, with acts of mourning and commemoration that include setting the dead adrift on a ship, exhuming their skeletons for a yearly dance, cremating bodies for at-home urns, building monuments and elaborate tombs for their interment, and leaving the deceased to be devoured by animals.[14] Often these events draw people together, even those without strong personal connections to the person who died, for purposes of tradition, respect, comfort, and group solidarity. Religion, too, can be a strong motivation.

Religion is unique and universal among humans.[15] Generally characterized as faith in the existence of supernatural powers and beings, no other living species has religion as we recognize it. Not every person is religious or learned religion in early life, but for many people around the world, it's a core component of their values, views, and decisions.

Among scientists, proposed explanations for how and why religion became a human universal are fiercely debated. Psychologist Paul Bloom sees religion as an evolutionary accident, a by-product of adaptations that arose under selective pressures for other functions.[16] Although culture is clearly one element, he suggests that religious beliefs emerged across human societies because of certain cognitive capacities of the human brain, such as our tendency to see agency and intention where none exists (which also explains our tendency to anthropomorphize microbes).[17]

Other researchers attribute religion to adaptation via natural selection, which means that it provided some reproductive benefit to earlier humans. Biologist Dominic Johnson and psychologist Jesse Bering, for example, argue that religious fears of supernatural punishment for selfish behavior would have promoted cooperation and thus survival.[18] I'm sorry to tell you that these debates won't be resolved here, although we'll revisit the evolution of human cooperative behavior and brain anatomy in later chapters. But as biologist Jeffrey Schloss points out, even if religion arose as a reproductive payoff for our predecessors, that doesn't mean that it came without costs for individual health.[19] These costs are what we're going to explore.

*   *   *

One of the most tragic features of the Ebola epidemic in West Africa was how many people got sick and died as a result of taking care of others. In a cruel paradox, the disease was spread by compassion. The pathogen preyed on love. Health care workers were disproportionately represented among EVD cases and deaths, with Guinea and Liberia losing 7–8 percent of their doctors, nurses, and midwives between 2014 and 2015.[20] And other people contracted EVD through caretaking in culturally significant ways, including during burial preparations for people who died.

Unfortunately, some of these final acts of farewell, guided by religious beliefs and mortuary traditions, contributed to further EVD transmission within communities. These behaviors existed long before EVD ravaged the region—that is, before they became routes of disease transmission. But they led to more suffering when combined with a pathogen of particular properties, and the Ebola virus was one of the worst possibilities.

The Ebola virus is transmitted between people primarily via direct contact with infected body fluids from symptomatic patients, such as blood, saliva, vomit, diarrhea, urine, breast milk, sweat, and semen, which can enter the body of an uninfected person through mucosal surfaces or skin abrasions. The R0 for the West African epidemic was 1.5–2.5, meaning that each patient infected one or two other people on average.[21] By comparison, an airborne respiratory virus like measles virus (with an R0 of 12–18) is far more contagious due to its route of transmission (as we learned in the previous chapter). Yet another reason for this difference is that unlike with measles, a person can only infect other people with Ebola virus after developing signs and symptoms of the disease, following an incubation period of two to twenty-one days. The virus can also remain infectious in people's body fluids for months or years after recovering from the disease, even when they no longer have symptoms of severe illness, such as in the semen of male survivors.

Typically beginning with nonspecific symptoms like a fever, headache, and weakness, early EVD can be difficult to distinguish from more common diseases such as malaria and typhoid fever without confirmation by a positive laboratory test. And despite the widespread idea of EVD patients in blood-gushing death throes (as depicted in Richard Preston's novel *The Hot Zone*), uncontrolled bleeding is rare. More commonly in the West African epidemic, patients experienced persistent and untreated dehydration from vomiting and diarrhea, and thus died from hypovolemic shock due to severe fluid loss. Although the average mortality rate for EVD in West Africa was around 50 percent, and varied between 25 and 90 percent in past outbreaks, early treatment and effective care was a big factor in survival outcomes. (As Farmer notes, most of the Europeans and North Americans who fell ill with EVD were able to survive because they were flown to other countries for medical care that could be delivered safely in a modern hospital with rigorous infection control.)[22] Since then, the development and use of EVD vaccines have helped control the spread of the disease in subsequent outbreaks, to the extent that the vaccines have been accessible and accepted by people at risk.[23]

But with EVD, death isn't necessarily the end of transmission.[24] The amount of virus in the body (known as the viral load) increases with disease severity and reaches its highest levels at the end of life.[25] The infectious virus may then persist in a deceased patient's body fluids and on their body's surfaces for more than a week.[26] Funerary treatments involving direct contact with the body are therefore highly risky. Also, along with the viral load, the quantity of a patient's close contacts may increase in their final days. No doubt, all over the world, there are few circumstances that compel people to gather and grieve together as disease and death do.

Unprotected contact with the bodies and fluids of EVD patients was common during the epidemic in West Africa, where family and community members often touch, kiss, and wash the bodies of loved ones in acts of comfort, sadness, and good-bye.[27] For many West Africans, these practices are intertwined with ideas about the supernatural world. In some cases, family members bathe their hands in a common bowl after touching the face of the departed in order to cement unity between the living and ancestral spirits. When the deceased is a prominent person, such as a traditional healer, people might lay on top of the body with the hope that some of the spiritual gifts will be transferred to them. Furthermore, failure to honor and respect the dead with an appropriate burial can represent greater risks than disease: some people believe that the deceased will return and even retaliate against the living if their transition to the afterlife was incomplete, or their burial treatment was unsatisfactory.[28]

During the epidemic, the postmortem viability of the Ebola virus set a vicious cycle in motion. Direct contact with one body led to more deaths, more funerary needs, and more transmission opportunities. The cycle crossed borders as it spun out of control. On May 25, 2014, Sierra Leone confirmed its first case of EVD: a young woman who was among hundreds of people linked to a funeral in Guinea.[29] Numerous other family members and healers in attendance subsequently became ill, and local authorities suggested that as many as 365 deaths from EVD could be traced to the ceremony.[30] In September, a three-day funeral in a rural and previously low-incidence district of Sierra Leone resulted in a sharp increase in EVD cases, including twenty-eight of the attendees from different locations—and 75 percent of whom carried or touched the corpse.[31] In December, another funeral ceremony in Guinea was linked to eighty-five confirmed cases, of which eighteen people (21 percent) had direct contact with the body of the deceased, a well-known midwife assistant.[32] Hence in 2014 alone, "traditional" funerary practices (a term that exoticized West African cultural behaviors in the international media) were linked to approximately 60 percent of the total confirmed cases in Guinea and 80 percent of those in Sierra Leone.[33]

From a public health perspective, it was clear that the behaviors that were spreading the virus needed to stop. In 2014, early action was bolstered by international outbreak experts, whose on-the-ground coordination with local governments and health authorities formed an alphabet soup of emergency medical responders within an epidemiological combat zone. Ebola Treatment Units were built to isolate and treat EVD patients throughout the region, and professional teams were trained for a variety of EVD prevention and control measures, including collecting samples from and the bodies of possible EVD patients who died at home.

Unsurprisingly, biomedical approaches that ignored cultural and social values didn't work. Many EVD patients were buried by cemetery management teams in ways and places deemed safe by public health protocols, but they excluded the families and communities of the deceased. After surrendering caretaking duties to these inscrutable strangers, covered head to toe in personal protective equipment and armed with disinfectant, some families never saw their loved ones again. In numerous instances, their last glimpses were unmarked body bags being loaded into a truck, possibly destined for an unmarked, mass grave.[34]

Already-battered communities grew angry, suspicious, and defiant. Many people distrusted the Ebola Treatment Units, perceived as shadowy centers

---→

Figure 4.1

Transmission of EVD among funeral attendees. The virus spread among twenty-eight people, whose contacts led to eight additional confirmed cases, after attending a single three-day funeral in Sierra Leone in September 2014. Three-quarters of the attendees carried or touched the deceased, and eight of these patients died from EVD within two weeks. *Source:* K. G. Curran, J. J. Gibson, D. Marke, V. Caulker, J. Bomeh, J. T. Redd, S. Bunga, et al., "Cluster of Ebola Virus Disease Linked to a Single Funeral—Moyamba District, Sierra Leone, 2014," *Morbidity and Mortality Weekly Report* 65, no. 8 (2016): 202–205.

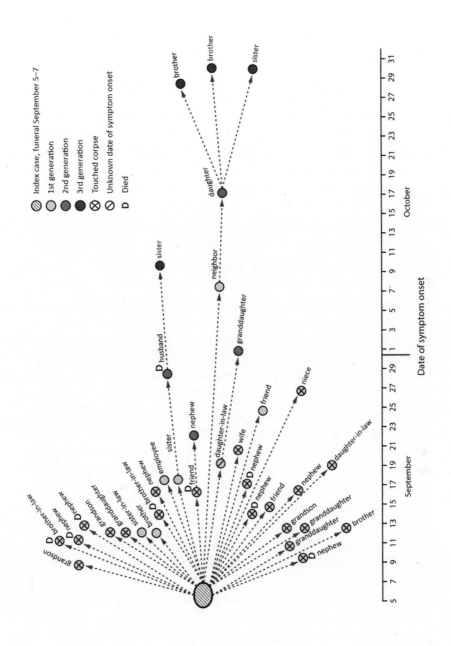

of unexplained disappearance and unseen death. And regardless of whether or not they understood the risks of EVD transmission, some people hid and buried bodies themselves in order to care for them more appropriately.

The cultural factors that were driving the epidemic required respect. Religious and traditional leaders thus became essential partners in developing and communicating about burial practices that were both safe and acceptable for families and communities. As a result, in October 2014, the WHO published a new protocol that involved religious rituals in burials of confirmed or suspected EVD patients.[35] Following these revised procedures, burial teams included a local religious representative and a communicator not wearing personal protective equipment, who worked with the deceased's family in planning a dignified burial that wouldn't commence without their consent. With separate guidelines for Christian and Muslim patients, the protocol empowered families to make specific requests concerning the burial (such as the clothing, symbols, grave markers, and grave site used) while limiting transmission risks. Families were allowed to participate in digging or preparing the grave, and alternatives to touching or washing the deceased (like sprinkling water over the body or performing a dry ablution) were offered for discussion and adaptation.

The protocol made a difference. Surveys revealed a 300 percent increase in the acceptance of safe burial practices after the implementation of faith-based interventions, along with a more than 60 percent increase in appreciation by bereaved families.[36] Some religious leaders and local faith communities also helped with public engagement and education concerning EVD control and prevention, promoting messages of support for the public health response to the epidemic.

In the months that followed, the behavior changes and the communities that adopted them made a critical difference that finally broke the epidemic curve. But its downslope was a difficult journey that stretched for another year, until the epidemic was officially declared over in Guinea and Sierra Leone in November 2015, and in Liberia in January 2016. By the end, more than 11,300 people lost their lives to EVD. Many more are counted among those who survived and those left behind.

*   *   *

As a case study on the role of mortuary practices in the spread of infectious disease, the Ebola epidemic in West Africa draws many parallels with previous epidemics in other parts of the world. And one feature that can't go unmentioned, as the most heavy-handed and culturally violent intervention enacted in Liberia, was forced cremation.

In August 2014, Liberia made the cremation of people who died from Ebola mandatory in Monrovia. It was a drastic measure because cremation violates the burial practices by which most Liberians, and West Africans generally, venerate their ancestors and mourn the deceased. Essentially, it's not part of the culture. Yet thousands of bodies were incinerated in a matter of months with the aim to avoid tampering with the dead and contaminating water sources, according to Liberian president Ellen Johnson Sirleaf at the time.[37]

Liberians resisted the mandate to the extent that Ebola Treatment Units were half empty, even as people died by the hundreds each week. Opposition to cremation became a major motivator in people's decisions to conceal a loved one's death.[38] Some Liberians even resorted to the black market for fake death certificates with a non-EVD cause of death so that funeral parlors would take their loved ones for burial.[39] After the mandatory cremation of more than three thousand EVD patients, the practice was abolished on December 30, 2014.

Among those whose family members were cremated, the violation may anguish them to this day. Families were left without graves to visit, clean, and adorn on Decoration Day, a national holiday in Liberia for honoring the dead.[40] As the absence of their relatives stretched on, they had nowhere to go to grieve. At the memorial service for her cousin who died of EVD, one woman spoke about the potential for cremation to prolong the trauma of families: "It is going to linger in the minds of people that your loved one died and you could not see the body."[41]

Although cremation had never been forced on Liberian people before, the idea wasn't new. More than a century prior to the Ebola epidemic in West Africa, similar measures were introduced to control a plague outbreak in Manchuria (a historical term for a region that includes present-day Northeast China and parts of the Russian Far East). It was the largest outbreak of pneumonic plague in history, killing as many as sixty thousand people within a few cold months of 1911–1912. And it prompted perhaps the first mass cremation in China.[42]

Leading the response by the Chinese government, physician Wu Lien-Teh arrived in the city of Harbin to see thousands of coffins and corpses on the snow-covered ground of the Chinese quarter of Fuchiaten.[43] There was plenty of space and workers to bury them. But it was impossible to dig graves in the frozen hard soil.

Fearing the thaw of the coming spring, when rats might gnaw on unburied bodies and spread the *Y. pestis* bacterium, Wu decided that cremation was necessary for public health. Yet similar to Liberia in 2014, cremation was a serious religious transgression in the Confucian culture of China during the early twentieth century. Among the Chinese residents of Harbin especially, for whom ancestor worship and caring for ancestral tombs were acts of filial piety, Wu knew that burning the bodies would be regarded as a sacrilege.[44] Nonetheless, he gained support from local officials and successfully petitioned an Imperial Edict for his iconoclastic plan.

On January 31, 1911, hundreds of workers began the days-long task of incinerating the dead of Harbin, with kerosene-fueled fires that blazed through the night. Neighboring towns and other parts of the country soon followed, cremating thousands of recent and older bodies of plague patients, some of whom were exhumed from their graves to be cremated. By spring, the epidemic had ended and an International Plague Conference was convened in the city of Mukden, where dozens of foreign delegates met to deliberate measures for plague control and prevention worldwide, including cremation as "the quickest, fastest, and most economical mode of disposal of the dead."[45]

There's little mention of public resistance to the mass cremations of 1911 in the report produced by the Mukden conference, for which Wu served as chair. According to the subsequent report, in some cities people didn't oppose it. In other places, however, Wu wrote that "the prejudices of the people outweighed their common sense."[46] In Mukden, the dead were thus buried in deep pits after being properly coffined with lime according to the customary Chinese method. In later writings, Wu acknowledged that cremation wasn't a realistic option everywhere due to religious beliefs and other cultural customs that require burial. "It would not be wise to embitter the population by insisting on it," he concluded. Yet Wu insisted that the Chinese agreed philosophically to cremation in times of epidemics, even if they abhorred the practice in ordinary times.[47]

Perhaps Wu was correct in his assertions, but we have only his word for it. The people of Manchuria are silent in his stories, never named and always generalized, voiceless about their harrowing sacrifices and survival under the threat of epidemic disease. During the Manchurian plague epidemic of 1920–1921, cremation was again employed, with apparent success. But it's notable that fear of cremation ran rampant in San Francisco's Chinatown during the bubonic plague epidemic of 1900–1904. The local Chinese paper *Chung Sai Yat Po* reported that the bodies of plague patients were to be burned by city health officials, who complained that residents of Chinatown hid their dead as a consequence.[48] Still, there were good reasons for them to distrust a public health campaign driven by US xenophobia— another pandemic liability that we'll discuss in chapter 6.

Commensal Connections

As social primates who rely on each other for just about everything, humans tend to have a lot of companions. Most of us think of a companion as someone with whom we do things. A companion can be a lifelong partner or short-term sidekick, a person who lives in your home or maybe somebody who travels with you. Companions aren't always human, such as pets whom you care for or service animals who care for you. Sometimes we talk about objects as companions, the same way that artists might describe feelings (according to Persian poet Rumi, his only companion was love). Basically, in common usage, it's a flexible term.

The literal meaning of companion is pretty specific, though. Derived from the Latin words *com*, meaning "together," and *panis*, meaning "bread," a *companion* is most closely translated as someone who shares bread with you. A looser interpretation is a person with whom you have meals. Later, in the form of the Old French word *compaignon*, the term became used for a colleague or friend. Which is to say, the meaning didn't change all that much.

Humans really like to share food with each other, generally speaking. We share food more than any other primate species, with family, friends, and even people we've just met. But what really sets us apart as a species is how much we share food between adults, compared to nonhuman primates who mostly share food between mothers and their offspring. Among human foragers, past and present, this pass-the-plate strategy has worked as a buffer against food shortfalls given the unpredictable returns of hunting and gathering. By transporting food to a central place and sharing widely with group members, our early ancestors could forage according to their best abilities, and then pool their profits for a greater total yield and better production efficiency.[49] In this way, food sharing became an integral part of the human foraging lifestyle—the kind of cooperative strategy that underlies the divisions of labor across human societies today.

For the majority of us who aren't foragers, food sharing remains central to our lives. Regardless of any formal exchange or reciprocity in resources, the human habit of eating and drinking together is a bedrock behavior of culture and sociality. And it too has a precise term: *commensality*. Again from Latin, the combination of *com* and *mensa*, meaning "table," literally means eating at the same table. In chapter 2, we applied this term to the friendly microbes that inhabit our bodies. But in its broader meaning, commensality describes eating and drinking together in a common physical or social setting. Not all people use a table for meals, after all, but eating is a social activity in every culture around the world. That's because commensal acts are essential for the integration of human society, from everyday gatherings to religious rituals to commemorative feasts.[50]

Commensality, like food sharing, is a powerful means by which we create, express, and reinforce feelings of mutual trust, intimacy, and kinship.[51] Bottom line, it helps us bond. Universally across human cultures, anthropologist Claude Fischler writes, there's a perception that "you are what you eat" and so people who share the same food become more like each other.[52] In other words, you are with whom you eat.

It makes sense that similarities in consumption might signal a shared identity or group membership, since cultural groups define themselves partly through cooking traditions and religions often impose food restrictions on their followers. Yet there's good evidence that people who share the same food then *feel* closer to one another, even if they have nothing else in common. In a series of experiments, researchers found that eating similar foods (as directed, not by preference) generated feelings of closeness and trust, and increased cooperation between strangers.[53] Furthermore, eating from shared plates—especially one plate of food, served centrally—led to more cooperation between both strangers and friends.[54]

The earliest discussion of commensality, written by theologian William Robertson Smith in his book *Lectures on the Religion of the Semites* in 1889, examines this phenomenon in a cultural context. "Among the Arabs," he observes, "every stranger whom one meets in the desert is a natural enemy. . . . But if I have eaten the smallest morsel of food with a man, I have nothing further to fear from him." He explains that if there is "salt between us," then the man is bound not only to do him no harm but also to help and defend him as if he were a brother.[55] (And here I'm reminded of an old Moroccan proverb: "By bread and salt we are united.") The principle extended so far into ancient times, according to Smith, that a famous warrior in the days of Mohammed (AD 570–632) refused to slay a camel thief who had drunk from his father's milk bowl.

This principle, Smith argues, proves that a social bond is created by food itself, and "the essence of the thing lies in the physical act of eating together."[56] Religion, however, can strengthen it. During sacrificial meals, he suggests, the gods and worshippers are commensals, meaning that they're all participants in the commensal act. In the Old Testament of the Bible, for instance, we find many cases of a covenant being sealed by the parties eating and drinking together. The Last Supper of Jesus Christ and his disciples is a striking image of religious commensality, and the Christian rite of Holy Communion reenacts this commensal union with God today.[57]

Although symbolic food sharing with gods isn't part of every religion—in the Chinese worship of deities and ancestors, anthropologist Tan Chee-Beng points out, the worshippers eat only after the spirits have done so—religious feasting is nonetheless socially significant by bringing worshippers together to honor them. Religion thus provides fellowship, Tan asserts, reinforced by commensality.[58] For example, among Muslims everywhere, Eid al-Adha, or the Feast of Sacrifice, is celebrated with prayers in congregation and the sharing of food (traditionally meat from the animals sacrificed) among relatives, friends, neighbors, and those in need.

Celebrations, whether or not they have a religious purpose, often call for some form of commensality. Whether they bring together close kin or a broader community, the sharing of food fortifies social relations and group solidarity. Weddings are typical occasions for joyous feasting, especially among families, which may host the meal at a home or more frequently nowadays in a location with a professional food service. I challenge any reader to think of a wedding where food was not involved.

For funerals, another rite of passage, a meal offers an opportunity to express feelings about the deceased and give social support to the bereaved as the process of adjusting to life without them begins.[59] Anthropologist Arnold van Gennep, who made the first study of celebrations associated with *rites of passage* (a term he coined) in his book *Les Rites de Passage* in 1909, viewed the purpose of the funeral meal as reuniting all the surviving members of a group "in the same way that a chain which has been broken by the disappearance of one of the links must be rejoined."[60] For Cantonese people in Hong Kong, for instance, it's typical for the family of the deceased to go to a restaurant after a funeral in order to console each other while sharing food and drink. It's so typical, in fact, that restaurants usually have standard menus for it.[61]

But for all the needs and benefits that commensality serves, there are some dangerous downsides. For one, foodborne illnesses—caused by food contaminated with harmful pathogens, parasites, or chemical substances—sicken about one in ten people a year worldwide.[62] Social eating carries these risks, as more than half of all foodborne disease outbreaks reported to the CDC are associated with eating in restaurants or delicatessens.[63] Dirty hands, as we learned in chapter 2, are another culprit. But recently an even greater concern is the involvement of commensality in the human-to-human transmission of disease. In these cases, it's not about the food; it's about the behavior.

*   *   *

On January 23, 2020, a sixty-three-year-old woman and her family left the city of Wuhan in China, the day that an unprecedented lockdown of the region went into effect. After hundreds of infections of a novel coronavirus (soon to be named SARS-CoV-2) had been confirmed in the population, the residents of Wuhan were informed that all public transport would be suspended immediately. Also, nobody could leave the city without permission from the authorities.

The notice came two days before the Lunar New Year, or Spring Festival—China's biggest holiday. Travel for the holiday is the world's largest human migration, an event called *Chunyun* by the Chinese, when hundreds of millions of people depart the major cities for rural areas. For many of them, especially migrant laborers who are born in the countryside but move to cities to work, it may be the only time all year that they'll return home. To be with their families for the Lunar New Year, a celebration of commensality and ancestor worship, some of them journey for thousands of miles.

The woman and her family were part of an exodus from Wuhan, as an estimated five million people fled the city before the lockdown began.[64] The family took a train about six hundred miles south to the city of Guangzhou, and the next day the woman went to the hospital with a fever and cough. She was subsequently diagnosed with COVID-19. But prior to show-ing symptoms of illness, she went to a restaurant with her family for Lunar New Year's Eve lunch.

Within two weeks, nine other diners in the same restaurant also became ill with COVID-19. Four of them were family members who ate with the woman, but the rest belonged to other families seated at neighboring tables. A subsequent study showed that these people were most likely infected by the woman (identified as the index patient) during the lunch.[65] The proba-ble route of transmission, they concluded, was exhaled respiratory droplets containing virus particles and spread by air-conditioning in the restaurant.

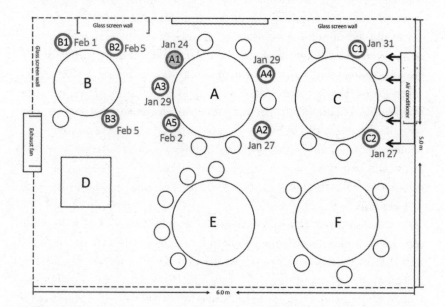

Figure 4.2
COVID-19 transmission in a restaurant. When a woman with COVID-19 (Patient A1) had lunch with her family (Patients A2–A5) in an air-conditioned restaurant on Janu-ary 24, 2020, nine other people became ill with COVID-19 within ten days. Although the woman was asymptomatic during the lunch, researchers concluded that she infected at least one of the patients in two other families (Patients B1–B3 and C1–C2). Given that they were seated more than three feet (one meter) from Patient A1, the transmission of the virus between the tables likely occurred via respiratory droplets spread by air-conditioned ventilation. *Source:* J. Lu, J. Gu, K. Li, C. Xu, W. Su, Z. Lai, D. Zhou, et al., "COVID-19 Outbreak Associated with Air Conditioning in Restaurant, Guangzhou, China, 2020," *Emerging Infectious Diseases* 26, no. 7 (2020): 1628.

A second study of the outbreak presented more startling findings.[66] The exhaust fans in the walls were turned off and sealed during the January 24 lunch, providing no supply of outdoor air into the restaurant. Plus the restaurant was busier than usual, with added tables to accommodate the increased number of customers on Lunar New Year's Eve. In this poorly ventilated, crowded environment, the researchers estimated that some of the people infected by the index patient were seated up to fifteen feet away from her. Under such conditions, they determined that long-range aerosol transmission had probably occurred.

This meal is a powerful demonstration of the infectious disease risks of commensality, particularly related to COVID-19. At the time of the restaurant outbreak in Guangzhou, the WHO insisted that SARS-CoV-2 wasn't airborne and recommended a safe social distance of one meter (three feet)—a range over which large respiratory droplets were thought to fall to the ground.[67] More contradictory evidence followed, including a study from South Korea showing that SARS-CoV-2 could be transmitted at a distance of *seven meters* and within *five minutes* of exposure between two people, both of whom engaged in maskless conversation with their respective companions in a restaurant that lacked windows and a ventilation system.[68] But nearly two years passed before the WHO stated clearly that the virus is airborne, with an ability to spread widely and linger in the air through tiny aerosols.[69]

In the meantime, probably millions of people caught COVID-19 while eating and drinking with other people indoors. Over a period of four months in 2020, for example, 14 percent of the COVID-19 outbreaks reported in Washington, DC, were traced to restaurants and bars.[70] Throughout the United States, adults who tested positive for COVID-19 were about twice as likely to have reported dining at a restaurant in the two weeks before becoming ill than those who tested negative.[71] And in 2021, the reopening of restaurants for on-site dining was followed by local rises in COVID-19 cases and death rates after forty days, especially when mask mandates weren't in place.[72]

The social nature of dining out is a huge amplifier of droplet and aerosol transmission, beyond the airflow and head count in a venue. Eating is hard to do with a mask, and it's far less fun to do without conversation. But as we learned in chapter 2, respiratory pathogens like SARS-CoV-2 are highly transmissible via human speech, and our speech tends to get louder and more forceful as we drink alcohol in particular. We may also increase our volume, and potentially the viral load of our respiratory emissions, in crowded places that are noisy from all the other chatting going on. And depending on how much we enjoy the conversation, the food, and social bonding that transpires with our companions, the meal may last for some time, while our potential to inhale more pathogens grows.

Of course, restaurants have upsides too. They've become important sites for organizing commensality in modern times since their birth in eighteenth-century Paris. In cultures around the world, as Tan notes, celebrations in restaurants are common and even prestigious, as expensive food can express wealth and status as lavish feasts once did.[73] Restaurants also solve the problem of limited space in urban settings as well as deficits in time, resources, and skill that at-home commensality requires.

Commensality is not something that human beings can give up. It's more or less inextricable from our cultural and social existence, although that doesn't mean that we can't modify our interactions. One clear way to lower the infectious disease risks of commensality is to eat and drink together outside and in small groups, as many people started doing more and more during the COVID-19 pandemic. These are simple controls of the physical environment, and restaurants around the world built open-air spaces and improved indoor ventilation to accommodate safer dining. But we can also adjust our commensal behaviors, as when restaurants in Hong Kong responded to the SARS epidemic in 2003. In Chinese restaurants where people eat family style from shared platters of food, it became popular for diners to use serving chopsticks (*gongkuai*) to transfer food from each dish to their own bowl rather than using their own chopsticks to pick food from a common plate.[74] This practice is now a rule of proper etiquette, serving society in more ways than one.[75]

Dangerless Liaisons

There are countless ways that culture affects infectious disease transmission beyond mortuary and commensal behaviors. For instance, physical touching—hugging, kissing, and hand holding—is another means by which we foster social bonds, similar to how other social primates groom each other. And the customs differ for people everywhere, depending on how they learn and make meaning of particular acts.

I have a burning memory of my first cultural faux pas of the COVID-19 pandemic, when I greeted someone in France with kisses on the cheeks in the age-old tradition of *la bise*. French public health authorities had advised against the habit in order to reduce transmission risks, just as handshakes were replaced by elbow bumps in many countries. But in the moment of the encounter, my ingrained cultural impulses overrode my common sense. I realized too late (and with utter horror) what I had done, as the previously polite act had become a totally wrong one in 2020. The culture, in ways small and large, had adapted to new dangers. (And by 2021, *la bise* made a comeback.)

That's because culture isn't static. It constantly evolves with our environments, often as a buffer against stressors and the unexpected challenges that they can bring. Can we keep up? Of course we can: we're humans. Adaptation is how we got here.

But as we think about cultural changes in how people respond to disease threats, we shouldn't underestimate their potential impacts. If behaviors need to be altered for public health purposes, most reasonable people will accept a reasonable explanation for it. Modifications are most likely to be successful, however, if they continue to serve the essential needs and functions as the original practice. Some acts are far more significant than they might appear on the surface, and they might be doing a lot more work than one assumes. The people who best understand the significance of the practice are most qualified to suggest culturally appropriate alternatives. Sometimes these people are anthropologists. Yet I firmly believe, as demonstrated with the Ebola epidemic in West Africa, that members of the affected community are the ideal individuals to develop and communicate these changes. Like in all matters related to public health and policy, multiple different messengers can reach the most people and make the greatest difference.

We also shouldn't expect anybody to make a change that we wouldn't accept or follow ourselves. Political scandals erupted in cities and nations around the world during the COVID-19 pandemic when government leaders were caught in disregard of behavior changes that were required for everyone else. For instance, in the United Kingdom, government and Conservative Party staff enjoyed social gatherings at the prime minister's official residence at 10 Downing Street, Conservative Campaign Headquarters, and in other government buildings during strict COVID-19 lockdowns. Some of these parties were attended by Prime Minister Boris Johnson himself.[76] But outside of Westminster, millions of people sacrificed and suffered to follow the laws set by Johnson's government, which kept Britons from leaving their homes freely, holding or attending funerals with more than a few mourners, and spending final moments with dying loved ones in hospitals.

The public did their best to carry on. Deprived of the commensality provided by pubs, a community-serving cornerstone of British life, people tried to stay socially connected in other ways. Occasionally I joined "virtual pubs" during the lockdowns in England, organized by my friend Nader, where we often discussed the latest COVID-19 measures over at-home beverages. Unknown to anybody on my computer screen, the rule makers were eating and drinking (and *dancing!*) together in person. Moreover, two of the Downing Street parties took place the night before the funeral of Prince Philip, whose widow Queen Elizabeth sat masked and alone during the service in compliance with the COVID-19 restrictions.[77] The UK public was rightly outraged when the shameless hypocrisy of the partying politicians was discovered, and Johnson's premiership was ultimately destroyed by it. Indeed, when he was finally held accountable by the UK Parliament for lying about the violations, Johnson decided to resign as a Member of Parliament rather than face the very real prospect of being defeated in a recall election in his constituency seat of Uxbridge and South Ruislip. "Partygate," as it had become known, had left Johnson's personal reputation in tatters. By this time though, as Nader told me with satisfaction, there were no Downing Street cleaners to deal with the mess.

The Partygate scandal carried a theme of illicit commensality found in other countries too. While Johnson and his associates gathered for wine, cheese, and cake, government officials in the United States and France chose to violate local COVID-19 lockdowns at expensive restaurants.[78] I don't think for a second that the social necessity of sharing food led to these double standards. Rather, I think that the power of their positions led the participants to behave as if they could do what they wanted, pandemic or not.

In the next chapter, we're going to consider the role of power in the spread of infectious diseases. Yet we're going to look at its effects on a broader scale than individuals and groups. As a species, humans have not only dominated each other but also other animals and environments to the extent that we've caused global change. And in so doing, we've ushered in an era of pandemic threats.

5   People Power: Domination and Disease

Agriculture, urbanization, and other Earth-altering activities have made *Homo sapiens* the dominant force of global environmental change today, as we exploit and modify the natural world in support of our endlessly expanding species. By seizing a status previously held by meteorites and volcanoes, and thus becoming the first species to single-handedly shape the Earth, we are the authors of this current chapter in our planetary history book.[1] In 2000, atmospheric chemist Paul Crutzen and limnologist Eugene Stoermer proposed that the chapter's opening paragraphs were already written in stone, as the beginning of a new geological epoch called the Anthropocene.[2]

Not everyone agrees that the Anthropocene should be formalized by the scientific community or that it even exists. But among its proponents, the biggest issue of contention is how and when to pinpoint its start. By convention, every geological time unit in the geologic time scale requires a beginning marker (that is, a Global Stratotype Section and Point [GSSP], also called a golden spike) in the geological record of Earth's 4.6-billion-year-old existence. Approved by the International Commission on Stratigraphy and ratified by the International Union of Geological Sciences, the marker serves as an end boundary for the previous time unit, corresponding to global events or processes that caused geologically identifiable changes worldwide. Furthermore, the marker should be an enduring one. If we can identify GSSPs from millions of years ago in today's geological record, then a GSSP for the present epoch should be recognizable millions of years from now, right? Imagining the geological record in the far distant future, how would an anthropogenic epoch—which should last for millions of years by epochal standards—be recognizable? Or as pondered by paleoclimatologist Simon Lewis and plant ecologist Mark Maslin, can we even conceive of environmental changes driven by us that will last longer than our species has existed?[3]

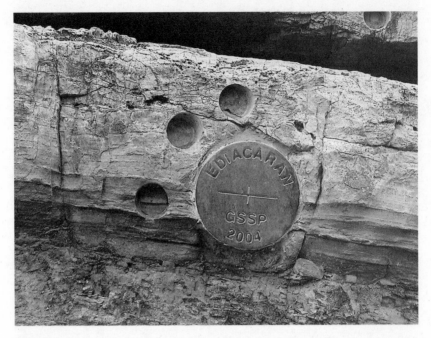

Figure 5.1
The golden spike, or GSSP, marking the beginning of the Ediacaran period around 635 million year ago. The spike is placed at the base of a chemically distinctive carbonate layer in the geological record, characterized by fossils of the earliest widespread communities of complex (multicellular) organisms. The Ediacaran period thus records Earth's transition from a planet dominated by microbes to one filled with animals. *Source:* "Bahudhara," CC BY-SA 3.0, Wikimedia Commons, accessed April 30, 2023, https://commons.wikimedia.org/wiki/File:Ediacaran_GSSP_-_closeup.JPG.

The International Commission on Stratigraphy's Anthropocene working group has long considered the optimal starting point of the Anthropocene as the mid-twentieth century, marked by radioactive fallout from the first nuclear bomb tests.[4] But many other markers have been proposed. When Crutzen and Stoermer first coined the term, they suggested that the late eighteenth century would be an appropriate starting point, coinciding with the increase in atmospheric concentrations of greenhouse gases during the Industrial Revolution. Some archaeologists, on the other hand, have argued that the Anthropocene is coeval with the Holocene, when humans began to domesticate plants and animals as well as develop agricultural economies and landscapes, and therefore could replace or be merged with it.[5]

However it's defined, many scientists have pointed out that the Anthropocene concept is a powerful tool to affect public opinion and policymaking on environmental issues as well as raise awareness about particular historical events and processes such as colonialism.[6] In this sense, the golden spike is likewise symbolic: the selected starting point will serve as a strong statement on the impacts of whatever human activities are related to it.

In this chapter, we'll examine how pandemics are not only a feature of the human species but also the age in which we live. Proposed markers of the Anthropocene that relate directly to disease emergence are useful frames for this discussion, helping to make the connections between the causes and consequences of epidemics and pandemics on a larger-than-life scale. We're going to focus on two of them here: the decimation of the Indigenous peoples of the Americas due to European colonization in the fifteenth to sixteenth centuries and the creation of the broiler chicken through the industrialization of poultry farming in the twentieth century. They may seem like an odd pairing, but both events draw attention to dramatic ecological changes through which human have spread disease threats worldwide. And by seeing these problems from such a vast vantage point, the potential solutions are within sight too. With more knowledge about the scope of our influence on Earth's history, we should all feel more empowered to control its future course.

Sickness and Suffering in the Americas

The American continents, comprising most of the land in the Western Hemisphere, were the final frontier of human dispersal around the world. On reaching them, *Homo sapiens* graduated to a truly global species. When exactly this first happened and how is still unclear, as remarkable findings and discoveries continue to emerge from new experiments, excavations, and collaborations. But with growing evidence, twenty-first-century science has at least knocked down the long-standing theory that the first Americans followed an ice-free corridor into the plains of central North America around 13,000 years ago.

No doubt, ice posed a significant challenge to people migrating across continents over the past hundreds of thousands of years. In the Earth's northern region, glacial ice was an obstacle to human migration from Asia into North America during the Late Pleistocene, after *Homo sapiens* had already set foot on most other lands across the planet. Scientists estimate that this frozen barrier was at its fullest extent between about 26,000 and 19,000 years ago (known as the Last Glacial Maximum), without a viable path through it until around 12,500 years ago.[7] But a coastal route along the Pacific Rim, with ice-free stretches of shoreline rich in aquatic and terrestrial resources, could have been a promising path for earlier human arrivals in the Americas at least 16,000 years ago.[8]

The coastal migration theory lines up with a lot of archaeological and genetic evidence. Human occupations have been identified near central Chile's Pacific coastline at least 14,500 years ago and throughout the United States between roughly 16,000 to 14,000 years ago.[9] For people to have settled as far south as Patagonia and as far east as the Florida Panhandle during this time, most archaeologists agree that initial American colonization began as early as 17,000 to 16,000 years ago. Furthermore, as anthropological geneticist Jennifer Raff discusses in her book *Origin: A Genetic History of America*, other significant clues have come from DNA analyses of ancient human remains. For example, genetic evidence suggests that there was a population boom among ancestral Native Americans around 16,000 years ago, when the coastal glaciers along the northwest Pacific coast rapidly retreated.[10] According to Raff, this is "exactly what we expect to see in the genetic record when people move into new territories" with more resources and less competition during a southward expansion along the coastlines of the Americas.[11]

Also important, the first ancient Native American genome to be completely sequenced (from the remains of an infant dated to about 12,600 years ago) represents a major branch from a split between northern and southern Native Americans that occurred shortly after the Last Glacial Maximum and south of the ice sheets.[12] The infant belonged to the southern Native American branch, which became, as Raff notes, the ancestors of many Native peoples in and south of the present-day United States.[13]

It's possible that people entered the Americas even earlier than 17,000 years ago, but the matter is still up for debate. In New Mexico, for example, undeniable human footprints have been dated as early as 21,000 to 23,000 years ago, although some researchers think that they could be several thousand years younger than that.[14] Yet none of it changes the fact that Native American history is deeper and more complex than many non-Indigenous scholars have previously contended and most history books have portrayed. This is crucial to remember—the many millennia over which Native people lived and settled in the Americas—when considering how much European colonizers and their diseases destroyed. But it's also important to recognize how much history survives in Indigenous knowledge systems, including stories, practices, and beliefs that "preserve, communicate, and contextualize Indigenous relationships with culture and landscape over time."[15] In Indigenous narratives about ancestry and origins, land- and waterscapes are not places through which people and their molecules move and settle, Kim Tallbear explains in her essay "Tell Me a Story: Genomics vs. Indigenous Origin Narratives." "An environment/human divide is presumed in the genomic narrative that is absent from the Indigenous narrative," she writes.[16]

*   *   *

Words can't describe the amount of human suffering that resulted from the fifteenth century arrival of Cristóbal Colón (better known as Christopher Columbus) and his fellow voyagers in the Americas, whose Indigenous inhabitants were soon decimated by violence, malnutrition, and disease. In raw numbers alone, even the deaths can't be counted with precision. One reason is that it's unclear how many people were living in the Americas when Europeans began to colonize them in 1492. Over a thousand languages were spoken across the continents, but as many Indigenous people didn't have writing systems, the most detailed (and unquestionably distorted) documentation of their population sizes is found in European colonial narratives at the time of contact.[17] Diaries, journals, letters, and published accounts of European observers were thus used almost exclusively in early reconstructions of precontact population sizes of the Americas.[18] More recent approaches have incorporated archaeological information from settlement patterns, residential structures, and skeletal remains as well as ecological considerations of constraints on population growth. As a consequence, the estimates have varied widely over decades among so-called high and low counters.

In North America, for example, one early estimate was 18 million people at the time of European contact, yet in the *Handbook of North American Indians* in 2006, biological anthropologist Douglas Ubelaker put the number near 2.3 million people. North American population densities were minimal compared to those in some parts of central Mexico and South America, although Ubelaker accounted for considerable variation across regions of the North American continent, estimating nearly 600,000 people in the Southeast and less than 40,000 people in the Great Basin.[19]

Likewise, the total estimate for the entire contact population of the Americas has ranged widely, between 8 and 112 million people. While the precise number will never be known, Lewis and Maslin suggest that these various approximations equate to a reasonable range of 50 to 80 million people in total. Demographer Massimo Livi Bacci argues that a still smaller number of around 30 million people is plausible.[20]

In any case, the Americas were far from undiscovered when Norse explorers first encountered them in the eleventh century and certainly by the time that Spanish ships made landfall centuries later. And their human history was much deeper than perhaps any of these newcomers supposed. But to be clear, this human history was intertwined with the natural history of the continents, not separate from it. The earliest Americans embraced astounding biodiversity across the vast and varied landscape of the Late Pleistocene and throughout the Holocene, with never-ending challenges in local environments that constantly evolved over millennia.[21]

Indigenous people weren't passive additions to ecosystems, nor did they make negligible impacts on the structure and composition of their natural surroundings. As archaeologist Bruce Smith writes in the *Handbook*, "To the contrary, they played an active and through time an increasingly substantial role in changing and shaping their environments in a wide variety of large and small ways that were designed to benefit those plant and animal species that were important to them, and in so doing improved and enhanced their own place or niche in the world."[22] Indigenous people did this through intensive foraging, plant and animal domestication, vegetation burning, and other landscape modifications.[23] And across thousands of years, as Indigenous societies grew and diversified, the environment remained a central and fully integrated core of their existence—an essential part of their cultural identity that influenced all aspects of their beliefs, behaviors, and relationships with the other organisms with which they coexisted.

This kind of ecological ethos is reflected in sustainable strategies used by Indigenous communities in countless different environments, such as those along the Atlantic coastal region of the modern-day United States. Around the Chesapeake Bay, as shown by researchers including archaeologist Torrey Rick, people have lived and fished for more than 13,000 years since the Late Pleistocene. Due to sea-level rise, preservation conditions, and limited archaeological research in the region, only a few shell middens are known to date to much earlier than 3,200 years ago. But from this period until contact with Europeans about 400 years ago, the Native American oyster fishery of the Chesapeake Bay was largely resilient and stable, with limited variability in oyster size and abundance, and no systematic evidence for a size decline through time.[24]

Even though ecological awareness permeated Indigenous life throughout the Americas, not all societies operated on a small scale. The majority of people at the time of European contact lived in the tropical zone of the continents, and perhaps two-thirds of them were concentrated in Mesoamerica and the Andean region.[25] This is where empires grew. In a vast area of southeastern Mexico and northern Central America, including the Yucatán Peninsula, the Maya civilization began with thousands of years of mobile ways of life, combining hunting, gathering, and fishing with the cultivation of maize and other crops, followed by increased sedentism and eventually monumental architecture as early as 3,000 years ago.[26] Maya cities emerged by 750 BCE, forming an urban network that linked dozens of population nodes, some as large as 50,000 to 200,000 people at their peak density.

The Mayan people had returned to mostly village-dwelling farming life by the time that Europeans encountered them, having suffered major political collapse in the ninth century. But others were still at the height of their power. By the fifteenth century, three city-states to the north, Tenochtitlan, Tetzcoco, and Tlacopan, ruled the region of the Valley of Mexico in the Triple Alliance (more commonly known today as the Aztec Empire). The Inca Empire also grew rapidly during the fifteenth century, centered on the Andean mountains, but incorporating much of western South America. Preceded by the Tiwanaku and Wari Empires, the Inca Empire reached an unprecedented expanse in the Americas, including up to twelve million people at the apogee of its dominance. Relatively few of them would survive the new threats that came across the Atlantic, though, unrecognized even by the colonizers who carried them.

* * *

Everything changed after Columbus made boot prints in the Caribbean sands of an island haven known today as the Bahamas. Barely five weeks after he and around a hundred people set sail in three ships from Spain in 1492 on a quest for a shortcut to Asia and its riches, the Europeans came ashore on foreign lands with no true understanding of where they were. After exploring the unfamiliar region, whose native Taíno people were called *indios* by Columbus (because he believed that he had reached India), the voyage ended when his flagship ran aground off the northern shores of an island that Columbus declared as La Isla Española ("The Spanish Island," later renamed Hispaniola).[27] There, on Christmas Day, he began his fledgling attempt to colonize the Americas with a Spanish outpost named La Navidad in honor of the Christian holiday. And then a continental collision of culture and biology, unlike any the world had ever seen before, got underway.[28]

The preliminary attempt at European settlement at La Navidad failed. As writer Charles Mann describes in his book *1493*, Columbus left about forty people to build an encampment from their shipwreck while he sailed back to Spain, taking a haul that included several kidnapped Taínos. He returned almost a year later, no longer with the aims of an exploratory economic venture but rather with a plan to colonize and Christianize the whole place.[29] Leading a fleet of seventeen ships and more than twelve hundred people, and naming other islands along the way, he arrived at La Navidad to find the marooned Spaniards dead and their fort destroyed. Some of the Taíno people, who recounted rapes and murders by the would-be conquerors, had effectively ended the experiment. The second Columbian voyage therefore sailed forth to a different part of Hispaniola, where the town of La Isabela was founded by Columbus in the name of Queen Isabella I of Spain in January 1494. But the town was also short-lived, lasting only four years. Actually, to paraphrase Mann and many others, it was a catastrophe.

The earliest American epidemic, as it's been called by medical historian Francisco Guerra, was probably brewing before the Spanish ships dropped anchor at Hispaniola in December 1493. From almost the moment they landed at the site of their doomed outpost, a wave of severe illness spread rapidly through the Spaniards and Taínos alike, striking even Columbus, who didn't recover for five months. Described in historical accounts as an acute infectious disease leading to excessive mortality, with symptoms including fever, chills and sweating, and fatigue, the epidemic apparently affected the whole island and those beyond it. In a letter to Spain during the following month, Columbus reported sudden sickness and suffering among most of the colonial contingent, for whom he requested "sustenance they were used to in Spain" in order to preserve their health.[30]

The likelihood that the Spanish were already weakened by malnutrition is supported by skeletal evidence from some of the individuals buried in the town's churchyard, suggesting that scurvy made them more susceptible to pathogen attack in their first few months of American life.[31] These findings also corroborate the failure of the European colonizers to take advantage of the locally available foods rich in vitamin C. According to archaeologists Kathleen Deagan and José Maria Cruxent in *Columbus's Outpost among the Taínos*, excavations found a scarcity of animal bone and plant remains at La Isabela, despite an abundance of cooking and eating utensils.[32] Possibly suffering from starvation as well as disease, many of the Spanish died soon after settling in. Yet so did the Taínos.

The causal pathogen of the epidemic was unknown at the time, and remains a mystery to this day. Influenza was hypothesized by Guerra, although he later proposed epidemic typhus as another possibility. Other suggestions, with varying plausibility, have included malaria and smallpox.[33] Retrospective diagnosis is difficult for a number of reasons, including the overlapping symptoms of many acute illnesses, ambiguous and inexpert descriptions of historical observers, and multiplicity and concurrence in which different diseases can spread. But one near certainty is that the epidemic's source was in the continents of the Eastern Hemisphere, from which the Columbian cohort brought microbes and more.

The European colonizers had the advantages of acquired immunity against the germs among which they had lived since birth as well as hard-won familiarity with the risks and responses associated with them. By contrast, the Indigenous people on whom they descended, who may have never come up against European agents and hosts of infectious disease, lacked any cultural or biological preparation for the assault. Moreover, zoonotic diseases weren't nearly as common in the Americas, as relatively few animals in the Americas were domesticated (namely, llamas and alpacas, dogs, turkeys, and guinea pigs). The Europeans weren't invulnerable to these pathogens, but the Indigenous Americans were more or less defenseless.

The most compelling element of the influenza possibility is the role of livestock in the Columbian Exchange, the name by which historian Alfred Crosby called the transatlantic transposition of biota that started in the fifteenth century. Influenza A viruses, the type that cause pandemics, are the greatest concern for people because they have the most zoonotic potential for cross-species transmission. Their primary reservoir is wild aquatic birds, but these viruses infect a diverse range of mammalian species besides humans, including pigs, horses, dogs, cats, and chickens. All of these animals were passengers on the 1493 voyage, along with cattle, goats, and sheep.[34] Almost none of them existed in the Americas before then, with the notable exceptions of dogs and possibly chickens (which we'll get to later). The pigs (*Sus domesticus*) in particular got Guerra's attention, however, because of the legitimate threat of swine flu to human health.

Swine-origin influenza A (H1N1 subtype) viruses don't normally infect people, but it happens most commonly after close proximity to infected pigs, whose coughs and sneezes can spread virus-laden droplets through the air and into the human body. People can then infect each other if the virus is well adapted to its human host, leading to flu-like symptoms that most of us have known at some point in our lives. Swine influenza viruses have been circulating in pigs in the Americas for a long time, yet only recently received worldwide attention in 2009, when a novel virus of swine origin emerged in humans and caused the first pandemic in more than forty years.[35] And arguably, it all goes back to Columbus, who brought eight sows from the Canary Islands to La Isabela in 1493.

Guerra suggests that swine flu is the most likely cause of the earliest American epidemic because it broke out right after the landing of hogs who'd been in the bottom of the ships. Although this is pure conjecture, it's possible that influenza virus spread throughout the Americas as the porcine population grew. More than any of the other imported animals, pigs prospered in the Caribbean environment, helped by the fact that they will eat almost anything, including human garbage and other refuse.[36] "One now sees innumerable pigs here," Columbus wrote in 1499, "all of them descended from those eight, which I brought on the ships at my own expense except for the purchase price."[37] Within decades, their numbers had reached tens of thousands.[38] And as a critical food source for the Spanish, their indirect contribution to the destruction of Indigenous people can't be understated, even if their involvement in disease transmission is unclear.

Typhus, as another candidate for the earliest American epidemic, highlights the inadvertent extras that came with Columbian introductions to the Americas. "The Iberian undoubtedly imported dozens of kinds of insects and animals that he would have preferred leaving behind in the Old World," writes Crosby, pointing out that the black rat would have been an effective carrier of typhus.[39] As we learned in chapter 3, the human louse can transmit *R. prowazekii* in all kinds of crowded and unsanitary conditions where typhus quickly spreads, and historian Noble David Cook concurs that both rats and lice probably came on board the ships that conveyed well over a thousand people to Hispaniola in 1493.[40] He doubts that typhus would have spread so extensively among the Indigenous population, however, due to cleanliness and a lack of clothing. (According to Deagan and Cruxent, the Spanish were fascinated by the absence of clothing among the Taínos, who supposedly could smell the Spaniards, clad in heavy wool and leather garments, amid the tropical heat.)[41] In any case, Europeans continued to transport lice and rickettsia as they moved through the Americas, helped by the fact that viable *R. prowazekii* can survive for months in the dried feces of the body louse and lay dormant in a person for years to decades after the initial infection.

Smallpox is a dubious suspect for the epidemic at La Isabela due to a lack of historical documentation. Its highly distinctive symptoms would have been recognizable to most Spanish people in 1493, and almost certainly to the physician who accompanied Columbus on the second voyage, given that the disease was well established in Spain and throughout Europe by the fifteenth century.[42] In fact, ancient DNA genomes of the causal pathogen (variola virus) have been recovered from northern European human remains dated to the Viking age, suggesting a pan-European presence of variola viruses since the late sixth century.[43]

Ancient variola virus strains differ genetically from modern ones, meaning that the epidemiological features of modern smallpox may have developed somewhat recently.[44] If the manifestations of the disease were the same in the fifteenth century, however, its severe and most common form (called variola major) could have progressed as follows: after an asymptomatic and noninfectious incubation period of seven to nineteen days, the initial stage of symptoms included high fever and body aches for several days, followed by an early rash of small red sores that started on the tongue and in the mouth, and then spread to over all the skin, followed by a pustular rash in which the sores developed into pus-filled blisters that lasted for about ten days before they scabbed and fell off, leaving the patient with scars and lifetime immunity to reinfection.[45] Many people wouldn't have made it to the scab stage, as the death rates for variola major were around 30 percent on average (although 1 percent or less with the less common form, variola minor). Still, it was highly contagious, spreading exclusively between human hosts through virus-laden respiratory droplets as well as contaminated objects and materials.

Despite these features, identifying smallpox in historical records and human remains, without genetic verification, is tricky business. Other diseases, such as measles, can manifest in similar symptoms, and the written descriptions can be misleading. Apparently Columbus recognized smallpox in some of the Taínos whom he took to Spain from his first voyage and brought back to Hispaniola on the second. He wrote, "I put ashore one of the four Indians that I had taken from there last year, who had not died as the others from smallpox on the departure from Cádiz."[46] Based on this document, Cook asserts that some of the Taínos who traveled on the ships were exposed to smallpox prior to embarkation from Spain. And if so, he argues, then it's possible that some of the passengers of the returning Columbian flotilla were carriers of the disease. Yet he acknowledges that there are no accounts of smallpox among the Taínos on the island in 1493 and 1494.[47] Furthermore, as Livi Bacci points out, nobody afterward ever mentioned smallpox scarring on the surviving individuals.[48]

Whatever the cause, the epidemic at La Isabela encapsulates the experiences that followed Spanish colonization of the Americas over the next centuries. Writings at the time estimated that perhaps as many as one-third of the Spanish died from the epidemic at La Isabela, and the next four years were full of hunger, violence, rebellion, and continuous disease. The Spaniards expanded their explorations of the island, and Columbus established other forts, as more ships replenished the colony with provisions and people. Yet the town deteriorated from chronic food shortages and massive mortality, and finally was abandoned in 1498. After Columbus established a new settlement at Nueva Isabela (later renamed Santo Domingo), the only remaining survivors were the masses of feral pigs who roamed freely in the area.[49]

It's unknown how many Taínos inhabited Hispaniola at the time that Columbus found it, with most estimates varying wildly between sixty thousand and eight million people.[50] Recent genetic evidence suggests that there were only several thousand individuals.[51] But the archaeological record indicates that the Taíno were among the most densely populated and complex prestate, sedentary societies in the Americas, with settlements ranging from small hamlets to large towns and sustained by an intensive agricultural system.[52]

The number of Taínos who survived Columbian colonization is less debatable: half a century after the first Columbian voyage, there were only a few hundred of them left. The ones who didn't die of disease were killed by weapons, famine, forced labor, and social disruption. They weren't fully erased, for millions of living Caribbean people inherited components of their genomes, languages, and culture.[53] But the devastating effects of European colonization are undeniable.

What happened in the Caribbean was repeated throughout the Americas in various ways for centuries. Viruses and violence were the theme. Smallpox has received much of the blame for enormous demographic collapse along with the fall of the Aztec and Inca Empires in the 1500s, although many more diseases were in the mix: measles, chicken pox, mumps, influenza, polio, malaria, scarlet fever, and whooping cough are a short list. In the end, an estimated 90 percent of Native peoples had died from these diseases and other impacts of European colonization by the end of the sixteenth century.

Making Marks in Earth History

The massive mortality resulting from European colonization of the Americas has been called the Great Dying of the Indigenous Peoples of the Americas by some scholars, in reference to another event that occurred about 252 million years ago. The first Great Dying was the largest extinction episode in Earth's history, claiming around 90 percent of the planet's species.[54] Because this event marks the geological boundary between the Permian and Triassic periods, the two Great Dyings have more in common than the decimation of diversity; the one that involved the genocide of peoples is a proposed geological boundary marker between the Holocene and Anthropocene.

This potential GSSP for the Anthropocene, put forward by Lewis and Maslin, pinpoints a pronounced and unusual decrease in atmospheric carbon dioxide (CO_2) after the Columbian voyages, beginning slowly in 1520 and dropping to a low in 1610 before rebounding. As detailed in their book *The Human Planet*, carbon isotopes in Antarctic ice cores indicate that the lowest level of the CO_2 dip was caused by the sequestration (that is, capture and storage) of carbon by the land rather than by the oceans.[55]

And what caused the sequestration of carbon by terrestrial ecosystems? A continental regeneration of plant life, according to the authors. They argue that the colossal death toll of Indigenous people (at least fifty million individuals by their estimation between 1492 and 1650) led to the removal of thirteen billion tons of carbon into quickly regrowing tropical forests on abandoned agricultural clearings, whose Indigenous stewards were no longer alive to maintain them. The deaths meant, in their assessment, that "farming across a continent collapsed." They also note that the decline in atmospheric CO_2 would have resulted in significant global cooling, which appears to have happened from 1594 to 1677 based on the geological evidence.[56] And the event more or less ended by 1650, possibly because carbon uptake by recovering farmland was offset by increasing human population growth elsewhere in the world.

Lewis, Maslin, and others have championed the global CO_2 dip in 1610 as a golden spike to define the start of the Anthropocene, which they called the Orbis spike in reference to the reuniting of the Eastern and Western Hemispheres through the Columbian Exchange (because *orbis* means "world" in Latin). The transoceanic movement of species is part of the conceptual package, as this permanent change to Earth's systems would mark the planet's last cool period before the long-term global warmth of the Anthropocene.[57]

The Orbis spike nevertheless has detractors, with some substantial evidence that goes against it. The crucial claim of extensive pre-Columbian deforestation by Indigenous peoples of the Neotropical realm, suggesting that they slashed and burned the natural vegetation into submission, has been challenged by recent research using ancient plant and charcoal remains. In Peru, for example, archaeologist Dolores Piperno led a reconstruction of 5,000 years of vegetation and fire history in the Amazon Basin, which showed the forests weren't cleared, farmed, or otherwise significantly altered in prehistory.[58] Rather than transforming the community composition and structure of the species-diverse forests over thousands of years of use, Indigenous societies appeared to have been a positive force in maintaining forest integrity and biodiversity over the long term.

Likewise, other research using remote sensing technology has identified many ancient earthworks associated with domesticated tree species across the Amazon, indicating landscape modification without large-scale deforestation for millennia.[59] The bottom line, therefore, is that vegetation recovery after the genocide of European colonization wasn't so widespread and intense as to have contributed significantly to decreasing atmospheric CO_2 levels.

But at least one aspect of the Orbis spike proposal is undisputed, and that's the Columbian consequences of biotic homogenization (that is, sameness in species) that are still visible on both sides of the Atlantic Ocean. Until they started to drift apart around 200 million years ago, the American and Eurasian continents were physically continuous with Africa and each other as a gigantic supercontinent known as Pangaea. Yet transcontinental shipping by the sixteenth century and later aviation in the twentieth century played the same role as plate tectonics in redistributing life on Earth.[60] Thus, with species no longer limited by geographic barriers or natural ranges, thanks to human-mediated movements, humans have created another Pangaea of sorts. And for this reason, almost a decade before the Anthropocene debate kicked off, ecologists were suggesting that our epoch could be called by another name: the Homogecene.[61]

Humans have been relocating plants and animals through long-distance travel, trade, and dispersal for millennia. The major transportations have been species that we domesticated, crops and livestock, with the first animal being the domestic dog (*Canis familiaris*) during the Late Pleistocene.[62] Early Americans brought dogs from Siberia to North America beginning around 10,000 years ago, but people didn't introduce any truly transformative species to the Americas until the Columbian voyage from Europe to the Caribbean in 1493. Except, some have postulated, for one. This is the part where we get to chickens.

*   *   *

Domesticated chickens (*Gallus gallus domesticus*) were essential cargo for the European colonists of the Americas, having been a well-established food source in Europe for millennia. Columbus brought them to Hispaniola with his second fleet, and their quantities were listed by the hundreds in requests for food supplies from Spain to La Isabela.[63] And by many accounts, the chickens did awfully well in the Caribbean environment. Chickens, like pigs, will eat almost anything. Also like pigs and other types of European livestock that sailed overseas with the Spanish, chickens grew bigger and faster, reproduced at higher rates, and often ran wild around the tropical terrain.[64]

There's no question that humans bred and brought the chicken around the world, but the dates and routes of their dispersal are controversial. A recent study of 863 chicken genomes has identified a subspecies of red jungle fowl (*Gallus gallus spaedicus*), native to Southeast Asia, as the most likely progenitor of the domestic chicken.[65] Hence the process of chicken domestication probably started among people there, though perhaps not as early as long believed. According to a study of chicken bones from more than six hundred archaeological sites in eighty-nine countries, the earliest unambiguous domestic chicken bones thus far known were buried in the graves of rice farmers in central Thailand between 3,250 and 3,650 years ago.[66] Based on new and revised data sets, the researchers suggest that chickens were incorporated into human societies as domestic birds by about 3,500 years ago in peninsular Southeast Asia, and then rapidly spread south into Island Southeast Asia and west across South Asia and Mesopotamia to Europe and Africa.

The possibility of a pre-Columbian introduction of chickens to South America by Polynesian seafarers has been debated for decades in a swirl of questions and claims. Based on interpretations of archaeological chicken bones, some scientists have proposed that the bird was first introduced to the Americas by Polynesian contact with the Indigenous people of present-day Chile, perhaps at least 70 years before initial Spanish contact with the Taínos.[67] Others, however, have argued in favor of a post-Columbian date for these remains.[68] Furthermore, both modern and ancient genetic sequences of South American chickens are consistent with European and Asian origins, favoring an introduction during the Columbian era after all.[69]

If the Spanish were shocked by how their imported chickens became fast-growing, meatier, and more numerous within decades, then their bearded jaws would have dropped at the ones found in supermarkets today. In 2018, a study led by geologist Carys Bennett showed that bones of the broiler chicken (the name for chickens bred and raised specifically for food production) are significantly larger in size than those of its progenitors in the wild and the archaeological record.[70] Startlingly, some bones of young broilers are three times larger than the same ones found in adult red jungle fowl. Their growth rate has also become three times higher since the 1960s, even though broilers only live for a few weeks and red jungle fowl can live for up to 11 years. And if we dare to count our chickens, their numbers are absolutely staggering. In 2018, there were an estimated *23 billion of them* across the planet at any time. As such, broiler chickens are possibly the largest-standing population of a single bird species in Earth's 4.5-billion-year history and certainly the most numerous terrestrial vertebrate species on the planet right now.[71]

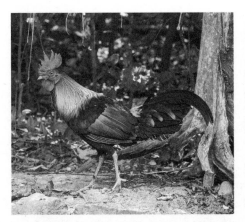 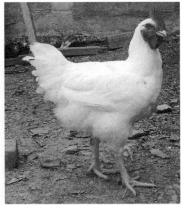

Figure 5.2
Left: The wild red jungle fowl. This tropical, ground-living bird of Southeast Asia is the
most likely ancestor of the domestic chicken. *Source:* Francesco Veronesi from Italy,
CC BY-SA 2.0, Wikimedia Commons, accessed May 1, 2023, https://en.wikipedia
.org/wiki/Red_junglefowl#/media/File:Red_Junglefowl_(male)_-_Thailand.jpg.
Right: The broiler chicken. Domestic chickens are significantly larger than their wild
progenitors, with a growth rate three times higher, due to changes in industrial poultry
production since the 1960s. *Source:* Cros2519, CC BY-SA 4.0, Wikimedia Commons,
accessed May 1, 2023, https://upload.wikimedia.org/wikipedia/commons/b/b3/Pollo
_broiler.jpg.

That's way more than a chicken in every pot: for every one of us, there's
at least three of them. And not by accident, of course. Since the twentieth century, broilers have been farmed by humans on a massive industrial
scale, with mechanical production processes that maximize the quantity of
inexpensive meat that can be added to our diet. More than seventy billion
of them were slaughtered by the global agricultural industry in 2020 alone,
with the United States leading in the production of more than nine billion
broilers a year.[72]

For this reason, according to Bennett and colleagues, broiler chickens
symbolize the transformation of the biosphere to fit evolving human consumption patterns. And given the potential of broiler bones to endure in
the geological record by accumulating in settings conducive to fossil preservation, the authors argued that the broiler chicken could be a key indicator
species for the Anthropocene. Our human epoch would then begin in the
late 1950s, from which point the Earth's archives would be full of these

morphologically and genetically distinctive birds, whose sudden world-wide distribution and population sizes are unlike anything that nonhuman nature could have pulled off.

Placing the broiler chicken at the start of the Anthropocene is an interesting prospect, illustrating how the selection of a GSSP is a forceful comment on the human activities related to it. Bennett and colleagues have focused on the impacts of industrialized food systems and biotic homogenization in nominating the broiler chicken for the golden spike. Yet they don't mention, and I can't help but observe, that this animal is linked to another hallmark of modern humanity: pandemics. And thus I think I'd also like to propose the broiler chicken as a mascot for a new age of pandemic risks. Call it the Anthropocene if you want. The Pandemocine isn't as catchy.

*   *   *

As a selling point for the broiler chicken as a plausible biostratigraphic signal of the human age, Bennett and coauthors note that avian influenza outbreaks can create chicken carcasses in abundance in the form of mass burials at landfills. Specifically, they point to an outbreak of highly pathogenic avian influenza (HPAI) in South Korea in 2008, when more than ten million birds on fifteen hundred poultry farms were preemptively killed in order to contain the spread of the influenza A (H5N1 subtype) virus.[73] The euthanized birds didn't have any symptoms, but it was safer to destroy them rather than risk further infection and transmission even though only thirty-three birds tested positive for the virus. This incident was neither the first nor the last outbreak of bird flu in South Korea since the H5N1 strain emerged in Hong Kong in 1997 (after being initially detected in China in 1996), resulting in millions of dead poultry and the earliest documented human deaths from the virus. The story has repeated year after year in dozens of other countries, as numerous H5 and H7 strains of HPAI viruses have evolved and spread internationally.

Culling is part of multicomponent efforts to stamp out HPAI epizootics in agricultural systems. There are economic reasons for destroying healthy birds in an infected flock when a highly contagious and severe disease is perhaps only a few bodies away from its next casualty. If the pathogen has a nearly 100 percent case fatality rate, as H5N1 does in chickens, there's really no other choice. Public health and safety are critical considerations too, where the sacrificial birds can serve as a firebreak between poultry and other species like us.[74]

Because let's be clear: bird flu has nearly all the makings of a lethal pandemic. Although H5N1 doesn't easily infect humans or transmit between them (meaning that people mostly catch it from birds as opposed to each other), among the rare human cases—a total of 878 reported worldwide to the WHO between 2003 through August 2023—over half of them have led to death.[75] That's deadlier than the average case fatality rate for EVD, by the way, although some experts say that it's likely an overestimation because many mild or asymptomatic infections may go unreported. But even more concerning, only a few mutations are required for the H5N1 virus to acquire airborne transmissibility, as scientists demonstrated experimentally in 2012.[76] And given that influenza viruses are highly mutable when constantly replicating within and across hosts, we face the serious danger that H5N1 will evolve into variants that are better adapted to our species.

In fact, this has already happened. Since 2020, there's been a global increase in HPAI H5 outbreaks in poultry like broiler chickens and wild birds, with H5N1 outbreaks reported in fifty-four countries in 2021 and 2022—including the largest avian influenza outbreaks on record for Europe and North America. And in late 2022, H5N1 showed at least one favorable mutation for mammal-to-mammal spread.[77] The first mammalian outbreak began on an industrial farm of some fifty-two thousand American minks (*Neovison vison*) in the Galicia region of northwest Spain, where wild birds had died from H5N1 in the previous weeks. The minks were housed in partially open barns and fed poultry by-products sourced from the same region, either of which could have exposed them to H5N1-carrying fowl.[78]

The spillover didn't stop there. Within months, several more countries reported H5N1 outbreaks in other mammalian species, with a growing list of confirmed infections in Europe and the Americas that included bears, dolphins, ferrets, leopards, otters, and skunks. Most of the mammals probably became infected with H5N1 from eating sick or dead birds with high virus loads, and the source species is anyone's guess; in addition to commercial chickens, the virus has been detected in ducks, geese, gulls, pelicans, swans, and dozens of other species of wild birds.[79] By May 2023, a dozen people had caught the virus too, including a Chilean man in whom H5N1 contained *two* genetic mutations signaling adaptation to mammals—mutations that likely emerged through viral replication during the course of his infection.[80] And this is the most alarming part: if someone with human influenza also caught H5N1 at the same time, then the two strains could swap genes and potentially produce a more human-transmissible variant. In this worst-case scenario, bird flu could start spreading through people as fast as it does flocks.

To reduce the chances of a mutant H5N1 strain wreaking havoc on humanity, the mink farm in Spain slaughtered all of its nearly fifty-two thousand minks. Over a hundred million broilers and other birds in the United States and Europe were also euthanized or died in 2021–2022 due to the HPAI H5 outbreaks. Reducing pandemic risks through such measures is unfortunately necessary in the twenty-first century.

Eliminating animals, however, is like killing the messenger when the real problems lie with us. These problems are embedded in the human-created, industrialized conditions in which billions of broilers are bred and fed. Wild birds are the natural reservoirs for avian influenza viruses, and migratory waterfowl often get all the blame for infecting poultry populations with these pathogens. But the blame is no longer justifiable, according to virologist Rob Wallace, who argues that industrial poultry farms have become their own reservoirs for bird flu, with circulating viruses that are well adapted to their flocks.[81] Consequently, intensive poultry operations have been called "factory farms of disease" and breeding grounds of the next pandemic, which could quickly travel the world as the H1N1 virus did in 2009.

Pathogenic threats are essentially built into the model of industrialized food production that started in the United States in the 1930s, by which huge numbers of genetically homogeneous chickens are raised at single sites under highly controlled and confined conditions. By the 1990s, almost all broiler facilities in the United States housed more than a hundred thousand live birds at a time (whereas in the 1950s, none of them had such large populations).[82] With thousands of susceptible hosts in close and constant proximity to each other, there have been few limits on the extent to which viruses can transmit and evolve among them. And flock-to-flock transmission can just as easily occur as people move infected birds and contaminated equipment from one feather fest to another. Poultry workers in particular are at high risk for occupational exposure to avian influenza viruses, which can be highly concentrated in bird feces and respiratory secretions. And again, the more often that humans are infected, the more likely that a new human-adapted influenza virus will emerge.

Unfortunately, viruses aren't the only kind of worrisome pathogens associated with the poultry industry. Bacteria are a huge concern because the tools used to treat and prevent bacterial infections in livestock—that is, antibiotics—have been overused to the extent that new and more dangerous germs have become abundant. Why the overuse? One big reason is that antibiotics have long been a special ingredient for making big chickens. Today a broiler chicken's slaughter weight is twice what it was seventy years ago and reached in half the time—an achievement made possible by growth promoters in the form of daily antibiotic doses that began in the 1940s.[83] Doses soon became overdoses through routine additives to food and water because the physical results were so economically enticing. The antibiotics helped animals to gain weight more quickly and build muscle more efficiently while providing protection against bacterial infections in the crowded captivity of industrialized livestock facilities. And one downside of these miracle drugs for poultry production is an evolutionary one. By exerting selection pressure on bacteria to become more resistant to antibiotics, the overuse of antibiotics has led to the worldwide emergence of antimicrobial-resistant (AMR) and multidrug-resistant pathogens.

These so-called superbugs can infect people via occupational exposure to broilers and other poultry as well as through contaminated food products from them. In addition, AMR bacteria can exchange their antibiotic-resistance genes among diverse bacterial species, creating more pathogenic threats by a microbial mechanism called horizontal gene transfer. And another problem is the still-active antibiotics that flow into the environment from the animals who receive them. As journalist Maryn McKenna explains in her book *Plucked*, the body doesn't use and ultimately excretes up to 25 percent of any antibiotic dose, and the remainders that enter the waste system could end up pushing resistant bacteria to evolve further, in unpredictable ways.[84]

Globally, over 70 percent of the antimicrobials produced on Earth are used in animal production, although some countries are worse offenders than others.[85] While the European Union has banned the use of antibiotics for growth promotion in livestock, there's far less regulation throughout the rest of the world. In the United States, for example, food animals account for around 80 percent of the nation's annual antimicrobial consumption, and two-thirds of these drugs are also used to treat illnesses in people.[86] That means that some common bacterial infections in people are becoming harder to treat with existing antibiotics. As bacteria grow resistant to antibiotics and outcompete those that are killed off by them, health metrics scientists like Christopher Murray and Mohsen Naghavi have sounded the alarm: infections that were previously curable with a few days of antibiotics could become incurable.[87]

In 2022, Murray, Naghavi, and their AMR collaborators published the first and most comprehensive analysis of the global burden of AMR to date.[88] Their findings were deeply troubling, especially the death counts: in 2019 alone, they estimated that there were almost 5 million deaths associated with bacterial AMR. And if all drug-resistant infections were replaced by drug-susceptible infections, the authors point out, then 1.27 million deaths could have been prevented.

These deaths aren't going to leave a pandemic-related signature in Earth's geological records. But big chickens just might.

Shaping Our Future

For all the debate about the Anthropocene, there's at least one thing that its proponents agree on: we're already in it. Humans have already made dramatic changes to the planet, and in a geological blink of the eye. Many of these changes have increased our pandemic risks, leaving little uncertainty that more pandemics are ahead of us. But at the beginning of this chapter, I assured you that there are things that we can do about it. And in my view, they come down to actions, priorities, and changes in mindset.

To address the growing problem of AMR, which the WHO identifies as one of the top global public health threats facing humanity, there are several steps that can be taken by individuals, businesses, and governments. One of the most important steps in the way forward, according to the WHO's *Global Action Plan on Antimicrobial Resistance*, is prevention: every infection prevented is one that needs no treatment.[89] Handwashing, vaccination, and sanitary practices are some of the most effective ways that we can avoid getting sick or transmitting diseases. If you do become ill, though, you can play a positive part in the AMR challenge by using antimicrobics only when and how they're prescribed by a health professional.

Always complete the full treatment course, even when you feel better, and never use leftover antibiotics or share them with others.

Other steps go beyond our individual choices. Health care workers have a vital role in preserving the power of antimicrobial medicines, the WHO states, by not prescribing and dispensing them inappropriately. This applies to both human and animal patients, and extends to people involved in agriculture and raising animals. The WHO also emphasizes that sustainable husbandry practices, including the use of vaccines, can reduce infection rates and dependence on antibiotics as well as the likelihood that antibiotic-resistant organisms will develop and spread through the food chain. Furthermore, in all countries and regions of the world, reducing AMR will require the political will to adopt new policies, including controlling the use of antimicrobial medicines in human health and animal and food production. In addition, governments can enact and enforce laws to ensure that medicines are of assured quality, safe, effective, and accessible to those who need them, using a One Health framework. And we, the public, should demand it.

More broadly, we can all think and act with a priority on sustainability in how we interact with the environment. Archaeological studies, such as those from the coastal United States and Amazon Basin of Peru, offer lessons on how Native and Indigenous people managed ecosystems for thousands of years, without degrading or dominating them. They prove that human land use isn't inherently destructive. Research by environmental scientist Earle Ellis and colleagues has shown that people have been shaping and sustaining diverse habitats across most of Earth's terrestrial biosphere—more than 95 percent of temperate and 90 percent of tropical woodlands—for the past 12,000 years, with a global acceleration of intensive use beginning in the late nineteenth century.[90] Our trend toward more extractive and industrialized uses of land for food and resources, leading to global warming, pollution, and biotic homogenization, is therefore a relatively recent phenomenon. But human-environmental interactions are not. And efforts to conserve and restore ecosystems, they argue, won't succeed without embracing the kind of cultural and social connections to nature and biodiversity that Native and Indigenous people have always held. This really comes down to a significant change in perception, where humans are part of nature and not separate from it. It's a message that I repeated at the

United Nations headquarters in 2023, during a forum about using science, technology, and innovation for sustainable development.

In his essay "Thinking Like a Mountain in the Anthropocene," paleobotanist Scott Wing offers ideas about how we can change our mentality in this human-dominated age. Making a case for a broader horizon, he writes,

> We need to instill a sense of geologic time into our culture and our planning, to incorporate truly long-term thinking into social and political decision making. This is what "thinking like a mountain" should come to mean in the Anthropocene. If we succeed in transforming our culture, residents of the later Anthropocene will look back on the early twenty-first century as a time of human enlightenment, when people learned to truly think like mountains by anticipating their long-lasting and complex effects on the world.[91]

In his view, the biggest challenge facing humanity is that our political, social, and economic systems lack foresight. For humans, long-term planning is restricted to years or decades, but our global impacts will play out long past our lifetimes, across centuries or millennia, if not more.

Human perception is a powerful thing, never more so when pathogens are in play. In the next chapter, we'll start to examine the kind of pandemic risks that relate to how we humans see ourselves within society and even within our species. Some of these ideas and perspectives can be particularly harmful in the ways that they rationalize the discrimination of certain groups, putting all of us in peril.

6   Foreign Foes

Humans, like virtually all other organisms, are built to recognize and retaliate against difference. In fact, our health and survival depend on it. So when disease-causing microbes breach the biological barriers of our bodies, they aren't just pathogens anymore. They're invaders. And when the first line of defense against them fails, we rely on the cells and proteins of our innate immune system to rally. This nonspecific strategy of protection, with ancient origins reflected in all classes of plants and animals, is a quick way that our bodies can destroy germs. To identify and remember specific invaders, vertebrates like us also have an adaptive immune system that reacts more slowly and precisely. But as an immediate response, innate immunity is an important safeguard against disease.

The innate immune system only has to detect something foreign that represents a threat in order to attack. The primary basis of discrimination is self and nonself. From a biological perspective, one could also think of it as a simple distinction between *us* and *them*.

We're actually good at thinking about things in this way: us and them. People do it instantly and all the time, as they sort and organize the world into categories and types of their own creation. At the core of this project is a cognitive and social process known as othering, which draws the biggest divide between those within one's group and those outside it. Except we aren't macrophages. Socially, there's no rational justification to equate difference with danger. But unfortunately, the human mind has the capacity to make it seem so.

Whether one's group is a country or club, others can be literally anyone who isn't a member. The process continues as the others are ascribed traits in contrast to the in-group, usually negative ones such as inferior morality, intelligence, and sophistication. These socially created constructs can provide a permission structure for the mistreatment, marginalization, and exclusion of anybody who's deemed to differ. People can even make non-humans into others, or nature in general, with a mental separation that excuses our exploitation and destruction of all other life on the planet.[1] Yet most commonly, others are fellow *Homo sapiens*, whose membership in humanity is outweighed by social judgments that place them outside the norm or familiar.

We're not the only species that makes others of their own. As paleo-anthropologists Anna Belfer-Cohen and Erella Hovers have noted, some nonhuman primates seem to distinguish others based on reproductive net-works, such as when chimpanzee groups from different breeding pools will fight until one of them is annihilated. But among humans, they suggest, othering changed during the course of the Pleistocene as population sizes increased and social barriers grew between expanding groups, with bound-aries less defined by clear-cut geographic features.[2] Being an other may therefore be an innate trait of human sociality. Given that archaeological data tell us little about how prehistoric people structured their social rela-tions, however, to trace the origins of othering is speculative.

Nevertheless, there's abundant archaeological evidence of human group formation and diversification over the past thousands and thousands of years, as people developed different histories, religions, cultural traditions, and behavioral patterns. And some perceptions of others have become clearer in more recent history, recorded in written language and other sym-bolic representations. These perceptions seem to be clearest, as we'll explore in this chapter, when people are threatened by disease.

*   *   *

Disease tends to give extra meaning to the other, and vice versa, as people struggle to repair the disorder of sickness and death. The Antonine Plague of the Roman Empire in 165–180, described by historian Kyle Harper in his book *Plagues upon the Earth* as "the earliest truly intercontinental disease outbreak that we can follow in any detail from human testimony," provides some of the earliest evidence of how othering figured into explanations of the unknown disease.[3] Emperor Marcus Aurelius blamed and persecuted the Christian minority for the epidemic, which was seen as punishment by pagan gods for the Christian refusal to sacrifice. Christians were again blamed for another epidemic, the Plague of Cyprian in 249–262, as pagan philosopher Porphyry recounted: "And they marvel that the sickness has befallen the city for so many years, while Asclepius and the other gods are no longer dwellers among us. For no one has seen any succor for the people while Jesus is being honored."[4] But Christians were longtime others within the empire, whose pagan majority attributed a variety of false features to them. Anti-Christian accusations included cannibalism, incest, and a hatred of humanity according to Roman historian Tacitus. So when Roman society needed a scapegoat for epidemics, earthquakes, famine, or drought, the Christian community got the job.[5]

The concept of a *scapegoat* derives ironically from Judaism, whose adherents have been othered and scapegoated for millennia. The term originates from a description in the Torah of a Yom Kippur ritual in which a goat was symbolically burdened with people's sins and set into the wilderness to get rid of them. Defined in modern parlance as a person or group blamed for something they didn't do, scapegoats can be charged with anything. And they usually are. Jewish people, as a religious and cultural minority, had been persecuted for centuries by the time that the Black Death struck Europe in 1346. Accused of spreading the plague by poisoning wells, streams, and food, thousands of Jews were rounded up, tortured, and burned alive by the Christian majority between 1348 and 1351.[6] In total, more than two hundred Jewish communities were wiped out.

Yet this conspiracy theory actually preceded the Black Death in western Europe during the early fourteenth century, when Jews were implicated in an alleged plot by lepers to destroy Christendom by contaminating the water supply.[7] Similar rumors resurfaced with subsequent plague outbreaks in the late sixteenth century during the most intense period of witch-hunting in Europe, when suspected Satanic witches (who were exclusively female and often elderly) were arrested, tortured, and killed for supposedly spreading the disease. Here again, others in the form of scapegoats offered easy answers that allowed people to deny the real reasons for sociopolitical and economic crises, which were frequently made even more chaotic by pestilence.[8]

Far from only or always involving religion, the other is a roomy construct that combines numerous aspects of perceived difference. Xenophobia (from the Greek words *xenos* and *phobos*, meaning a fear of strangers) has been a first responder to outbreaks throughout history, often imprinting the name of a disease with a putative and disfavored foreign source. Syphilis, for example, was named "the French disease" by Italians in the late fifteenth century, when the first recorded outbreak of the disease occurred in Naples during a French invasion. The French, in response, called it "the Neapolitan disease." As syphilis spread to more countries, the disease acquired various other epithets depending on who was being blamed for it: it was "the Polish disease" in Russia, "the German disease" in Poland, the "Spanish/Castilian disease" in Denmark, Portugal, and northern Africa, and the "Christian disease" in Turkey.[9] This pattern is embedded in disease terminology even today. The influenza pandemic of 1918 remains widely known as "the Spanish flu," for instance—a name initially adopted by the British, French, and Americans based on early reports of the disease in Spain. But the Spanish called it "the French flu," possibly because of its perceived origins in France. And further from the theater of World War I, as journalist Laura Spinney notes in her book *Pale Rider*, people in other countries continued the practice of blaming the obvious other: it was the "Brazilian flu" in Senegal, "the German flu" in Brazil, and "the Bolshevik disease" in Poland, to mention just a few.[10]

Xenophobia can meet with racism in a particularly virulent reaction to epidemics. Whereas xenophobia is place-based prejudice, racism is rooted in the bogus claim that humans are naturally divided into biological types. It's like saying that buckets are a natural division of rain drops. The truth is that "races" such as white and Black don't exist in human biology, because our physical differences occur in ranges, not categories. And yet the Western concept of race has been socially, politically, and legally constructed over the last five centuries.[11] Which is to say, people made it up—and with the intention of keeping others down. Racial classification systems developed by early doctors and physical anthropologists, with their emphasis on continuous traits like hair texture and skin color, gave a scientific veneer to these human-made divisions. As a result, the socially constructed groupings of others into "races" have gravely misrepresented the unbroken diversity across our species. These damaging ideas went hand-in-hand with the historical expansion of European settler colonialism, white supremacy, and slavery, and they have been used to justify the exploitation, oppression, discrimination, and outright dehumanization of racial others ever since.

Although race isn't a biological fact, racism has real biological consequences. Racism produces systemic inequalities in access to health care, housing, food, education, wealth, and public services within and between populations, and those inequities have cascading effects on how the organs, systems, and processes of the human body develop, function, and respond to infections. As seen with COVID-19 in the United States and elsewhere, these social determinants of health are linked to disproportionate burdens of disease in communities of color, such as two to three times higher rates of COVID-19 hospitalizations and deaths among Black, Latino, and Native Americans than white Americans in 2022.[12]

The ways that xenophobia and racism can contribute to emerging disease risks are evident in the origins of the bubonic plague in the United States. The story is set in San Francisco, where Chinese immigrants were beset by nativist grievances and violence. Viciously miscast as economic, cultural, and medical threats, the Chinese residents of San Francisco, like Chinese people across the country, were targeted by discriminatory laws, policies, and practices to drive them out. In this case, xenophobia wasn't the first responder to an outbreak; it was already at the scene.

Hashtags and Hate Crimes

Today the singular beauty of San Francisco's Chinatown, a twenty-four-block district in the heart of the Bay Area of northern California, is a sight to behold. Passing through the green-tiled portals of the Dragon Gate, flanked by stone lions on guard against evil spirits, you encounter an urban habitat that is wholly distinct from all that surrounds it. Dozens of dragon lamps guide cars and pedestrians along sloping streets, as countless red lanterns sway overhead, drawing your attention to the pagoda roofs and curved eaves that shape the skyline. Dazzling murals adorn the brick walls of narrow alleyways, from which the wafting scent of freshly baked fortune cookies might lure a passerby. Chinese characters dominate the signs and banners that hang on every storefront, from fish markets to dim sum restaurants to souvenir shops.

Chinatown has been a top tourist destination in the city for generations, but visitors only add to the hubbub of people who live and work there. The community forms the largest Chinese enclave outside Asia, entirely within a little more than one square mile, making it the most densely populated area west of Manhattan in the United States.

Yet the protective statues at the gateway to Chinatown haven't kept its residents free from threats. Wandering the streets of the district, an upward gaze might fail to observe the hints of danger from without. On my last visit in 2022, as I walked the main thoroughfare of Grant Avenue, a small, black-and-white sticker caught my eye. Affixed to the padlocked door of an unleased property, among images of vibrant Chinese American scenes, the words were simple and in English: #stopasianhate.

The meaning of the sticker was obvious; it was a direct reference to the explosive rise of anti-Asian racism during the COVID-19 pandemic. China in particular was a target of blame by US president Trump, who stoked resentment and xenophobia by using the monikers "Chinese virus" or "China virus" for the causal pathogen. He deliberately drew on the old playbook of dubbing diseases for political purposes rather than using the official name of SARS-CoV-2 announced by the WHO in February 2020. The WHO's name followed 2015 guidelines that recommended neutral scientific terms, avoiding words associated with a specific place or group of people in order to reduce any unfair blame or discrimination for the disease's emergence.

Predictably, Trump's rhetoric did the opposite. Following his first use of "Chinese virus" in a Twitter (later renamed "X") post on March 16, 2020, there was an avalanche of anti-Asian sentiments on the social media platform. One study led by computational epidemiologist Yulin Hswen showed that Trump's tweet coincided with huge increases in tweets using #covid19 and #chinesevirus hashtags, about 797 and 17,400 percent, respectively.[13] The authors determined that approximately one in five hashtags with #covid19 were anti-Asian, whereas half the hashtags with #chinesevirus were anti-Asian. Although the authors couldn't assess the relationship between the hashtags and hate crimes, they noted that many of the tweets implied violence.

And violence ensued. From March 2020 to September 2021, a total of 10,370 hate incidents against Asian American and Pacific Islander (AAPI) people in the United States were reported to Stop AAPI Hate, a San Francisco–based nonprofit organization that started tracking racist attacks on the AAPI community as a result of the COVID-19 pandemic.[14] People who self-identified as Chinese reported the most incidents of any AAPI group—almost 43 percent of them. Based on a national survey conducted online in September to October 2021, Stop AAPI Hate also estimated that one in five AAPI people experienced a hate incident in the previous year. The narratives from the survey are gut-wrenching. One person recounted being in a grocery store where "a middle-aged man began yelling and

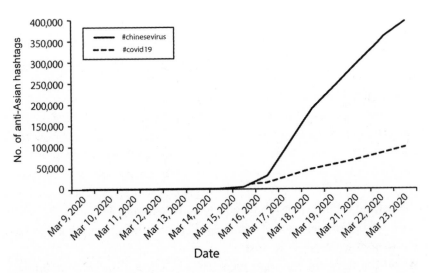

Figure 6.1
Timeline of anti-Asian Twitter hashtags in March 2020. The number of anti-Asian
hashtags rose by 797 and 17,400 percent, respectively, for #covid19 and #chinese-
virus immediately following the first tweet by President Donald Trump using the
phrase "Chinese virus" on March 16, 2020. *Source:* Reprinted, with the permission of
Sheridan, from Y. Hswen, X. Xu, A. Hing, J. B. Hawkins, J. S. Brownstein, and G. C.
Gee, "Association of '#covid19' versus '#chinesevirus' with Anti-Asian Sentiments
on Twitter: March 9–23, 2020," *American Journal of Public Health* 111, no. 5 (2021):
956–964.

blaming me for the 'Chinese Flu' and he told me to 'Go home! Go back
where you came from!'" Others described acts of physical assault, vandal-
ism, workplace discrimination, and online and verbal harassment. Sadly,
Stop AAPI Hate's data are consistent with many news reports of dramatic
increases in anti-Asian hate crimes as COVID-19 spread across the United
States and around the world.

As early as May 2020, UN secretary-general António Guterres urged governments to act responsibly as "the pandemic continues to unleash a tsu-
nami of hate and xenophobia, scapegoating and scare-mongering."[15] On
the heels of his statement, the international nongovernmental organization Human Rights Watch highlighted racial abuses being experienced by
people of Asian descent in many countries, some of whose government
leaders and senior officials directly or indirectly encouraged hate crimes,
racism, or xenophobia by using anti-Chinese rhetoric.[16]

In San Francisco's Chinatown, the discrimination was felt in more ways than one. In March 2020, before a mandatory shelter-in-place order went into effect in the Bay Area, the city's Chinese American leaders called attention to a big drop in foot traffic and business in Chinatown, concurrent with a big increase in xenophobia.[17] Unfortunately for the community of Chinatown, none of this was new. In 2003, Chinatowns in San Francisco and elsewhere, such as in New York City, took a huge financial hit from the SARS epidemic, with some businesses reporting a 90 percent drop in revenue.[18] Across the Bay, the University of California at Berkeley announced that it wouldn't accept summer students from the parts of Asia affected by the SARS virus, including mainland China, Hong Kong, Taiwan, and Singapore, out of fear that some of them might be infected. After receiving heavy criticism, the policy was revised.

But the story doesn't begin there. For as long as Chinese communities have existed in the United States, they've been accused and affronted with countless misperceptions about epidemic diseases. Nowhere more aggressively than in San Francisco, a port of entry to the United States for thousands of Chinese immigrants beginning in the mid-nineteenth century. Establishing the first Chinatown in North America, they created a place that still stands as a unique testament of Chinese American perseverance. And in trying to understand how xenophobia and racism can help to prolong a plague, there may be no better place to look.

Except, again, the story doesn't start with the plague. Because the ideas that spread the plague were already endemic in California, much earlier than the pathogen was.

Perpetual Aliens

In 1848, the lure of gold brought people rushing to California from all parts of the world. The first fortune seekers from China arrived on ships with visions of *gam saan*, the "Gold Mountain" that had been shouted from the ports to the provinces. Fleeing natural and economic disasters that devastated much of the Chinese population in the nineteenth century, many seemed willing to suffer just about anything for economic opportunities to help their families and communities back home. But for a lot of these Chinese voyagers, mostly young men, unimagined adversity lay ashore.

By the time the gold rush peaked in 1852, the Chinese population of California was already more than twenty thousand people and about 12 percent of residents of San Francisco, a city that grew from a thousand to thirty-five thousand people in just four years.[19] Yet Chinese dreams of the Gold Mountain were met with brutal conditions and meager rewards—the unexpected realities of an unwelcoming land where many Chinese could not read or speak the language. Unable to return to China or bring their relatives to California, many of them stayed to work, earn, and send money home, even as they were exploited for cheap labor.

From the 1850s to the 1870s, in addition to mining gold and silver, Chinese immigrants worked on farms as well as in fisheries and factories. They were critical to the construction of railways, such as the western part of North America's first transcontinental railroad, and in the reclamation of swamplands. Chinese laborers also created cultural landmarks such as Old Saint Mary's Cathedral, the first cathedral built in California. Established in 1854 by Father Henry Ignatius Stark, who aimed to introduce Catholicism to the Chinese community of San Francisco, the cathedral stood only steps away from the Chinese businesses that began to emerge and cluster on Sacramento Street. Called *Tongyan gaai* ("Street of the Chinese") by its occupants, this nexus of Chinese immigrant life began to take form as Chinatown while nativist animosity toward them grew.[20]

Anti-Chinese xenophobia was bad enough in a booming economy, but rose to a fever pitch with the inevitable bust. During times of recession following the gold rush, fears about unemployment and poverty fed into an all-encompassing hatred of Chinese people as a menace to US life. The coalescing anti-Chinese movement lobbied for federal, state, and local legislation to make it extremely difficult and expensive for Chinese workers to stay in California, if not force them to leave.[21] The Anti-Coolie Act, passed in 1862, imposed a monthly tax on anyone of Chinese origin who applied for a license to work or do business in California, and the Anti-Coolie Association, formed in 1867, coordinated boycotts of manufacturers that employed Chinese workers.[22]

Even then, the question of banning immigration from China persisted in politics and the press. When California fell into an economic downturn in the 1870s, which left at least one-fifth of its laborers out of work, the Chinese were blamed outright.[23] "Our people cannot compete with them," insisted US Senator John Hager to his congressional colleagues in 1874. Proposing modifications to the Burlingame Treaty, which would discourage further Chinese immigration to the United States, the California politician contended that "wherever labor is employed, there these Chinese are offered at lower rates than our citizens can afford to work for, and the result is that at this time there are thousands of our own people in the streets of San Francisco destitute of the necessaries of life, because they have been crowded out from all employments by this Chinese labor." He predicted a dire outcome where "either our white citizen labor will be entirely driven from every field of labor" or else a bloody race war would erupt between the Chinese and desperate white Americans faced with starvation.[24] Anti-Chinese sentiments also doubled as campaign ads for the California Workingmen's Party, formed in 1878, whose goal to rid the country of Chinese cheap labor was summed up with a simple clarion call: "The Chinese must go!"

The Chinese did not go. Not even as the Workingmen's Party formed vengeful mobs that attacked Chinese communities and businesses along the West Coast.[25] Not even when, a few years later, Chinese exclusion became the law of the land. In 1882, the US Congress passed the Chinese Exclusion Act, which singled out Chinese applicants for restricted entry to the United States. Never before had the United States so explicitly restricted immigration by a specific ethnic or national group.[26] The act also blocked Chinese immigrants already in the United States from US citizenship and basic rights. More than a hundred thousand people were thus made permanent aliens within the country where they lived, both foreign and disenfranchised in perpetuity.

Following the government's legitimization of Chinese exclusion from US society, the Chinese American experience involved a heightened state of resistance and endurance. Mass murders, roundups, and purges of Chinese people became horrifyingly frequent in the1880s, when almost two hundred towns in the Pacific Northwest drove out their Chinese residents.[27]

And yet the Chinese did not go. With support from the Chinese consul in San Francisco, the Chinese Consolidated Benevolent Association (also known as the Chinese Six Companies) was created to battle anti-Chinese legislation, resulting in thousands of cases and a high proportion of wins.[28] And by the early twentieth century, there were four major Chinese-language dailies in San Francisco, including *Chung Sai Yat Po*, which helped to mobilize the community for various political and socioeconomic causes and against anti-Chinese racism.[29]

Xenophobic discrimination didn't drive the Chinese out but instead drove them together. And it shaped how they lived. From the outset of the gold rush, San Francisco's Chinatown was a place of refuge in the hostile environment of California, where violence and discrimination were so thick that the Chinese had no other residential option.[30] Even so, these conditions brought other threats into their community, such as disease, which endangered the whole city.

Public Nuisances

In the late nineteenth century, Western media promoted anti-Asian tropes with zeal. Fearmongering cartoons, books, and films captured the xenophobic zeitgeist with exaggerated portrayals of Asian supervillains as an existential threat. The so-called Yellow Peril applied to all Asians, seen as unassimilable aliens who might destroy the West unless stopped. But the threat of disease was associated with the Chinese specifically. This notion predated the beginning of Chinese immigration to California, where the Chinese became an all-around scapegoat as politics and public health became intertwined.

Anthropologist Christos Lynteris has identified four main focal points in the Western projections of disease onto China and the Chinese during the late nineteenth and early twentieth centuries: origins, urban spaces, bodies, and culture.[31] Against a sociolegal backdrop of exclusion and discrimination, these themes played out in epidemic scenes that always cast the Chinese as the other.

First, China was perceived as the original source of the plague, the infamous disease that devastated Europe in the fourteenth century. In 1894, Hong Kong experienced the first outbreak of the plague with international press coverage, and newspaper headlines around the world announced the reemergence of the Black Death as a threat to civilization. And as they made clear, it came from China. Numerous other diseases, like cholera and smallpox, were likewise thought to originate in China, thereby giving a double meaning to its nickname as "the sick man of Asia" in the late nineteenth and early twentieth centuries. In the case of the latter, as Chinese media scholar Ari Larissa Heinrich notes, the Western idea of China being the cradle of smallpox was derived largely from a single document written by a French Jesuit missionary to China in the eighteenth century.[32]

And then in the late nineteenth century, there was an emerging theme of Chinese urban spaces and forms as the breeding grounds of disease.[33] From 1868 to 1887, across four successive smallpox epidemics in San Francisco, anthropologist Susan Craddock argued that the physical place of Chinatown was increasingly associated with disease and ultimately became synonymous with it.[34] In the 1868 epidemic, according to Craddock, public health officials didn't implicate Chinatown as the source of the contagion, nor did they attempt a racial framing of the disease.[35] But this changed during the 1876 epidemic, which coincided with a demographic shift in San Francisco: the Chinese community more than doubled between 1870 and 1871, and reached a peak of about 30,000 by 1876.

Hence the cause of the smallpox epidemic, wrote health officer John London Meares in 1877, was "the presence in our midst of 30,000 (as a class) of unscrupulous, lying and treacherous Chinamen, who have disregarded our sanitary laws, concealed and are concealing their cases of smallpox."[36] Meares repeated these claims in an 1890 report to the Board of Health of San Francisco, which consequently condemned Chinatown as a nuisance. Published by the California Workingmen's Party as a pamphlet titled *Chinatown Declared a Nuisance!*, the report described Meares's investigation of Chinatown in sordid detail, including offenses such as "a house of terrible filth, stink, and slime" and "piles of dirt, filth, stench and slime." Filth was mentioned to the point of redundancy as well as overcrowding and foul "Chinese" odor, consistent with the sanitarian ideology of the late nineteenth century.[37] As noted by historian Guenter Risse, *filth* and *stink* were code words intended to evoke disgust, "a powerful emotion that would demonize and isolate the undesirable 'other' living in a polluted material world."[38] An investigating committee of the Anti-Chinese Council of the Workingmen's Party added further vitriol to the pamphlet with recommendations to relocate the Chinese outside the city, and criminalize business and other relations with them.[39]

Meares's sinophobic rants failed to appear in the municipal report on the smallpox epidemic in 1887 because he fell ill and died (from unrelated causes) before it ended. Nonetheless, his successor, D. E. Barger, blamed Chinese passengers on steamships from Hong Kong as the sources of both the 1876 and 1887 epidemics.[40] Although it's equally, if not more, likely that these epidemics resulted from European and US travelers from the East, as Craddock argues, fingers pointed always to China.[41] And to the Chinese.

This is because Chinese people themselves, not just their places of origin or living, were inherently pathological in the Western imagination.[42] Like foreign invaders of a healthy body, whose innate immune cells recognize and attack something that is *not self*, it seems that the Chinese were simultaneously the agents and carriers of disease. Their cultural traditions, practices, and behaviors resisted assimilation, and their mortuary beliefs and customs in particular were blamed as an obstacle for epidemic control. Furthermore, as they were perceived as biologically different and inferior, Chinese people were ascribed all kinds of characteristics that made disease part of their being—not even a human being, in some views.

Thus in the *Chinatown Declared a Nuisance!* pamphlet of 1880, the descriptions of Chinese people read like a brochure for pest control. The Chinese were characterized as vectors of disease who existed only in modes of infestation. Basically like rats: "The honeycombed condition of Chinatown is perfectly well known; they (the Chinamen) can pass from one block to the other, from one house to the other, either by subterranean passages or above the roofs."[43] But the evocation of rodents wasn't simply racist. It was also foreboding of the plague to come.

And when the plague did arrive, the living conditions in Chinatown couldn't have been worse. Certain nuisance allegations in the public health reports probably contained some truth because they described the social and environmental consequences of anti-Chinese xenophobia and marginalization. Under exclusionary laws, most Chinese immigrants were renters with no legal rights to properties, and non-Chinese landlords weren't required to provide habitable conditions.[44] Without public sanitation services, along with poor housing and plumbing, many people lived in squalor.[45] Also, the legislation created an extreme sex ratio imbalance, with men outnumbering women almost twenty-seven to one by 1890.[46] Unable to bring their wives to the United States or marry US citizens, Chinese men were largely deprived of family and essentially formed a bachelor society by force. In order to return to China or support people there, they worked long hours at low wages and saved what money they could, spending little on food and belongings, and rooming with as many other men as possible.[47] These conditions were largely uncontrollable, but they were endured like so much else. And unfortunately, they were highly conducive to pests.

Plague and Plague Proofing

Bubonic plague struck San Francisco in two epidemics during the first decade of the twentieth century. The first epidemic, from 1900 to 1904, riddled Chinatown with fear and death as the district yet again shouldered all the blame. Yet the second epidemic, from 1907 to 1908, left the Chinese community largely untouched. In fact, Chinatown seemed to be the only neighborhood spared from the spread.[48] Notably, these epidemics occurred on opposite sides of a historic earthquake in 1906, when San Francisco shook and burned to the brink of annihilation. Almost thirty thousand buildings were destroyed and about three thousand people perished.

But the shift between 1900 and 1907 wasn't a tectonic one. And the epidemiological differences are only crude comparisons. Instead, the most significant change between the first and second epidemic of the bubonic plague in San Francisco was a factual understanding of the disease. As we will see, the die-hard bigotry that hampered the first response, possibly contributing to the ever-presence of plague in the United States today, gave way to ecological knowledge that informed antiplague measures years later. With a reoriented focus on other species as the source of the disease, rather than other humans, public health improved beyond disease control, particularly in Chinatown. In contrast, the counterproductive and damaging consequences of racial discrimination and xenophobia during the earlier years are all the more apparent.

*   *   *

Although plague was known by humans for centuries before reaching North America, relatively little was understood about its causes in the early twentieth century. There were ongoing debates about how people caught it as well as how to prevent and treat it. Germ theory was well established by the late nineteenth century, but many scientists and public health officials retained fourteenth-century ideas that plague was caused by miasmic vapors from decaying waste—the kind of atmospheric conditions created by poverty and filth.[49] Even after Swiss French bacteriologist Alexandre

Yersin identified the culprit as the bacillus *Y. pestis*, within weeks of the Hong Kong outbreak in 1894, scientists still struggled to fit the pieces together.

One popular theory proposed that plague was a soil-bred bacterial disease, whose bacilli could infect and lay dormant in the earth. British colonial doctors in Hong Kong and Bombay thus reasoned that walking barefoot or sleeping on soil caused human infections, implicating native laborers and women in pathological behaviors.[50] Eventually the soil theory of the plague lost ground as evidence mounted for a zoonotic etiology of the disease. But its decline was slowed where social and moral assumptions clouded scientific reasoning, as historian Myron Echenberg wrote in his book *Plague Ports*: "Their blinkered assumption that plague spread because 'barefoot Indians were infected from bacilli lurking in cow-dung floor' reflected the orientalist bias that India was intrinsically different from, and inferior to, the West."[51]

Dead rats, as it turned out, were a big clue to the mysteries of plague. In Hong Kong, Yersin observed dead rats lying all over the houses and streets of poor, plague-stricken neighborhoods, and found that many of the rats contained large quantities of *Y. pestis* in their organs. When he announced his discovery of the plague bacillus, he also speculated that rats were the main vehicle of the disease. Not even European houses were safe from plague, Yersin warned on seeing nearby dead rats, which were *"indices certains du très proche voisinage des germes infectieux"* ("sure signs of the very close vicinity of infectious germs").[52] Yet on the subject of insect vectors of plague, while Yersin mused about flies, he wrote nary a word about fleas.

Fleas, or rather their bites, were a final piece of the puzzle. In 1898, French physician Jean-Paul Simond published his discovery of *Y. pestis* in fleas from rats who had died of plague, along with experimental support for the flea-borne spread of plague among rats and humans. People in India who handled infected rat corpses, Simond suggested, contracted the disease when infected fleas abandoned their expired rodent hosts for living human ones. Nonetheless, skepticism prevailed for years, despite strong proof of the flea factor in plague transmission. "Only later understandings of the critical role of the flea vector," as Echenberg pronounced, "would explain so many of the conundrums presented by plague epidemics."[53]

One conundrum was why plague in San Francisco, a metropolis of nearly 350,000 inhabitants by 1900, resulted in fewer than 300 cases and

200 deaths in the end. Well, as it turned out, the most common rat flea on the California coast, and in other places where plague was mild during the third plague pandemic, was an ineffective vector of the *Y. pestis* bacteria.[54] And while the local flea (and rat) populations were studied and reported by public health officer Rupert Blue in 1909, the year after he led the elimination of plague from San Francisco, the vector efficiency of the different species was not.[55] It was a minor oversight, compared to his predecessor. Until Blue was on the case, the differences between people had gotten all the attention.

*   *   *

The first hint of bubonic plague in San Francisco was spotted on March 6, 1900, in the form of a swollen lymph node on a dead man's groin. The man was a Chinese resident of the Globe Hotel in Chinatown, and the textbook bubo triggered a panic. As autopsy samples were rushed to nearshore Angel Island, where Joseph James Kinyoun was in charge of the US Marine Hospital Service quarantine station, the city's Board of Health convened an emergency meeting. Not waiting for a bacterial confirmation of the cause of death, the board made a late-night decision to blockade Chinatown. Immediately.

Misguided by the mindset that plague was an Asiatic disease of filth, the board ordered brutish assaults on Chinatown by means of disinfection, isolation, and quarantine. By midnight, a cordon sanitaire of police roped off the district, with officers at every corner "to permit neither whites, Chinese, or Japanese in, and to allow no one but whites to pass out."[56] The police were also instructed "to search everywhere and to drive out any whites found," ensuring that only Chinese people would be trapped inside. By dawn, as one-fifth of San Francisco's residents awoke to a state of imprisonment, sanitation workers began to fumigate buildings such as the Globe Hotel while health inspectors went door-to-door in search of infected bodies, living or dead.[57]

News of the quarantine was covered by local papers, which informed public perceptions of the Chinese and often boosted racist public health rhetoric about the risks they posed to the city.[58] The *San Francisco Call* assured its readers that plague didn't threaten the white population. Quotations from top-ranked US medical authorities declared that plague was "a disease peculiar to the Orient, and seldom, if ever attacks Europeans," and flourished only where there was dirt and filth.[59] The paper pleaded for calm regarding the "Asiatic pestilence," asserting that "when these diseases appear they prove to be largely racial, as this plague is, and experience with it proves that Occidental races are but little subject to it." It therefore concluded that "no apprehension need be felt by our non-Asiatic population."[60]

As the city awaited Kinyoun's bacteriologic results, nobody was more anxious than its Chinese community. On March 7, a report in the Chinese newspaper *Chung Sai Yat Po* gave no comfort: "By Friday, it is hoped that we will know that this was not the plague. Otherwise what happened in Honolulu might happen to us."[61]

What happened in Honolulu was more than a tragedy. It was an erasure. In the final weeks of 1899, residents of Chinatown in Honolulu, Hawaii's largest city, started dying of plague. Similar to what happened in San Francisco months later, the Board of Health of Honolulu sealed off the fourteen-block district in order to inspect, disinfect, and isolate the community. The board twice imposed a quarantine on its five thousand inhabitants, and restricted travel in and out of Honolulu and between the Hawaiian Islands, but only for Chinese and Japanese people (the latter of whom represented about a third of Chinatown's population).[62] In response to concerns that these measures were too weak and might allow plague to linger for many economy-crippling years, the Board of Health then evoked emergency powers for extreme action: to forcibly remove Chinatown residents to quarantine camps and burn down their buildings.

The "sanitary fires" began on December 31 and continued for weeks, destroying Honolulu's Chinatown piece by piece. And then on January 20, 1900, one of the fires blazed beyond control. A wind-driven inferno swept through entire blocks of the district, destroying about one-fifth of Honolulu's buildings and leaving more than one-eighth of the city's residents without their homes, businesses, and personal property.[63] By late January, one-sixth of Honolulu residents were in detention camps.

In San Francisco, the residents of Chinatown had every reason to fear the same outcome. For as long as Chinatown had existed, nativists had schemed to force the Chinese out of the city and claim the real estate for white business interests. Public health claims provided a flimsy guise of legitimacy for these long-held plans. But the Chinese community wouldn't submit to elimination by expulsion.

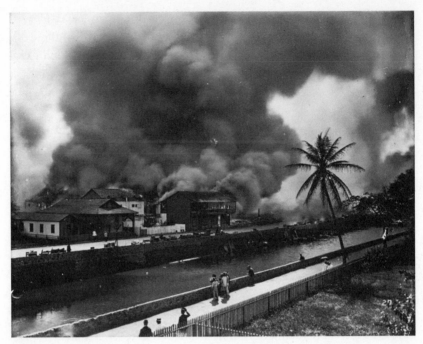

Figure 6.2
Honolulu's Chinatown fire of 1900. During an attempt by health officials to control plague in Honolulu by burning down buildings in Chinatown, an out-of-control fire ended up destroying most of the neighborhood. *Source:* Gabriel Bertram Bellinghausen, public domain via Wikimedia Commons.

The morning after Chinatown was quarantined, the Chinese Consul and the Six Companies protested the measures and vowed to end them.[64] The following day, on behalf of a Chinatown merchant, a lawsuit in an injunction was instituted in the US District Court against the health and police departments of the city, with the aim to declare the quarantine as unnecessary and injurious to the business interests of the Chinese community.[65] Before further legal steps were taken, the Board of Health moved to lift the quarantine.

Yet the battles didn't end there. Kinyoun soon confirmed that plague was indeed in San Francisco. Nobody was willing to accept it, however—not the Board of Health, nor the press, nor the mayor, nor even the governor. And the Chinese, who had no trust in any of them, certainly didn't believe it. As the epidemic grew and stretched over months, more attempts at racial quarantine failed in the courts. Kinyoun's efforts to mandate vaccination for Chinese residents was resisted and soon abandoned. And by the time that the presence of plague in San Francisco was affirmed by a visiting panel of experts, Kinyoun had made little progress in controlling it. Still facing denial and disrespect from all sides, he suffered the final humiliation of a transfer to Detroit, Michigan, in 1901.

*   *   *

After Blue stepped into Kinyoun's role, he ultimately found success with a target that had never before guided epidemic control measures in the United States. After years of battling uncontrolled plague, by 1903 he decided to "throw the burden upon the rat, and to base the campaign upon rodent eviction and eradication."[66] Leaving behind the racist philosophies of public health officials like Kinyoun, who continued to see and distrust the Chinese as the ultimate enemy of his efforts, Blue didn't view his challenges as people to be kept in or driven out. Rather, he aimed to "build out" plague from San Francisco by improving the urban environments where rats thrived.[67]

In places where Blue saw unsanitary conditions owing to defective construction, neglect of repairs, and general decay in buildings, he also found large colonies of rats in cellars, basements, walls, and ceilings, often in coexistence with crowds of people and their waste. In 1904, his program for "the breaking up of these relations" led to the first rat-proofing legislation, which required property owners to replace wood and cover soil with concrete on ground floors, and empowered the US Public Health and Marine Hospital Service to force the demolition and removal of unsafe structures. "Man was no longer to be held responsible for the crime," he later wrote. "In other words, it was a new orientation of the problem whereby isolation and quarantine, if practiced at all, would be applied to the potential rat carrier."[68] In addition, Blue hired workers to set rat traps throughout Chinatown and elsewhere, baiting the traps with poison made by federal doctors in Blue's laboratory. Blue and his colleagues dissected and tested thousands rats for evidence of plague, including those brought in by amateur rat catchers who took advantage of Blue's offer of ten cents per rodent, living or dead.[69]

His strategy worked. After months without any new cases of plague reported, Blue found that the city's overall death rate had fallen by 15

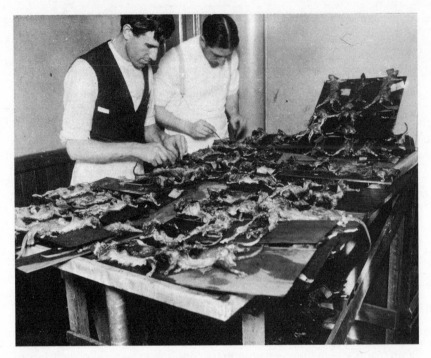

Figure 6.3
Rat dissection for antiplague measures in San Francisco in ca. 1907. *Source:* NIH
National Library of Medicine Digital Collections.

percent from the previous year, presumably due to the massive elimination
of rats from its streets and sewers.[70] The efforts continued until February
1905, even after plague hadn't been identified in a human or rat for more
than a year, when San Francisco was finally declared safe and Blue its savior.

San Francisco was then devastated by the earthquake and fire of 1906,
and its charred remains became a rat paradise. Plague returned to the
city in 1907, but not in Chinatown, which had gotten a head start on its
defenses. At a meeting with the Citizen's Health Committee in early 1908,
Blue showed maps of the city, spotted with the locations of human cases of
plague and captures of infected rats. And to the mortification of many of
the people present, Blue recounted, the only sanitary part of San Francisco
appeared to be Chinatown.[71] Indeed, as plague struck people all over San
Francisco until 1908, not a single one of them was Chinese. The formerly
plagued community was seemingly plague resistant.

Partnerships without Prejudice

For years, while Chinese people were made the scapegoats for plague in San Francisco, a different animal had already carried *Y. pestis* off into the wild. Infected fleas on rats, such as those who came ashore from ships at Bay Area ports, spread the pathogen to native rodents like California ground squirrels at some point during the first epidemic. In 1903, Blue became aware of a recent die-off of squirrels in the East Bay and investigated the possibility that sylvatic plague was spreading there.[72] He couldn't prove his theory by finding an infected squirrel, but he warned the US surgeon general of the potential risks for all of California.[73] Nonetheless, it wasn't until 1908, with the case of a plague-afflicted boy on an East Bay ranch, that Blue also confirmed infections in several squirrels in the area.[74] Within a year of the first evidence of a naturally occurring plague in the California ground squirrel, he and his colleagues found that more than 1 percent of the squirrel population of the East Bay carried the pathogen.[75]

Once *Y. pestis* became established in wild rodent populations, plague outbreaks of varying sizes took place in urban areas along the Pacific coast until 1925, ending in Los Angeles, where echoes of San Francisco's Chinatown resonated in an ethnic quarantine of the city's Mexican residents.[76] But the rural spread of *Y. pestis* continued, spanning approximately 2,250 kilometers in forty years as the pathogen became entrenched in several western US states.[77] By the mid-1940s, epizootics were documented in the wood rat (*Neotoma* spp.), deer mouse (*Peromyscus* spp.), ground squirrel (*Spermophilus* spp.), and prairie dog (*Cynomys* spp.) populations as far east as the US states of Oklahoma and Kansas.[78] And every so often, human cases still occur. In recent decades, an annual average of seven human cases of plague have been reported to the CDC in a part of the United States marked by a geographic limit known today as the Plague Line.[79]

As Echenberg and others have suggested, it's possible that the ineffective response under Kinyoun provided opportunities for zoonotic transmission that has made plague a permanent, if minor, danger in the United States today.[80] Of course, knowledge about plague ecology was limited at the time, but Kinyoun's xenophobic fixation on Chinatown certainly didn't help science or society. After being assured that plague was a disease of filthy foreigners, for instance, people in the East Bay resisted being diagnosed with plague because they resented the social implications.[81] While energies were spent on blaming the Chinese, and perhaps because of it, the real threat therefore took hold.

*   *   *

Xenophobia and racism can still impede our abilities to prevent newly emerging pathogens from becoming endemic across continents. The insults and allegations traded by US and Chinese government officials at the beginning of the COVID-19 pandemic led to one example of how this might happen. In March 2020, China's Ministry of Foreign Affairs endorsed a baseless theory that members of the US Army introduced the virus to Wuhan during a visit months prior to the outbreak.[82] The Trump administration retaliated with the "China Virus" mantra, a tried-and-true gimmick to deflect responsibility for the spread of SARS-CoV-2 within the United States, while distracting from the government's failures to contain it. Without presenting any evidence, Trump and his allies also suggested that the virus originated in a government laboratory in China—implicating the Wuhan Institute of Virology (WIV), where bat coronaviruses have been studied since the SARS epidemic in 2002.[83] Furthermore, Trump accused the WHO of colluding with China to cover up the outbreak in Wuhan and moved to withdraw the United States from the organization (a decision that President Joe Biden reversed on his first day in office in January 2021).[84]

As I write these words, three years later, it's still unclear how the virus emerged. Right now it seems like we may never know for sure. And while it's valuable to understand the evolutionary and ecological pathways that led to the pandemic, there's other important work to do—in monitoring and preventing the spread and mutation of SARS-CoV-2 and other pathogens, as well as reducing risks of spillovers with One Health policies and sustainable practices—irrespective of COVID-19's origins. Unfortunately, the pandemic whodunit turned into a political imbroglio that complicated these efforts. And with such a fixation on blaming China, a basic point of scientific consensus has been brushed aside: epidemics start because of human-induced ecological disruptions that bring people and livestock into closer contact with wildlife.

One of the two major theories about the source of COVID-19, endorsed by the Federal Bureau of Investigation and the US Department of Energy, is the "laboratory leak" theory that SARS-CoV-2 escaped from the WIV through a research-related accident.[85] This is plausible given that research-related infections of dangerous viruses (such as the causal agent of SARS) have happened in China and elsewhere. However, solid proof that this occurred with SARS-CoV-2 is yet to be seen. It's also worth noting that neither agency rated their assessments with high confidence.

The other major theory, which was favored by a WHO-China joint report in March 2021 and numerous other US agencies, is that SARS-COV-2 resulted from a natural zoonotic spillover, as happened with SARS-CoV-1 in China in 2002 to 2004. The report's authors declared that it was extremely unlikely that the virus had escaped from a laboratory, although critics—including a number of leading scientists—raised concerns about an unbalanced appraisal of evidence by the team and insufficient data sharing by the Chinese government.[86] In 2023, the WHO abandoned its plans for a second phase of studies, with epidemiologist Maria Van Kerkhove lamenting that "the politics across the world of this really hampered progress on understanding the origins."[87]

As of June 2023, the zoonotic spillover theory has the most scientific support, especially by scientists with expertise in emerging diseases and virology.[88] According to an international team of virologists, genomicists, and evolutionary biologists who analyzed genetic, spatial, epidemiological, and social media data from Wuhan in late 2019 and early 2020, the Huanan Seafood Wholesale Market was an early epicenter of SARS-CoV-2 transmission, and the virus likely emerged from live animals sold there.[89] Their findings showed that the majority of early COVID-19 cases were clustered around the market, where many of the patients worked or shopped in close proximity to potential hosts of SARS-CoV-2 progenitor viruses, such as common raccoon dogs (*Nyctereuntes procyonoides*)—the same kind of bandit-faced canine that was found to be infected with a SARS-CoV-1-related virus in a live animal market in 2003. Genetic material from a racoon dog was detected in SARS-CoV-2-positive samples from the Huanan market in 2023, which provided important evidence that susceptible animals were traded in the part of the market where SARS-CoV-2 was identified on surfaces. Even so, it doesn't necessarily mean that raccoon dogs were infected with the virus or that they had passed it on to humans.[90] Earlier events that might have brought SARS-CoV-2 into the market, along with the specific animals that spread the virus to people, remain unknown. However, it's widely suspected that the original source of the virus was bats, from which more than forty-eight hundred coronavirus sequences have been identified to date.[91] So far, the ones most similar to SARS-CoV-2 (up to 98.6 percent identical) are from Laos and Japan.[92] There is also a bat-borne coronavirus sequence with a

96.1 percent similarity to SARS-CoV-2 at the whole genome level, obtained through disease surveillance and sampling among wild bat populations in southern China.[93]

This discovery, led by WIV scientists, was exactly the kind of research that was blocked by Trump in an anti-Chinese furor. On the heels of his #Chinavirus tweeting in April 2020, the US president announced his intent to cancel National Institutes of Health funding for a collaboration between WIV and US-based nonprofit EcoHealth Alliance for the surveillance and study of bat-borne viruses in China.[94] A few days later, the National Institutes of Health abruptly terminated the grant, stating that the project's outcomes didn't align with the program goals and agency priorities. In response, seventy-seven US Nobel laureates in science called for a thorough review and rectification of the decision, asserting, "Now is precisely the time when we need to support this kind of research if we aim to control the pandemic and prevent subsequent ones. . . . The abrupt revoking of the award," they went on, "deprives the nation and the world of highly regarded science that could help control one of the greatest health crises in modern history and those that may arise in the future."[95]

But control of the virus was already lost. By 2022, the United States counted more than a hundred million cases and one million deaths due to COVID-19, reaching a point where the virus was considered by many as endemic in the US population. And like the spread of *Y. pestis* a century earlier, the transmission of SARS-CoV-2 among wildlife has become a sobering prospect for years to come. Humans infected a wide range of animals with SARS-CoV-2 during the course of the pandemic, and may have established a new natural reservoir in US wildlife, such as free-ranging white-tailed deer (*Odocoileus virginianus*). Approximately thirty million of these animals are distributed broadly across urban, suburban, and rural environments throughout the country, and their susceptibility to SARS-CoV-2 infection opened new evolutionary pathways, opportunities for transmission to other wildlife species, and possibilities of spill back to humans of novel variants that our immune system hasn't previously encountered.[96]

*   *   *

Xenophobic responses to COVID-19 made the pandemic worse for the targets of anti-Asian hate, directly and harshly. In the United States and around the world, people of Asian ancestry or nationality encountered everything from online attacks to verbal slurs to physical assaults. And it's possible that antagonism against Chinese researchers and their collaborators increased our pandemic risks by diverting attention and resources from scientific efforts to monitor as well as manage them—or by making these activities more onerous if not unworkable. In the wake of the COVID-19 origins debate in 2023, the National Institutes of Health announced a new policy to require foreign collaborators in grants—but not their US partners—to turn over all their relevant notebooks, data, and documents every few months.[97] With extra work and targeted scrutiny for scientists in other countries, the policy alarmed US scientists who feared that their foreign colleagues would sooner forgo collaborations than comply with it. There was also a concern that US scientists would sooner not collaborate with their international colleagues than offend or alienate them, let alone take on an added reporting burden without additional funds to to pay for it.

These othering instincts are part of a pattern across epidemics and pandemics, formed by some of the darkest and most destructive elements of humanity. We can address them by naming, exposing, condemning, and correcting harmful behavior where and when possible. But reducing them will take a lot more work, and it starts with education, activism, and embracing our commonalities. Because when we make and reinforce human differences through actions and words, we create vulnerabilities in society that help pathogens infiltrate and spread through the cracks. In the words of a banner that was carried through San Francisco's Chinatown in February 2020 and later displayed at the Smithsonian's National Museum of American History, "Fight the virus, not the people."

Pathogens are the antithesis of xenophobes. They don't recognize borders. They don't choose hosts. They're completely impartial in how and whom they cause disease, but they're not equalizers. They don't impact everyone and every community in the same way because of how humans see each other. These perceptions of people can extend to the disease itself, and how we punish others for real or imagined connections to it, as we'll investigate in the next chapter.

7 Diseased Deviants

Absolutely everyone gets sick at some point or for some period in their lives, usually without transforming how people see them or how they see themselves. If anything, illness should, and often does, elicit sympathy and care. But sometimes a disease has so much social meaning that it can alter a person's self- or social identity, becoming a characteristic that overrides others. Thus somebody who wasn't deemed deviant may become so, or someone who was already deemed deviant may become more so, in the experience of a socially unacceptable illness. And in the latter case, the compounding effects of social exclusion and rejection can make it even more difficult for a person to regain health. Furthermore, they make it even more likely that an infectious disease will continue to spread.

Social exclusion is a feature of human society around the world and through history, down to the roots of our evolutionary origins. Although we don't have extensive records of how the earliest humans behaved, some researchers spot clues among our closest living relatives today. Chimpanzees are social primates like we are, but as highlighted in chapter 6, they can attack difference when and where it matters. And they can ostracize each other too—not necessarily in the ways and for the same reasons as people do, of course. Human talents and tools for othering are unmatched. But at least when it comes to disease, some chimpanzee behaviors and social dynamics can hold a heartbreaking mirror to our own.

One haunting example of social exclusion in response to disease, described by primatologist Jane Goodall, took place at the Gombe Stream Chimpanzee Reserve in Tanzania in 1966.[1] A local outbreak of polio reached a village nearby the feeding area of the chimpanzees, where a spillover from humans may have occurred. The debilitating disease spread through the chimpanzee community, leaving some individuals with use-less limbs. And the most severe case was Mr. McGregor, an old male chimp who became paralyzed in both legs. Struggling with his sudden disability, he pulled himself along the ground and into trees using only his arms. Swarmed by flies due to incontinence from his condition, he dragged his stiff and soiled body parts until they bled. The worst pain, however, may have come from the reactions of his fellow chimpanzees. With a strange appearance, grotesque movements, and awful stench, Mr. McGregor was physically attacked by some of them. Those who got used to him simply kept their distance.

Deprived of social contact, Mr. McGregor finally attempted to join a ses-sion of mutual grooming by making a tortuous journey from his isolated nest to a tree where his former companions sat. But as soon as he managed to get close enough to extend a greeting hand to two males, they swung away and started grooming each other on the far side of the tree, without even a backward glance. "For a full two minutes old Gregor sat motion-less, staring after them," Goodall wrote. "And then he laboriously lowered himself to the ground." Only Mr. McGregor's likely brother, a younger male named Humphrey, showed an unwillingness to abandon him. Hum-phrey rested, nested, and groomed near his suffering sibling, assuaging the isolation of a social death. Mr. McGregor's biological death came within days, at the humane hands of Goodall and her colleagues, after he was ren-dered helpless by a dislocated arm. Humphrey alone seemed to mark Mr. McGregor's absence and remember their friendship for months to come.

The behaviors that Goodall observed in this account don't necessarily reflect any social meaning of polio in the minds of chimpanzees. In addi-tion to physical barriers to pathogen entry, like nasal hairs and mucus mem-branes, there are many behavioral adaptations that animals use to reduce disease in their communities, such as feather preening and fur licking, mud wallows and dust baths, and keeping their home sites clean.[2] A variety of animals also appear to avoid contacts with members of their species who may carry pathogens. Bullfrog tadpoles (*Rana catesbeiana*) seem to avoid close proximity to individuals infected with intestinal parasites, based on waterborne chemical cues.[3] Possibly for the same reason, healthy Caribbean spiny lobsters (*Panulirus argus*) avoid sharing dens with those who have viral infections.[4] Even socially complex insects such as leaf-cutting ants (*Acromyrmex crassispinus* and *A. rugosus*) may adjust their social interactions in order to reduce risks of parasite transmission.[5] And in writing about Mr. McGregor's experience with disease, Goodall even acknowledged that the avoidance of chimpanzees showing abnormal behavior may be highly adaptive since it reduces the likelihood of spreading contagious disease. Yet the fear, avoidance, and shunning of Mr. McGregor had human parallels, she noted, even if chimpanzee society didn't seem to be as sophisticated as human society in the social punishment of deviancy.[6]

Anyone who has ever felt or witnessed ostracism due to illness can relate to Goodall's story. Certainly, people who have been touched by polio might identify with some aspects of it. Polio was a highly feared disease for the majority of the twentieth century. And for some people, death from polio was a less frightening prospect than survival.[7] That's because the lifetime disabilities endured by a small proportion of polio patients, relying on braces, crutches, canes, and wheelchairs for basic mobility, came with social, economic, and psychological challenges.

In the 1940s, writes historian Daniel Wilson, there was a growing population of people in the United States who feared "the crippling of polio and the almost inevitable alienation, loneliness, pain, stigmatization, and loss of income or earning potential that followed."[8] Some of them sought assurances through letters to US president Franklin Delano Roosevelt, a famous polio survivor whose ostensible recovery gave hope to millions of people. But even Roosevelt was subject to polio's socially stigmatizing effects. His disability was entirely unknown to the public, when in fact he couldn't stand without heavy leg braces or walk without significant support. According to historian David Oshinsky in his book *Polio: An American Story*, "To be crippled in this era was to be viewed by many as a moral failing, a sign of inner weakness, a character flaw requiring the person's removal from normal society," which was a fate that Roosevelt apparently couldn't risk.[9] Hence by preventing any opportunities for the public to see the manifestation of polio in his body, he avoided the enormous stigma attached to it.

*   *   *

Polio is just one of the many maladies that convey social stigma, meaning that it carries negative attitudes and beliefs about the people associated with the disease. There are endless conditions or circumstances that can be stigmatizing, and not necessarily those involving infectious disease, such as mental illness, addiction, obesity, and poverty. The word *stigma*, from the

Greek language, originally referred to a mark cut or burned onto a person's body as a stamp of unusual or unfavorable social status, such as a slave, criminal, or traitor.[10] But in medical terminology, it's a term for evidence of disease. And in common usage, there's a lot more to it than that.

Numerous forms of stigma have been created by humans, reaching far beyond the social kind. Internalized (or self-) stigma is an insidious phenomenon in which a person places the blame and shame of social stigma onto themselves. And then we have structural stigma, which is the way that social stigma is embedded in systems of society, determining people's opportunities, safety, and access to health care. As Kellan Barker, executive director of the Whitman-Walker Institute in Washington, DC, has explained, "It all comes wrapped in the ways in which we, as a society, have developed norms, policies, and laws that decided whose lives matter and whose don't. Regardless of the form that it takes, stigma kills."[11]

The context in which Kellan spoke about stigma, for a public program in support of the *Outbreak* exhibit, was a conversation about the ongoing HIV pandemic. The HIV pathogen and the disease that it causes, AIDS, have been highly stigmatized for more than forty years. And it's partly because of this stigma that the pandemic continues. In the previous chapter, we examined how social constructs of foreign or racial others can intertwine with disease when people are misperceived as being the source or carrier of a particular pathogen. Here we're going to focus on how illness itself can be part of the othering process. And to do that, we're going to focus on HIV and AIDS. Although the pandemic is spread across continents, it's impossible to describe the experiences of every group of people in every place that's been impacted. Just one sampling of them, from the United States, is all that I can fit on these pages. But all over the world, over forty million people have died of AIDS, and nearly forty million are living with HIV. Make no mistake, this is not one country's story; it's a human one.

Deviant and Dying

The rumblings of the HIV pandemic were first published in the CDC's *Morbidity and Mortality Weekly Report* (*MMWR*) on June 5, 1981.[12] Brief and bare, the report gave no inkling of the quaking to come. Since October 1980, the authors wrote, five men in three different hospitals in Los Angeles were diagnosed with pneumocystis pneumonia (PCP), a serious infection found almost exclusively among people with severely weakened immune systems.[13] Despite being young and previously healthy, two of the men had already died. The report suggested a cellular-immune dysfunction related to a common exposure and a disease acquired through sexual contact, but offered no easy explanations of the cause—because at that time, there were none. Yet one link was implied: all the men were gay, described as "active homosexuals" in the opening sentence.

One month after the first *MMWR* piece, more cases of unusual illness caught the public's attention in a *New York Times* headline, "Rare Cancer Seen in 41 Homosexuals."[14] Dozens of gay men in California and New York City had been diagnosed with Kaposi sarcoma (KS), a type of cancer that was rare in the United States at the time (affecting two people out of three million, according to the CDC, and primarily men over fifty years old), as well as some with PCP.[15] KS can form tumors in the lymph nodes, mucous membranes, and other parts of the body, potentially damaging the immune system to the point of dysfunction or failure. Reddish-purple lesions can appear on the skin of people with KS, often on the feet but most noticeably on the face. More than forty years later, they remain the most physically recognizable and highly stigmatic symptom of AIDS.

Even more than these violet spots, the *New York Times* article emphasized the sexual behavior of the patients, which included as many as ten sexual encounters each night up to four times a week along with the use of drugs such as amyl nitrite and LSD to heighten sexual pleasure. All of them were identified as gay men, on average thirty-nine years old, and a CDC spokesperson was quoted as saying that there was thus "no apparent danger to non-homosexuals from contagion."[16] The best evidence against a contagious disease being responsible for the cancer, he said, was that no cases had been reported outside the homosexual community or in women.

Many more cases followed over the next year, in more reports, across the country and around the world. Soon it became clear that the mysterious syndrome was indeed contagious and potentially fatal, destroying the immune systems of those affected and allowing rare and opportunistic infections, such as PCP and KS, to attack their bodies. Much was still unknown about the syndrome, most critically its cause, but some facts were certain. If the public needed to know only one thing, it seemed, it was that homosexual people were sick and dying from it. In other words, straight people didn't need to worry.

As a case in point, the *New York Times* ran another article under the headline "New Homosexual Disorder Worries Health Officials" in May 1982. It did not bury the lede: "A serious disorder of the immune system that has been known to doctors for less than a year—a disorder that appears to affect primarily homosexuals—has now afflicted at least 335 people, of whom it has killed 136."[17] Thirteen of those affected were reported to be heterosexual women, while some others were suggested to be heterosexual injection drug users. Yet the title of the story, in big and bold letters, linked the syndrome to homosexuality alone.

Harmfully, the scientific community reinforced the association. Some researchers called the syndrome "gay-related immune deficiency," as the *New York Times* article noted, and even used the term in scholarly communications.[18] "Gay compromise syndrome" was another stigmatizing misnomer, which appeared in leading British medical journals for more than a year after the first reported cases.[19] The proposition of a "gay" disease, as historian Sarah Schulman noted in her book *Let the Record Show*, gave support to the contradictory ideas that homosexuality was an adverse biological condition as well as a transmissible one.[20]

*   *   *

Given how AIDS was initially reported, it's no wonder that people started calling the disease "gay cancer." And in these two words, the social condemnation was doubly weighted. Homosexuality was already abhorred by many people in the United States long before AIDS emerged. In a brazenly homophobic television program called "The Homosexuals" in 1967, anchor Mike Wallace reported that most people in the United States looked on gay people with disgust, discomfort, fear, or hatred. In one of the earliest representations of gay people on national television, he interviewed gay men who were cloaked in shadows and despair. No doubt these portraits of displaced deviants, outsiders to society, reflected the worst fears of every gay person who risked abandonment by family members, neighbors, and friends on the sole basis of their sexual identity.

But more than that, homosexuality was punished. In the United States, antisodomy laws had been inked and enforced since the colonial period of British rule, derived from church laws against nonprocreative and nonmarital sexuality.[21] Religious beliefs justified these legal bans on behavior, which the majority viewed as sinful and wrong. Until the US state of Illinois got rid of its antisodomy law in 1961, homosexuality was a crime everywhere in the country. Same-sex relationships between consenting adults remained illegal in all other US states until the 1970s, at which point some antisodomy laws were explicitly rewritten so that they only applied to homosexuals. These laws were used to rationalize the unequal treatment and marginalization of nonheterosexuals in many aspects of social life, such as marriage, raising children, and employment. Some of them were in effect until 2003, when the US Supreme Court finally stuck down all remaining antisodomy laws in the nation as unconstitutional.

And not only was homosexuality criminalized but it was also pathologized. Which is to say, it was defined and diagnosed as a disease by one of the highest medical authorities in the land. The American Psychiatric Association formally recognized homosexuality as a mental illness in 1952, using a classification of a "sociopathic personality disturbance" that was changed to "sexual deviation" in 1968. In the professional opinion of many psychiatrists, homosexuality was therefore a psychological disorder that should be treated and could be cured, with a normative state of heterosexuality as the end goal. As a consequence, socially nonconforming people were subjected to conversion (or reparative) therapy involving electromagnetic shocks, nausea-inducing drugs, and lobotomies. But these treatments were no such thing. Ineffective and harmful, they caused depression, anxiety, and self-destructive behavior.[22] Finally in 1973, after years of protests, the American Psychiatric Association decided that homosexuality was not a mental disorder and would cease to be described as one, on a day that gay rights activist Franklin E. Kameny joked "we were cured en masse by the psychiatrists."[23]

The fight for lesbian, gay, bisexual, and transgender (LGBT) rights in the United States burgeoned throughout the 1970s, catalyzed by the Stonewall uprising against a police raid in New York City in 1969. Gay men and women pushed back on antigay stigma as they sought to live openly and with pride. Yet they did so under constant threats of violence from bullies and thugs, emboldened by homophobic fearmongering from right-wing religious and political leaders. Horrific antigay assaults and murders were on the rise in major cities in 1981, as the assailants acted on societal permission to victimize anybody who was different.[24] And after a decade of painful progress, then came a "gay cancer." As a killer that preyed on gay people who were unashamed of enjoying sex, it was a medical metaphor for homophobia if ever there was one.

Ironically, cancer was the most feared disease before AIDS arrived on the scene. Like homosexuality, it too was highly stigmatized. As a cancer survivor herself, writer Susan Sontag was enraged by how much additional suffering was experienced by cancer patients who were blamed for their illness, having been assigned the responsibility for both falling ill and getting well. Rather than being just a disease, Sontag wrote in *Illness and Metaphor* in 1978, cancer was a disease with meaning: a curse, a punishment, an embarrassment. A death sentence. But she saw the onus of cancer lifted by the emergence of AIDS, "whose charges of stigmatization, whose capacity to create spoiled identity," was far greater. "It seems that societies need to have one illness which becomes identified with evil," she later wrote in *AIDS and Its Metaphors* in 1989, "but it is hard to be obsessed with more than one."[25]

In 1982, however, few people were obsessed with the mysterious new disease. After all, it was broadcast as an affliction of homosexuality and nearly exclusive to promiscuous gay men, whose very existence was rejected by the broader society. The *New York Times* only published six stories about the disease in 1981 and 1982, and none of them made the front page. In his book *And the Band Played On*, journalist Randy Shilts noted this widespread disinterest in the new disease, commenting that the media response to dead and dying homosexuals was "a collective yawn."[26]

And from the White House, there was absolute silence. That is, apart from bursts of laughter. In September 1982, when the CDC released the first case definition for the syndrome, with the official name of AIDS, there was an average of one to two cases diagnosed every day in the United States.[27] By then, almost six hundred cases had been reported and hundreds of patients had died. But at a White House press briefing the following month, Deputy Press Secretary Larry Speakes responded to questions about the AIDS epidemic with homophobic jokes. Joining in the chuckles around the room, perhaps his most serious statement on the issue was "I don't know anything about it." The callousness continued in press briefings over the next several years, memorialized in Scott Calonico's short film *When AIDS Was Funny*, while President Ronald Reagan himself said nothing publicly about AIDS until 1985.[28] Showing no concern for the plague on the US populace, Reagan kept quiet as the disease kept spreading. "To his everlasting shame," journalist Laura Helmuth wrote, "he was silent at a time when silence equaled death."[29]

Suffering from Stigma

When the words "Silence = Death" began to appear on posters around New York City in 1986, emblazoned under a fuchsia triangle on a black background, the AIDS epidemic in the United States had been spreading for five years. Researchers made strides in understanding the disease, such as the discovery of HIV as the causal pathogen of AIDS in 1983–1984 and the first HIV antibody test in 1985, amid mounting evidence that unprotected sex, blood transfusions, and shared needles were its primary routes of transmission.[30] Yet the White House had shown few gains in compassion. And without a single AIDS treatment approved by the US Food and Drug Administration (FDA), a diagnosis really was like a death sentence. Outraged by institutional indifference to this suffering, a consciousness-raising group created the arresting Silence = Death artwork as a product of its members' shared pain.[31] Soon the graphic became the touchstone of a growing social justice movement as well as the visual centerpiece of the activist group AIDS Coalition to Unleash Power (ACT UP).

Formed in New York City in 1987, ACT UP followed other grassroots organizations in the city, such as the Gay Men's Health Crisis and People with AIDS Coalition, in creating a community of people determined to fight for their own lives and those of others. Schulman described ACT UP as "simultaneously a place of decline and a place in defiance of loss" at a time when people with AIDS could lose everything: family and friends, jobs, income, homes, health, and social worth.[32] Composed of HIV-positive people and their allies, the group was particularly successful in transforming how AIDS drugs were tested, approved, and priced. With creative and media-savvy demonstrations, ACT UP forcefully challenged the bureaucratic and capitalistic systems that delayed and refused relief to so many.[33] To this day, physician Anthony Fauci, director of the National Institute of Allergy and Infectious Diseases (NIAID) from 1984 until 2022, has given these AIDS activists enormous credit for their effectiveness—even though some of them were harshly critical of him at times, including those who became his friends.[34]

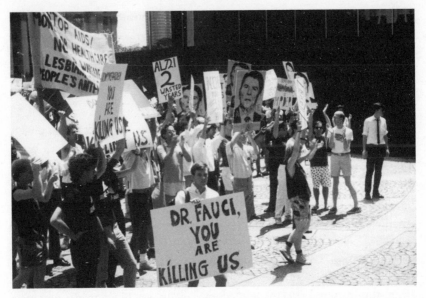

Figure 7.1
ACT UP protest at the National Institutes of Health in 1990. Protesters carried signs
with messages of "Silence=Death," referring to President Ronald Reagan's silence at
the beginning of the AIDS epidemic in the United States, and "Dr. Fauci, You Are
Killing Us," regarding the bureaucratic barriers to AIDS treatment by the National
Institute of Allergy and Infectious Diseases and others. *Source:* NIH History Office via
Wikimedia Commons.

But one downside of the media attention received by ACT UP, and especially its focus on a select few members, was a narrow narrative of AIDS in
the United States. Gay white men in large cities were the earliest cases and
the most visible activists, and some became icons of the epidemic. The
most famous face of AIDS was Rock Hudson, a white US movie star who
disclosed his illness (but not his homosexuality) months before his death in
1985. People who were unaware of the AIDS crisis finally took notice when
celebrities started getting sick and involved. Nonetheless, the struggles of
women and people of color were largely overlooked and untold.

For years women were left out of the studies and stories of AIDS, except
when they appeared as stigmatized others such as sex workers and drug
abusers, as detailed by investigative reporter Gena Corea in her book *The
Invisible Epidemic*.[35] Most women with AIDS couldn't even get validation

of their illness, let alone treatment for it. That's because for more than a decade, the US government defined AIDS by infections that occurred mostly in men, such as KS, and ignored gynecologic manifestations of immunocompromise, like cervical disease.[36] These criteria determined who was counted and received disability benefits as an AIDS patient as well as how much federal funding was given to cities for AIDS response.[37] In 1992, the CDC finally expanded its definition of AIDS after years of international advocacy by organizations like ACT UP, which hammered health officials with the slogan "Women don't get AIDS, they just die from it."[38] As a result, there was a huge increase in reported AIDS cases in 1993, more than doubling the number of women diagnosed in the previous year.[39] Also in 1993, the National Institutes of Health established a new policy that required clinical research and trials to include women, as well as ethnic and racial minorities. Until then, they had long been left out. But for many women with AIDS, like activist Katrina Haslip, it was too late. Haslip died of AIDS in 1992, only weeks before the revised classification was published, having fought for and never received the care that she needed. As fellow activist Terry McGovern lamented, she was a victim of the AIDS definition.[40]

Meanwhile, the epidemic was raging unseen in rural and Black communities, where heterosexual and mother-to-child transmission were much more frequent.[41] In August 1985, for instance, the agricultural community of Belle Glade in southern Florida became the AIDS capital of the world, with an infection rate four times higher than in New York City.[42] A subsequent study of HIV transmission in Belle Glade, published in *Science* in 1988, reported 93 cases of AIDS among its approximately 16,500 residents between 1982 and 1987.[43] Nearly all the AIDS patients lived in the same impoverished area, which was characterized by crowded living conditions and high rates of drug abuse, sexually transmitted diseases, and prostitution. All but one of the individuals identified as HIV-positive lived in the same area, and every one of these individuals was African American or Haitian. Furthermore, among the AIDS patients in Belle Glade, more women than homosexual or bisexual men were diagnosed. These findings didn't align with patterns reported in the nascent days of the AIDS epidemic, which shaped common assumptions about the typical profile of an AIDS patient and sensationalized initial reactions to the Belle Glade outbreak. But they did little to change the popular narrative about the disease.

*   *   *

Misperceptions and false assumptions about AIDS can be traced back to some of the earliest reports, which were based on limited knowledge at the time. The famous *MMWR* piece on July 5, 1981, for example, contributed to the widespread idea that AIDS was a disease of gay white men. The report's five gay men with PCP were indeed white—a fact implied but not stated by the authors. Yet there were two other documented cases of Black men with PCP, a gay African American and a heterosexual Haitian, who weren't mentioned. Lead author Michael Gottlieb, when questioned by journalist Linda Villarosa in a *New York Times* article titled "America's Hidden HIV Epidemic" in 2017, said that the cases were discovered after the report was finalized.[44] "But in retrospect," he said about the African American patient, "I think it would have made a difference among gay Black men" to have included the case. Villarosa agreed, given that African Americans became and remain the demographic group most affected by HIV in the United States, with half of Black men who have sex with men (MSM) projected to be diagnosed with HIV during their lifetimes, according to a CDC analysis in 2016.[45] "Including gay black men in the literature and understanding of the origins of the disease and its treatment," she suggested, "could have meant earlier outreach, more of a voice and a standing in HIV/AIDS advocacy organizations, and access to the cultural and financial power of the LGBT community that would rise up to demand government action."[46]

In contrast, Haitian people suffered greatly, and wrongly, for their inclusion in early reports and articles on AIDS. One year after Gottlieb's report, in July 1982, another *MMWR* article described thirty-four diagnoses of opportunistic infections in Haitian residents of five US states since April 1980.[47] More reports followed, with additional cases of Haitians in the United States and Canada, mostly recent immigrants, showing similar symptoms of immunodeficiency. Unlike other North American patients, however, the Haitian patients for the most part denied any involvement in homosexual activity, injection drug abuse, or blood transfusions. Thereby ungroupable according to known risk factors of AIDS at the time, Haitians were thus categorized as a separate high-risk group by the CDC in 1983, rounding out the so-called Four-H Club of the majority of AIDS patients: homosexuals, heroin users, hemophiliacs, and Haitians.[48]

Haitians carried the same risks as anybody else, no more and no less. In 1984, Haitian physician Jean William Pape and colleagues reported that known risk factors were present in most of the AIDS patients diagnosed in Haiti, interpreting their reported absence among Haitians with AIDS in the United States as a greater willingness of Haitians to provide reliable responses to personal questions in their native country and language.[49] Yet by defining Haitians as a high-risk group based on nationality rather than behavior, the CDC implied that all Haitians were potential carriers of the disease.[50]

As a result, all Haitians faced immediate and outright discrimination. Haiti's tourism industry collapsed, as the whole country was stigmatized by AIDS.[51] People of Haitian origin or ancestry in the United States encountered an onslaught of aggressions in which children were bullied, families were evicted, businesses were bankrupted, and even casual touches were withheld. After relentless protesting by Haitian community groups and allied activists, the CDC finally removed Haitians as a high-risk group for AIDS in 1985. But the stigma couldn't be erased, and Haiti's economy never recovered. And the discrimination continued, as the FDA still banned blood donations from Haitians until 1990.

One of the most persistent prejudices against Haitians was the suspicion that AIDS not only spread but also originated from them. Conveniently, Haitian Americans already filled the role of a diseased deviant, being Black and typically poor immigrants associated with exoticized religious practices, as noted by anthropologist Paul Farmer in his book *AIDS and Accusation*. AIDS therefore reinforced existing stigma in a combination of racism and xenophobia not unlike the Chinese American experiences discussed in chapter 6, fueling origin stories involving voodoo rites, sacrificial animal blood, the eating of cats, and ritualized homosexuality.[52] Still today, Haitians live with the damaging consequences of being blamed for AIDS, as scientists continue to explore the evolutionary history of the HIV pandemic.

In 2007, for example, when a genomic study suggested that the predominant form of HIV-1 outside sub-Saharan Africa—that is, HIV-1 group M subtype B—was introduced into the United States from Haiti around 1970 (following an introduction into Haiti from Central Africa around 1966), Pape and colleagues challenged this conclusion with epidemiological data that showed no evidence of AIDS in Haiti until the late 1970s. Moreover, without naming the CDC or FDA, they also cautioned that "scientists need to carefully consider the great harm that can result from asserting dubious claims of causality."[53] In a response led by evolutionary biologist Michael Worobey, the study's authors defended their conclusions, reinforcing that the arrival of HIV undoubtedly preceded the recognition of AIDS in Haiti by several years, just as it did in the United States, Africa, and elsewhere. Worobey and colleagues also noted that the exportation of blood products from Haiti in addition to US visitors returning from Haiti were plausible entry routes of the virus that emerged in the United States in the late 1960s or early 1970s.[54]

But first and foremost, the scientists insisted that they had no intention to assign blame. In a subsequent study in 2016, Worobey and colleagues didn't speculate about the specific involvement of Haiti or Haitians in the early history of HIV/AIDS in North America, despite providing more evidence that HIV-1 group M subtype B moved from the Caribbean to the United States, not the other way around.[55]

Another scapegoat of the AIDS epidemic was exonerated by the same study, however. Worobey and his collaborators sequenced eight complete HIV-1 genomes from US serum samples dating back to the late 1970s, thereby revealing a series of key founder events in the form of HIV that caused the earliest reported cases of AIDS in the United States: the epidemic spread from Africa to the Caribbean by about 1967, from the Caribbean to New York City by about 1971, from New York City to San Francisco by about 1976, and then involved extensive geographic mixing in the United States and beyond. And one of the genomes came from an AIDS patient who had been blamed for HIV-1's introduction to North America.

This person was the original *patient zero*—a term that only emerged with and because of AIDS. He started as the "non-Californian" in a *MMWR* report of nineteen gay men with KS and PCP in Los Angeles and Orange County in 1982, but eventually became "Patient 0" in a study published in 1984.[56] The 1984 study reported that Patient 0 had sex with eight AIDS patients in Los Angeles and New York City, and was possibly a carrier of the infectious agent. To illustrate possible transmission routes of the disease, the study included a sociogram of sexual contacts between different patients, with Patient 0 in the center. And above the sociogram was a label of "0 = Index patient" that implicated him as the origin of all the AIDS cases therein. Fascinated with the study, Shilts discovered and published the identity of Patient 0 in his 1987 book, vilifying him as a promiscuous French Canadian flight attendant who may have been "the person who brought AIDS to North America."[57] Named Gaëtan Dugas, the man didn't live long enough to defend himself against the allegation. But the virus that killed him held the truth: he had nothing to do with it.

The story of Dugas is sad for a number of reasons. From a scientific perspective, one sees clearly the potential pitfalls of early research on a newly emerging disease. Most critically, the 1984 study estimated the latency period of HIV-1 infection as 10.5 months on average. But subsequent findings indicate that the average incubation period is closer to *10 years* than 10 months, meaning that someone who starts to show symptoms could have been infected with HIV-1 up to a decade earlier. As Worobey and colleagues concluded, the 1984 sociogram almost certainly depicted the sexual contacts of men who were already HIV-positive. The man placed at its center therefore didn't infect any of them. His innocence was bolstered by the fact that the HIV-1 genome from his serum sample was typical of US strains at the time and in no way indicative of a founding role in the spread of HIV-1 group M subtype B in the Americas.

In the exploitation of that man's life, there's also a sobering demonstration of how media narratives can create and reinforce disease stigma. Shilts's imagining of the 1984 sociogram on an international scale was groundless, making his blaming of the perceived perpetrator even worse. Ironically, his book's central thesis was that US institutions failed to respond to the AIDS epidemic because of prejudice, ignorance, rejection, and fear. And yet the patient zero storyline was the book's core marketing strategy, filled with fodder for conservative media outlets to attract readers with lurid headlines. Shilts even suggested that Dugas knowingly infected his many sexual partners—a charge that Dugas's friends refuted in the 2019 documentary *Killing Patient Zero*. Incidentally, Shilts was a gay man himself (who was later diagnosed and died with AIDS), and was focused on ensuring accountability for the epidemic, particularly among those who were supposed to prevent it. But in making Dugas a scapegoat among scapegoats, and by creating a stigmatizing story frame for all the patient zeros who followed, he showed that anybody is a potential participant in these sinister social processes.[58]

Lastly, this cautionary tale speaks directly to the dangers of stigmatization as a force that can perpetuate and magnify a pandemic. The 1984 study, which helped to establish AIDS as a sexually transmissible disease, used personal information from Dugas to arrive at its findings. The authors

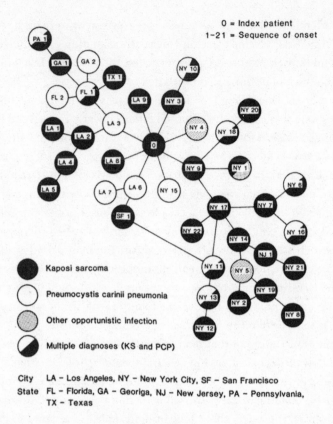

Figure 7.2
Sociogram from 1984 study of sexual contacts among a cluster of AIDS patients.
With the description that "0 = Index patient," the authors wrongly identify "Patient 0" as the source of HIV transmission within the cluster. After journalist Randy Shilts publicized his identity, "Patient Zero" was blamed for spreading AIDS in the United States. *Source:* Reprinted, with the permission of Elsevier, from D. M. Auerbach, W. W. Darrow, H. W. Jaffe, and J. W. Curran, "Cluster of Cases of the Acquired Immune Deficiency Syndrome: Patients Linked by Sexual Contact," *American Journal of Medicine* 76, no. 3 (1984): 487–492.

relied on the ability and willingness of AIDS patients to share data on their sexual contacts, which Dugas did more than anyone else (thus creating a sampling bias that helped to center him in the study). Yet he was punished for his cooperation, not rewarded it. And he was only vindicated after decades of suffering by his family and loved ones, thanks to the serum sample that he also provided for scientific research. What happened to Dugas could, and perhaps did, dissuade countless people from seeking HIV testing, treatment, or research participation for fear of mistreatment like he received. And for as long as this happens, we will all be living with HIV.

Ending a Pandemic

People truly started living with HIV rather than dying from it more than twenty years ago. But death was forcefully and necessarily associated with AIDS in the 1980s. It became the leading cause of death among young adults in the United States, claiming more than a hundred thousand lives by the close of the decade. By 1991, one million people in the country were HIV-positive, and as many as one-fifth of them were expected to die within two years.[59] Having witnessed the rapid and fatal decline of countless others, many people with HIV were convinced that the same thing would happen to them. Activists staged die-ins to hold US institutions accountable for the massive mortality, lying in the street with paper tombstones in symbolic displays of their impending fate. They needed medication that worked against the virus and didn't have time to wait.

Death often came quickly back then because many people didn't even know that they were HIV-positive until the virus had been reproducing in their body for years. By the time that they found out, frequently by showing severe symptoms of AIDS, there wasn't a lot that doctors could do or offer for them. AIDS is the final and most severe stage of an HIV infection, when the immune system has become damaged to the point of dysfunction due to a precipitous depletion of certain white blood cells (called CD4 cells) that are infected and destroyed by the virus. At that point, a person is left with few natural defenses against opportunistic infections—the kind that are rare in healthy people but serious threats to the immunocompromised. And for this reason, AIDS isn't technically a disease but instead a condition (or syndrome), which is signaled by and predisposed to a large number of illnesses. An HIV-positive person only becomes an AIDS patient after years of passing through earlier stages of infection, acute and chronic, where symptoms are mild or absent. Being HIV-positive, then, isn't the same thing as having AIDS. And when effective treatments for HIV infection were finally discovered in the 1990s, AIDS was no longer an inevitability.

An early glimmer of hope was the first FDA-approved medication for AIDS: a chemical compound called azidothymidine (AZT) that became available in 1987. Soon other anti-HIV drugs were on the market, but few patients felt saved. Many experienced severe side effects from AZT, if they could afford and had access to it. Furthermore, the virus developed resistance to AZT and all the other early antivirals when used as monotherapies (that is, one at a time). By the early 1990s, two-drug combinations showed more promise, and AZT was proven to significantly decrease the mother-to-child transmission of HIV. But rates of new infections and AIDS-related deaths continued to rise globally.

The breakthrough came in 1996 with highly effective combination antiretroviral therapy (ART), which blocked the virus from replicating in the body and suppressed its levels below detection. In many cases, the effects were simply miraculous, although access to the costly therapy was highly unequal across countries. HIV-positive people saw their viral loads diminish and their immune systems regenerate, while AIDS patients rose from their deathbeds and walked out of hospital wards.[60] By the end of 1997, AIDS-related deaths fell by 50 percent in the United States, marking the largest single-year decline for a major cause of death ever recorded.[61] After receiving and adhering to an effective and continuous ART regimen, HIV-positive people with undetectable viral loads regained a nearly normal life expectancy. Plus they couldn't transmit the virus to their sexual partners—a fact referred to as "undetectable equals untransmittable," or "U = U." In the absence of a vaccine or cure for HIV, these treatments became and remain critical to HIV prevention, along with other interventions such as condoms and preexposure prophylaxis (a daily medication also known as PrEP). Together they provide a powerful tool kit to end the HIV pandemic once and for all, and underpin the strategies to make it happen.

Building on the lifesaving promises of ART, an ambitious plan for an HIV-free world was launched by the United Nations Programme on HIV/AIDS (UNAIDS) and its partners in 2014. To end the pandemic by 2030, it laid out "90-90-90" targets for counties and municipalities all over the world: by 2020, 90 percent of people living with HIV would know their HIV status,

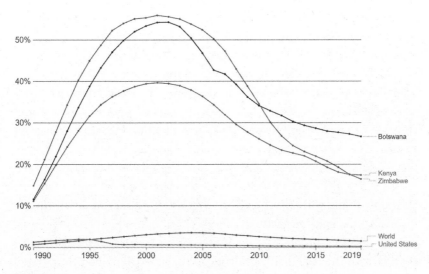

Figure 7.3
Share of deaths from HIV/AIDS, 1990–2019. By 1997, the AIDS-related death rate in the United States fell below 1 percent and remained less than half the global rate. In regions and countries of the world without equal access to lifesaving treatments, however, the death rates climbed for several more years, reaching 40–56 percent in Botswana, Kenya, and Zimbabwe in 2001. Soon after, affordable ART and funding initiatives like the President's Emergency Plan for AIDS Relief (PEPFAR) helped these and other resource-limited countries make major strides in preventing and treating HIV infections—although some still vastly exceed the global rate. *Source:* Data published by Global Burden of Disease Collaborative Network, *Global Burden of Disease Study 2019 Results* (Seattle: Institute for Health Metrics and Evaluation, 2021), via Our World in Data.

90 percent of people diagnosed with HIV infection would be receiving ART, and 90 percent of people receiving sustained ART would be virally suppressed.[62] If successful, this three-part testing and treatment cascade would result in the viral suppression of 73 percent of all people living with HIV, greatly reducing the chances for the virus to keep spreading. In addition to treatment, the plan included other core strategies for HIV prevention, such as condom and PrEP use, voluntary medical male circumcision, harm reduction services for people who inject drugs, and focused programming for people with higher risks of infection or transmission. Additionally, there was an emphasis on the critical need to eliminate stigma, discrimination, and social exclusion related to HIV/AIDS.

But the plan fell short. Globally, at the end of 2020, nearly thirty-seven million people were living with HIV, but only 84 percent of them knew it. Among the people who were diagnosed with HIV infection, only 87 percent were receiving ART, while 90 percent of those receiving ART were virally suppressed. Although a few percentage points might seem like trivial deficits, they translated to more than one-quarter of HIV-positive people worldwide who weren't being treated for it and about one-third of them with transmissible levels of viral loads.[63] And the gaps were unequally distributed across places and populations. Almost twenty countries reached their 90-90-90 targets or an equivalent 73 percent viral load suppression among all people living with HIV by 2020, demonstrating success across diverse income levels, epidemic settings, and sociocultural norms in Africa, Asia, Europe, and the Middle East. In South Africa, though, a middle-income country with the largest HIV epidemic in the world, only 66 percent of all people living with HIV were virally suppressed. And in the United States, success was variable[64] Notably, some cities did better than others. New York City, the original epicenter of the HIV pandemic, was the first US city to meet its 90-90-90 targets. In contrast, Washington, DC, the nation's capital, didn't even come close.[65]

There are varying reasons for these disparities and failings across communities, which tend to hit the hardest where people are underserved and historically marginalized. Around the world, HIV intersects with other stigmatized characteristics and behaviors, with a 25–35 percent higher risk of HIV infection for MSM, female sex workers, transgender women, and injection drug users in 2020.[66] Yet social and internalized stigma related to HIV can transcend all socioeconomic variables as a ubiquitous and pervasive barrier at every point along the HIV continuum of care.[67] Fear of ostracism and feelings of shame, based on prejudice, stereotypes, and discrimination against people living with HIV, can be impediments to even getting tested. For example, among men and women in sub-Saharan Africa, studies have found that the prospect of an HIV-positive diagnosis can stir fears of job loss, partner abandonment, and familial or social rejection due to negative misperceptions about AIDS.[68] In India, research shows that HIV-related stigma can also reduce adherence to HIV treatment as patients are afraid of taking pills in front of family members, asking for transportation to clinics, receiving phone reminders about appointments, or being seen refilling their prescriptions at pharmacies.[69] In South India specifically, many fears are compounded by the belief that only "perverted" and "sinful" people have HIV/AIDS.[70] Around the world, in fact, people fear wrong assumptions or suspicions about how they contracted HIV, which remains strongly associated with stigmatized behaviors involving sex and drugs.

As a form of structural stigma, certain laws can keep people away from HIV testing and treatment services as well. A study led by global health scholar Matthew Kavanagh found that countries with less success in reaching their 90-90-90 goals have adopted a criminalizing approach to groups that have higher-risk behaviors for HIV infection and transmission.[71] Among countries reporting data to UNAIDS in 2019, 69 of them criminalized same-sex sexual activity, 129 of them criminalized some aspect of sex work, and 111 of them criminalized the use or possession of drugs for personal use. Countries that criminalize same-sex sexual acts had on average 11 percent lower knowledge of HIV status among people living with HIV, and the rates of viral suppression were on average 8 percent lower. The criminalization of sex work and drug use was also associated with significantly lower levels of knowledge about HIV status and viral suppression, with 18–24 percent worse outcomes in countries where all three behaviors were criminalized. In contrast, countries with national laws on nondiscrimination, independent human rights institutions, and gender-based violence did much better. In light of these findings, a new UNAIDS strategy for 2021–2026 prioritized the elimination of legal obstacles to HIV testing and treatment as well as social ones in order to get the world back on track to an HIV-free future.[72]

Significantly, some of these legal obstacles carry specific punishments for people living with HIV. And many of them are holdovers from the pre-ART era of the pandemic, when AIDS was poorly understood, largely untreatable, and frequently fatal. At least 92 countries in the world criminalize HIV exposure, nondisclosure, and/or transmission, and 48 countries or territories continue to block people living with HIV from entry, stay, or residence. It wasn't until 2010 that US president Barack Obama finally lifted a twenty-two-year ban on immigration and travel to the United States by non-US citizens living with HIV. Yet half of US states still have HIV-specific criminal laws.[73] Furthermore, blood donation restrictions on MSM were in effect until 2023 after 40 years of MSM-specific bans intended to keep HIV out of the blood supply. France has had similar restrictions in place since 1983, and the French government only lifted them entirely in early 2022 at the peak of a deadly wave of COVID-19 across the country. The timing was ironic. Due to the latest novel virus sweeping the country, patients needed the blood.

COVID-19 has overlapped with the HIV pandemic in numerous ways, including as another hindrance to the global HIV response. Critical HIV services were disrupted during the COVID-19 pandemic, and according to UNAIDS, it blew the world's HIV progress way off course.[74] The response could be set back further, perhaps by a decade or more, if the disruptions continue.

But stigmatization has been a problem from the start. No other pathogen has led to or reinforced so much othering on a global scale. Our human abilities for creating and enforcing stigma are terrifying because they can allow epidemics to become pandemics, and pandemics to continue for generations. We have the tools to end the spread, but not until we break the cycle of perpetuating the same harms against the same groups of people over and over again.

8   Distrusted Authorities

Trust is generally defined as having confidence in someone or something. Trusting someone usually means that you don't think they'll do you wrong. It's the perception of a certain future.

We're far from the only species who thinks this way; the identification of trustworthy partners is important for any species that relies on cooperation for survival. Chimpanzees, for example, are more likely to voluntarily place food at the disposal of another chimpanzee, and thus wager on a payoff in the form of reciprocity, if that individual is a friend.[1] This behavior suggests that chimpanzees may have evolved strong forms of trust toward their close social partners, allowing for cooperative relationships amid threats of exploitation and nonreciprocity. The same can be said for humans. But even fish seek trust in situations where they need to work together. In a study of interactions between cleaner fish (*Labroides dimidiatus*) and client species, researchers found that clients gravitated toward cleaners whom they observed being cooperative rather than those whom they hadn't observed at all.[2] The reason may be that an unknown cleaner seems more likely to "cheat" a client (by feeding on its mucus) instead of providing a service (by removing ectoparasites) like it's supposed to do.

The flip side of identifying a trustworthy partner is being attuned to potential threats. Perhaps one of the most serious threats is an individual or group that means to do you harm. As a consequence, the tree of life is filled with adaptations that assist with the recognition and avoidance of predators. These are valuable assets, and some are finely tuned to classify predators into different categories based on the nature and level of risk associated with them. In Amboseli National Park in southern Kenya, for instance, African bush elephants (*Loxodonta africana*) encounter people such as the

Maasai, cattle-herding pastoralists whose young men demonstrate virility by spearing elephants, and the Kamba, agriculturalists and village dwellers who pose little threat to elephants.[3] The elephants differentiate the Maasai and Kamba as high and low dangers, respectively, and react accordingly to visual and olfactory cues. In a series of experiments, elephants showed greater fear when they detected the scent of garments previously worn by Maasai than by Kamba men, and reacted aggressively to red cloth, the color of traditional Maasai clothing. Interestingly, fear of the Maasai wasn't specific to elephants who had personal experience with spearing. These findings suggest that knowledge of Maasai people and the emotional responses associated with them are transmitted via social learning throughout the local elephant population. I also suggest that these emotional responses are comparable to mistrust and distrust.

Mistrust and distrust are often used interchangeably as terms, but they're not quite the same thing. While mistrust is a general sense of someone or something being unreliable, such as the way that I feel about horoscopes, distrust is a feeling of mistrust based on specific past experience. It's a projection of a previous betrayal into present interactions and those yet to occur. This is how I feel about bicycles.

In humans, trust isn't just a relationship between individuals; it's effectively a social glue that holds human society together. And according to sociologist Jonathan H. Turner, societies don't exist and humans don't survive without institutions. In his book *Human Institutions*, Turner defines social institutions as "population-wide structures and associated cultural (symbolic) systems that humans create and use to adjust to the exigencies of their environment."[4] These structures, which include polity (or government), law, economy, and education, are universal and fundamental to the viability of our species. Moreover, they require the public trust to function. Institutional distrust is therefore unique to humans and uniquely harmful to them.

It's a privilege to live without a lot of distrust because many people are beset by it. They may have good reasons to not consider a particular person, group, or entity as trustworthy. Usually these people have been exploited and harmed in some way, and sometimes for no better reason that they were seen as lower, less, or simply other. As we've discussed in previous chapters, epidemics and pandemics can often be the optimal setting for this kind of mistreatment. Ironically, they can also be occasions when trust is most needed.

In this chapter, we're going to examine some instances of how distrust has impeded or complicated efforts to control infectious diseases. First, we'll explore the history of some medical and public health practices that are part of infectious disease response and prevention, and rely on a social contract of trustworthiness. Then we'll take a close look at some particularly egregious examples of how the public trust was violated. Finally, we'll discuss how work can and is being done to build or repair trust in communities in order to improve health and well-being for them as well as all of us.

Containment and Control

In the ancient town of Cavaillon in southeastern France, on grounds filled with Greek and Roman ruins, a pink stucco mansion preserves some fascinating parallels between ancient and modern attempts at disease control. In 2021, before I ventured across the threshold of the historic Hôtel d'Agar with my colleague Marianne, we took notice of a small sign displayed near the front door. Alongside a drawing of a cloaked figure in a birdlike mask wielding a long wooden stick, there was a stern warning: "*Contre la peste-Covid, le port du masque est obligatoire!*" To protect against plague *and* COVID-19, the sign told us, wearing a mask was required.

The drawing was the portrait of a plague doctor in 1721, modeling a costume that would make more sense at a Halloween party than a hospital nowadays. In it, the long beak of the mask was filled with perfumes and pleasant-smelling herbs in order to protect the wearer against the foul odors of bad air, the so-called miasmas that were blamed for diseases like bubonic plague. The stick allowed the doctor to examine the bodies of patients without touching or getting near them as well as keep living people at a bay. Indeed, before there was a word for social distancing, there was tool for it. The entire spooky ensemble was supposedly developed by French doctor Charles de L'Orme when Paris was hit hard by bubonic plague in 1619 during the second plague pandemic, and it endures as one of the most famous symbols of the disease—even though there's no proof that it was actually worn in real life.

Masked by twenty-first-century standards, without the beaks, we were welcomed by the Morand family into a home and museum steeped in antiquity. Open to the public for guided tours, the labyrinthine Renaissance building is chockablock with artifacts, sculptures, paintings, and records spanning the history of France since the Neolithic. But we came

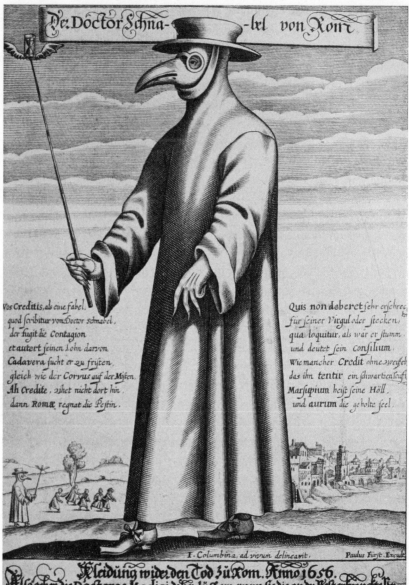

Der Doctor Schna-   -bel von Rom

Vos Creditis, als eine fabel,
  quod scribitur vom Doctor schnabel,
    der fugit die Contagion
    et autert seinen Lohn darvon.
  Cadavera sucht er zu fristen,
  gleich wie der Corvus auf der Misten.
  Ah Credite, sehet nicht dort hin,
  dann ROMÆ regnat die Pestin.

Quis non deberet sehr erschrec,
  für seiner Virgul oder stecken,
    qua loquitur, als wär er stumm,
    und deutet sein Consilium.
  Wie mancher Credit ohne zweifel,
  das ihm tentirt ein schwartzen Teuffel
  Marsupium heist seine Höll,
  und aurum die geholte seel.

I. Columbina, ad vivum delineavit.   Paulus Fürst Excud.

Kleidüng wider den Tod zü Rom. Anno 1656.
Also gehen die Doctores Medici daher zü Rom, wann sie die an der Pest erkranckte Personen besüchen, sie zü curiren und fragen, sich wed em Gifft zü sichern, ein langes Kleid von gewaxtem Tuch ihr Angesicht ist verlarvt, für den Augen haben sie grosse Crÿstalline Brillen, wider Nasen einen langen Schnabel voll wolriechender Specereÿ, in der Hände welche mit Handschühern wol versehen ist, eine lange Rüthe und darmit deuten sie, was man thün, und gebrauche soll.

with a specific interest, which was shared by our hosts, a couple of doctors who bought the nine-hundred-year-old Hôtel d'Agar in the 1990s. We were there to see relics of plague.

The Morand family has assembled an immense collection of objects and documents related to the last major outbreak of bubonic plague in western Europe, the Great Plague of Marseille in 1720–1722. Over the course of two years, the disease spread throughout Marseille and killed at least half of its inhabitants, claiming the lives of around a hundred thousand people within and beyond the city.[5] As testimony to its rampage, the Hôtel d'Agar had depictions of dramatic scenes of mass death on the walls and detailed epidemiological records laid out on display.

I wandered over to one document, lying on a small table with a number of others exactly like it. Dated 1720, they were multiple copies of a blank certificate bearing two coats of arms, one of the nearby village of Aubignan and the other of Pope Clement XI. The document was a travel authorization for the holder, who was verified as plague free by the alders and health council of Aubignan. Each copy had blank spaces for the holder's name, age, height, hair color, and destination.

Lying next to them was a modern analog, which our hosts had used themselves the previous year. Dated 2020, it was a travel certificate required for people everywhere in France during the first wave of the COVID-19 pandemic when there was a mandatory lockdown throughout the country. For nearly two months, anyone leaving their home was required to fill out the form by declaring a valid reason for going outside, such as travel to their place of work. Around a hundred thousand police officers were deployed nationwide to ensure compliance with the confinement, and people caught breaking the rules were fined more than €100.[6]

Figure 8.1
A plague doctor. Named Doctor Schnabel (meaning "Doctor Beak" in German), the figure in this engraving is wearing the costume of a physician treating the plague in the seventeenth century, including a fragrance-filled beaked mask, long and heavy cloak, wide-brimmed hat, and stick for keeping patients at a distance. *Source:* Eugen Holländer, *Die Karikatur und Satire in der Medizin: Medico-Kunsthistorische Studie von Professor Dr. Eugen Holländer*, 2nd ed. (Stuttgart: Ferdinand Enke, 1921), 171, fig. 79.

From the outset there was strong support for the new rules among the French population, according to a study conducted ten days after the lockdown was implemented.[7] For the majority of the respondents, however, their support was tinged with critical views of the public health strategy by French authorities, who seemed unprepared to offer any better alternative. Notably, criticism or limited support of the lockdown was more frequent among the low-income respondents, who were more likely to experience financial difficulties, unemployment, and crowded living conditions because of it. This finding lined up with previous research showing that lower socioeconomic status was correlated with less trust in public health authorities in general.

Examining the two documents, separated by three hundred years, I was reminded of the ancient history of public health measures in human society. Isolating the sick from the healthy is a timeworn practice, with references in the Bible that include the physical separation of lepers from everyone else.[8] But the first form of institutionalized public health began with antiplague measures in the fourteenth century in response to the Black Death, the start of the second plague pandemic that lasted in France until the devastation of Marseille.

The Black Death wiped out as much of a third of the European population between 1346 and 1353, but Mediterranean port cities suffered the most, as ships transported the pathogen along with trade goods.[9] In 1348, the Republic of Ragusa (present-day Dubrovnik in Croatia) suffered the greatest loss of life in its thousand-year existence, according to medical historian Zlata Blažina Tomić and translator Vesna Blažina in their book *Expelling the Plague*. They also detail how in 1377, after decades of recurring outbreaks, Ragusa enacted the first quarantine legislation in the world. Based on the belief that plague was contagious, the legislation required thirty days of isolation (*trentino*) for people arriving from plague-infected areas for the purpose of disinfection. During the next eighty years, similar laws were introduced in Marseille, Venice, Pisa, and Genoa, and the isolation period was extended from thirty to forty days. Renamed as *quarantino*, such restrictions on the movements of people, animals, and merchandise have remained a pillar of modern disease control.[10] In English, they're called quarantine.

The neighboring cities of northern Italy likewise initiated health measures that spread through Europe and around the world. In 1374, Milan and

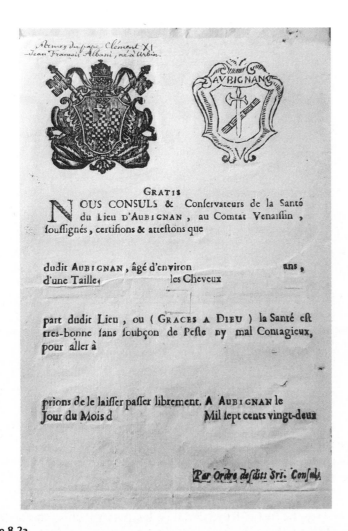

Figure 8.2a
Travel pass for French citizens during the Great Plague of Marseille in 1720. Plague-
free travelers were required to show an authorization form that included their name,
height, hair color, and destination.

ATTESTATION DE DÉPLACEMENT DÉROGATOIRE

En application de l'article 1ᵉʳ du décret du 16 mars 2020 portant réglementation des déplacements dans le cadre de la lutte contre la propagation du virus Covid-19 :

Je soussigné(e)

Mme / M.

Né(e) le :

Demeurant :

certifie que mon déplacement est lié au motif suivant (cocher la case) autorisé par l'article 1ᵉʳ du décret du 16 mars 2020 portant réglementation des déplacements dans le cadre de la lutte contre la propagation du virus Covid-19 :

☐ déplacements entre le domicile et le lieu d'exercice de l'activité professionnelle, lorsqu'ils sont indispensables à l'exercice d'activités ne pouvant être organisées sous forme de télétravail (sur justificatif permanent) ou déplacements professionnels ne pouvant être différés;

☐ déplacements pour effectuer des achats de première nécessité dans des établissements autorisés (liste sur gouvernement.fr);

☐ déplacements pour motif de santé;

☐ déplacements pour motif familial impérieux, pour l'assistance aux personnes vulnérables ou la garde d'enfants;

☐ déplacements brefs, à proximité du domicile, liés à l'activité physique individuelle des personnes, à l'exclusion de toute pratique sportive collective, et aux besoins des animaux de compagnie.

Fait à ...., le ..../..../2020
(signature)

Figure 8.2b
Travel certificate used during the COVID-19 lockdown in France in 2020. People were required to fill out their name, birth date, address, and reason for leaving their home.

Mantua were the first cities to declare a temporary ban on travelers from plagued places, and in 1423, Venice established the first plague hospital on a nearby island known as a lazaretto or lazaret. In 1400, Milan was also the first city to use a river as a natural barrier to keep potential plague-infected pilgrims from Germany and France outside the urban centers.[11]

These tactics caught on in Marseille, with the first lazaret in 1526 and a quarantine system that lasted from 1620 to 1830. Many documents at the Hôtel d'Agar attest to the countless ways that people and their property were controlled for the sake of public health during the epidemic of 1720–1722. In an attempt to protect the rest of France from infection, one-quarter of the French Army formed quarantine lines (cordons sanitaires) across much of Provence, the largest single exercise of state power ever mounted against plague.[12] Their defenses included the construction of a stone wall that was two meters high and twenty-seven kilometers long, with guard towers and ditches along it. Some portions of the wall are still standing, although today they can't even keep out tourists, much less disease.

These measures were unpopular with the public at the time. And fair enough, it wasn't obvious how they were effective against a disease that was poorly understood. The rationale for the forty-day quarantine period is a total mystery, for example, and may relate to the Christian observance of forty days of Lent or other events of biblical significance.[13] It definitely didn't correspond to the incubation period of the plague, which is typically one to six days, although nobody knew it back then. But even as knowledge improved, plague quarantines remained pressure cookers of distrust into the twentieth century, as we saw in the case of San Francisco's Chinatown in chapter 6.

*   *   *

Quarantines have been used for numerous other diseases since the plague pandemics, such as in response to the West African Ebola epidemic in 2014. And debates over their potential benefits and problems have continued. When cordons sanitaires were used to seal off an area of West Africa where 70 percent of EVD cases were found, which meant that the police and military wouldn't let anyone leave (whether or not they were infected), CDC quarantine expert Martin Cetron expressed concerns. "It might work," he said when the plan was announced, "but it has a lot of potential to go poorly if it's not done with an ethical approach. Just letting the disease burn out and considering that the price of controlling it—we don't live in that era anymore."[14]

It did go poorly. The mobility restrictions created an actual humanitarian crisis within the isolation zone, as the disruptions in access to food and health care increased the risks of infections.[15] In fact, research suggests that they may have accelerated disease transmission and led to more cases within the cordoned area.[16]

Things went from bad to worse when two weeks later, the Liberian government imposed another cordon sanitaire around the poorest quarter in its capital city. As the oldest slum in Monrovia, West Point has been targeted for urban renewal for decades, with residents living under the constant threat of forced relocation and demolition.[17] Yet despite its overcrowded and underserved population, with at least sixty thousand people crammed onto a squalid sandspit near the city center, West Point had just become the site of Monrovia's first holding center for suspected EVD patients.[18] Some residents of West Point saw the center as an attack on the neighborhood—a deliberate effort by a distrusted government that wanted to infest and erad-icate West Point with the Ebola virus.[19] Others doubted that the disease was real and shouted "There is no Ebola!" as they descended on the center.[20] (Remember, there had never been an EVD epidemic in West Africa before.) Hundreds of locals broke through the center's gate, looting supplies and driving out patients.[21] The facility was forced to close within days.

Shortly thereafter, barricades of razor wire went up around West Point without any warning or information about the quarantine. Armed police and soldiers announced that the neighborhood was under total lockdown, with no passage in or out, cutting off all of its inhabitants from their live-lihoods and loved ones.[22] Probably anyone would panic at the involun-tary confinement given that EVD spreads via infected body fluids and the sanitary conditions in West Point were abysmal. (In 2009, there were only four public toilets in the entire neighborhood, used by hundreds of peo-ple a day.)[23] And being trapped with EVD patients inside the cordon, not knowing if or how the government would provide supplies, the residents immediately fought back.[24] Some tried to break through the barricades, as soldiers fired live rounds to drive them back, killing a fifteen-year-old boy. "The quarantine is going to worsen the spread of Ebola," said physician and Ebola expert Jean-Jacques Muyembe at the time. "Putting the police and the army in charge of the quarantine was the worst thing that you could do. You must make people inside the quarantine zone feel that they are being helped, not oppressed."[25]

Rather than fighting the quarantine, other people found ways to bypass it. They climbed over, under, or around the blockades, with or without cooperation from the guards, or even swam out of the neighborhood. The West Point quarantine was soon called off by the Liberian government, only ten days after it was announced. It was, in the words of anthropologist Danny Hoffman, an obvious failure.[26]

None of this is to say that isolation and quarantine can't be effective public health measures for some diseases, when communicated and imple-mented appropriately. They absolutely can be, although the paradox of public health is that you never know what you've prevented when it works. But people have to be trusting enough to submit to them. And broken trust can be hard to repair. In Liberia, fourteen years of brutal civil war and oppressive rule helped to solidify the public's distrust of government authorities, particularly among its poorest citizens, more than a decade before the country's first Ebola outbreak in 2014. The state of emergency powers declared by Liberian president Ellen Johnson Sirleaf, by which she ordered the quarantine of West Point, possibly recalled the authoritarian measures of previous regimes. And by framing citizens as a population that needed to be controlled rather than people deserving of care, as journalist Aaron Leaf argued, she created more distrust in the country at a time when cooperation was needed most.[27] So when people resisted, who could blame them? Tragically, the measures may have contributed to the further spread of the disease too, as there was an exponential rise in new EVD cases in Liberia around the same time that the cordons sanitaires were implemented.[28]

*   *   *

As the French were building barriers to contain the bubonic plague in 1721, the British were discovering strategies to prevent smallpox. That year, the practice of variolation (also known as inoculation), which involved inserting powdered scabs or fluid from smallpox pustules into a small cut in a healthy person's skin, was introduced to England by one Lady Mary Wortley Montagu. She learned about the procedure in Istanbul (then Constantinople, the capital of the Ottoman Empire), where the Turks used it to induce immunity to the variola virus through a milder, localized infection. There and elsewhere, such as in China, India, and Africa, people had been practicing some form of variolation for centuries. Of course, it wasn't entirely fail-safe—2 to 3 percent of those treated ended up dying as a result of the intentional infection—but many Europeans saw better odds in variolation than in natural infection.[29] That's because at least 20 percent of people with natural infections died from the disease, with around four hundred thousand European deaths on an annual basis during the eighteenth century. You could count on a certain level of immunity if you survived, but you might wind up blind and likely disfigured nonetheless.[30] During the Revolutionary War, smallpox was an even greater threat to native-born colonial soldiers, most of whom lacked immunity to the disease from childhood exposure, unlike their British opponents. For this reason, in 1777, Commander in Chief George Washington mandated variolation for all the vulnerable soldiers in the Continental Army.[31] It was the first mass military inoculation in history, and by all accounts it worked out well.

By then, both royalty and regiments embraced the practice. In 1774, after a smallpox outbreak at the Palace of Versailles led to the demise of King Louis XIV of France, the next king started off his reign with Lady Montagu's trick. King Louis XVI and his younger brothers were inoculated at the same time as he was, thereby giving the entire line of succession protection against smallpox. (Protection against revolution, not so much.)

The same year, however, another method of smallpox protection was developing in England. In 1774, cattle breeder Benjamin Jesty successfully defended his family from smallpox by inoculating his wife and two children with pustular matter from cows infected with cowpox, a zoonotic disease caused by cowpox virus. (I imagine that there was a lot of trust in the Jesty household.) Closely related to the variola virus, the pathogen can infect humans and produce a mild infection that confers immunity to smallpox—without actually giving a person smallpox. This phenomenon was apparently well-known in the dairy counties of eighteenth-century England, and Jesty had experienced it himself. His experiment succeeded, as his children remained immune to smallpox, even when they were variolated fifteen years later.[32]

Enter Edward Jenner. The British physician suspected that cowpox not only protected against smallpox but also that the pustules in a person with cowpox could be used to produce smallpox immunity in another person. In 1796, Jenner gave it a try, transferring fluid from a cowpox blister on a milkmaid to an eight-year-old boy. Two months later, he inoculated the boy again, but with fluid from a fresh smallpox lesion. Since no disease developed, Jenner determined, the protection was complete.[33] He published his findings from this case and others in 1798, coining the term *vaccination* for the process (after the Latin word *vacca*, meaning cow). By 1800, vaccination had been picked up throughout England and other European countries. The British government passed the first Vaccination Act of 1840, making variolation illegal and providing free vaccinations for the poor. With the Vaccination Act of 1853 and until the end of the century, vaccination was made compulsory for infants and children. But not everyone was happy about it. Soon after the Vaccination Act of 1867, which included threats of coercive cumulative penalties for noncompliance, people began to resist on a large scale.[34]

Although Jenner's vaccine seemed safer than variolation, since cowpox is a much less dangerous disease for humans than smallpox, it still posed risks. Person-to-person vaccination could easily transmit *other* pathogens between people, in addition to the variola virus, at a time when nobody even knew about microbial agents of disease. And so the next major advance toward a safer and more consistent vaccine came with Pasteur's work on fowl cholera in the 1870s.[35] By developing a weakened form of the causal bacterium in his laboratory, he laid the groundwork for his human rabies vaccine and many others that followed.

There are numerous types of vaccines today, with many variations in how they're made and work, even though they all do essentially the same thing: help the body's immune system to recognize, remember, and destroy a specific pathogen, and thus protect against the disease that the pathogen might otherwise cause. The human virus vaccines created in the nineteenth century (namely Jenner's variola vaccine and Pasteur's rabies vaccine) were live vaccines that used a whole weakened form of the target pathogen. At the same time, scientists developed several inactivated bacterial vaccines for typhoid, cholera, and plague, which used pathogens incapable of replication due to heat or chemical treatment. Beginning in the twentieth century, both live and inactivated vaccines continued to be produced, along with subunit vaccines that use specific components of the pathogen rather than the whole germ, such as toxins, proteins, sugar molecules, and genetic material (that is, DNA or RNA). Recent advances include messenger RNA (mRNA) vaccines, which use a subtype of RNA that teaches human cells to make proteins that trigger an immune response against the target pathogen, and viral vector vaccines, which use a modified version of a different virus to provide protection. Both of these types of vaccines were among those developed to provide protection against COVID-19 in 2020, and proved to be highly safe and effective, despite receiving a lot of public skepticism (which we'll discuss further in chapter 10). In fact, the 2023 Nobel Prize in Physiology or Medicine was awarded to scientists Katalin Karikó and Drew Weissman for discoveries that enabled effective mRNA vaccines against COVID-19—and thus saved tens of millions of lives.

For as long as vaccines have existed, people have been distrustful of them. These concerns are rooted in a number of issues where the question of safety looms large. And to be fair, long before the rigorous standards, requirements, and ethics of modern clinical research, people had good reasons to worry about the safety of vaccines and medicines. The first laboratory-created human vaccine, developed by Pasteur for rabies in 1885, encountered an immediate outcry from the public, horrified by the deliberate injection of a deadly agent into a person's body.[36]

Pasteur's decision to treat nine-year-old Joseph Meister with his rabies vaccine, after the asymptomatic boy was badly bitten by rabid dogs, was objectionable even to Pasteur's close collaborator. Physician Émile Roux was conspicuously absent from the Meister case, possibly because he refused to participate in the boy's treatment based on insufficient experimental evidence of the vaccine's safety and efficacy.[37] He also would have known about the contents of Pasteur's laboratory notebooks, which recorded two prior (and unpublicized) human rabies vaccinations that resulted in one death. Roux left Pasteur's laboratory in protest of Meister's vaccination, only to return for unknown reasons months later. Possibly he was reassured by the success of the rabies vaccine in almost all subsequent human cases as well as by the growing favorable evidence from animal experiments. Yet as anesthesiologist Henry Beecher stressed in 1966, "An experiment is ethical or not at its inception; it does not become ethical *post hoc*—ends do not justify the means. There is no ethical distinction between ends and means."[38]

Ethical and rigorous experimentation is a big part of how safety of a substance is determined. And in Beecher's 1966 article "Ethics and Clinical Research," he called attention to ethical lapses in research carried out and published by the leading physician-scientists of his day. Perhaps the most influential paper ever written about experimentation involving human subjects, his article was a catalyst for federal rules governing the conduct of human experimentation in the United States.[39] Unfortunately, this kind of research was long overdue for regulation, as human experimentation has been documented for over a thousand years. In the tenth century, Persian physician Abu Bakr al-Razi (known as Rhazes in the West) described the first-known use of a control group in a human trial when he tested the efficacy of bloodletting in treating the symptoms of meningitis by dividing patients into groups that either did or didn't receive the treatment.[40] Then in the eleventh century, another Persian physician named Abu Ali al-Husain ibn Abdullah ibn Sina (known as Avicenna in the West) wrote the earliest treatise on clinical trials in *Kitab al-Qanun fit-Tibb* (*The Canon of Medicine*). In it, he identified seven conditions necessary for testing drug treatment using the basic building blocks of the scientific method. And the final condition on his list was that in order to understand the strength and effect of a drug, it must first be tested on a human being.[41]

It wasn't until the twentieth century, in the aftermath of some shockingly unethical practices by doctors and government scientists, that testing requirements and restrictions on drugs and vaccines took their modern form. But even then, mistakes and wrongdoings still occur. And when they do, the impacts can be far-reaching and hugely damaging, resulting in a distrust of institutions that exceeds a mistrust in the health protections or treatments that they may offer.

Broken Trust

During the nineteenth century, cholera spread to almost every part of the globe. Yet in the 1830s, the first wave of cholera in Europe sparked furious violence. The violence had little to do with the disease, an acute diarrheal infection of *Vibrio cholerae* bacteria, often due to drinking water or eating food contaminated with feces.[42] Rather, cholera riots in various European cities as well as on the East Coast of the United States sprang from ground seeded with discontent.[43] Invariably, the rage was directed at the elite and dominant classes of society—such as doctors, soldiers, aristocrats, and government officials—by the impoverished and dispossessed people who distrusted them. From attacks on cordons sanitaires and military officers in Saint Petersburg, to the sacking of castles and massacre of nobles in Hungary, to the burning of property in response to sanitation measures in Paris, there were ubiquitous suspicions that cholera was a cover story to exterminate the poor.[44] In the British Isles and especially the English city of Liverpool, however, the distrust was linked more closely to real events than conspiratorial imaginings.

In 1832, the cholera riots in Liverpool coalesced around patients, doctors, and hospitals, all easy targets at which large mobs hurled objects and abuse over the course of ten days. The insults and accusations were peppered with some odd words that hinted at the source of their anger: doctors were called "Burkers" and accused of wanting to "get the poor into their clutches to Burke them."[45] The slang referred to William Burke, one of a pair of men who went on a killing spree in Edinburgh in 1828. Their victims were murdered for the value of their corpses, which Burke and his accomplice, William Hare, sold to a local anatomy teacher for dissection.[46] At the time, there was a clandestine and lucrative business in the United Kingdom of body snatching, which illegally supplied medical schools with human bodies for surgical training and research. Burke and Hare brought a new level of disgrace, and public outrage, to the transactions. They also inspired a copycat cadre of London Burkers who did the same thing in 1831.[47] In Liverpool the following year, when rioters demanded that hospitals "Bring out the Burkers!" it was clear that the public believed that doctors were killing cholera patients in order to use them for anatomical dissection.[48]

The timing of the European emergence of cholera undoubtedly exacerbated this fear. In the midst of the epidemic and expedited by the crimes that preceded it, the UK Parliament passed the Anatomy Act of 1832. The legislation provided physicians, surgeons, and medical students with legal access to bodies if the deceased didn't formally dissent to dissection during life or if their spouse or nearest known relative failed to claim them for burial within forty-eight hours of death.[49] If you think that doesn't sound fair or consensual, you're right. Nonetheless, the unclaimed poor became a convenient stock of "specimens" for anatomists, hardly making the lower classes of Liverpool feel any safer. At the same time, the poor were most likely to be infected by cholera and die from it because many of them inhabited overcrowded cellar dwellings with virtually no clean water supply or sewage disposal.[50] Thus they probably weren't comforted by the news that deceased cholera patients had been removed from cemeteries and sold to dissecting rooms in London mere months earlier.[51]

The cholera riots in Liverpool ended when the Catholic Church intervened with a statement reassuring its congregations that cholera was real and physicians were doing their best to care for cholera patients, who wouldn't be dissected after death. And when cholera declined and disappeared in late 1832 (only to reemerge in subsequent years), physicians Sean Burrell and Geoffrey Gill note that dissection also faded from public attention. Yet during the brief time when these two social events coincided, they argue, the riots unquestionably contributed to a fearful and chaotic atmosphere of possibly the worst disease epidemic to affect Britain since the Great Plague of London in 1665.[52]

In England, the use of human bodies, organs, and tissues for medical research is now governed by the Human Tissue Authority, under the Human Tissue Act of 2004. The act was motivated partly by another medical scandal in the late 1990s and early 2000s, when the public became aware that the Alder Hey Children's Hospital in Liverpool (and others within the National Health Service) had retained organs and tissues from patients following postmortem examinations, and without knowledge or approval from their families. As a consequence, the parents of deceased children had no idea that they had buried only some of their children's remains while the rest were stored by the hospital.[53] Although the crowds that gathered at the hospital gates didn't escalate to unruly mobs, the moral uproar was ear-splitting. Most of all, it was another blow to the already shaky confidence that many people held in the medical profession.

*　　*　　*

As a steward of museum collections that include human remains, I'm familiar with the long-term labor of building relationships with people and communities that have good reasons to distrust doctors and scientists. My field, biological anthropology, was born from medicine during the eighteenth century, when scientists began to study "racial" differences among human beings in reinforcement of white supremacy. Early curators thus amassed huge collections of human skeletal remains, especially skulls, in order to measure, compare, and categorize every aspect of physical variation among them. Many of these remains were collected from archaeological excavations and surveys, while others were purchased or donated. Yet some of the largest collections of human skeletal remains at the NMNH, for example, were created from unclaimed bodies that were dissected at medical schools in the late nineteenth and early twentieth centuries, and later transferred to the Smithsonian Institution for research purposes.

That's right, the United States did it too. In 1831, US states began passing anatomy laws similar to the Anatomy Act of 1832, starting in Massachusetts. By 1913, almost every state with medical schools had passed a law that allowed them to appropriate people's unclaimed bodies for dissection. The anatomy lobby claimed that the arrangement was beneficial for all, as historian Michael Sappol explains in his book *A Traffic of Dead Bodies*. Paupers could posthumously repay their debt to society with their dead bodies, and everyone would profit from the advances in medical practice and knowledge.[54]

But that was, as the Brits say, nonsense. While it's true that medical and anthropological science has been built upon these bodies, it's wrong to assume that their study has resulted in significant health gains for communities and descendants of the deceased. I would challenge anyone to say as much about the historical anatomical collections at the NMNH, which are largely composed of individuals most marginalized in US society, such as recent immigrants, people with mental illness, and people of color.[55] The Smithsonian restricted research access to these and all human remains in its museums in 2023. It was only the start to a reckoning with our responsibilities toward these people and their descendants, whose stories are intertwined with a broader phenomenon of exploitation and dehumanization of others in the name of science.

The most egregious event in the history of medical distrust in the United States is the Tuskegee Syphilis Study. Conducted by the US Public Health Service from 1932 to 1972, this forty-year horror show did nothing but harden African American attitudes toward the US biomedical community. "No scientific experiment," writes author James Jones in his book *Bad Blood*, "inflicted more damage on the collective psyche of Black Americans than the Tuskegee Study."[56] And fifty years later, during the COVID-19 pandemic, the experiment still encapsulates the negative public health consequences of distrust in institutions because in many people's eyes, not enough has changed.

The Tuskegee experiment didn't try to help its participants. Over a span of four decades, the purpose of the experiment, which apparently lacked any formal protocols, was to observe and document the effects of untreated, late-stage syphilis in Black men. (It's therefore not entirely accurate to call it a study, in fact, when the lack of research design and documentation is completely antithetical to the scientific process.) All the syphilitic patients, around four hundred Black men in total, were selected to showcase the ravages of the infection (caused by bacterium *Treponema pallidum*) when left unchecked until death. The experiment was conducted around the town of Tuskegee in Macon County in the US state of Alabama because there were so many available subjects in the area. Macon County was not only filled with syphilitic African Americans but many of them had received little or no medical care for their condition either.

The doctors who proposed the experiment were fixated on the idea that syphilis was an entirely different disease in white and Black patients, with a greater attack on the neural system in the former and cardiovascular system in the latter. Although a previous study had suggested that there were no clinical distinctions, the researchers were determined to find some.[57]

Beyond its racism, the Tuskegee experiment was monstrous in its ethical offenses. There was no informed consent, meaning that its potential risks and benefits weren't explained to the participants. The participants weren't even told by Tuskegee clinicians that they had syphilis but instead merely "bad blood." Nor were the men offered penicillin when it became known as an effective treatment for syphilis in the 1940s. Instead, they were given free meals, medical examinations, and burials—a pitiful compensation that reflects the poverty of some participants as well as how little they knew about the experiment and how much they trusted the people conducting it. Many participants died of complications from syphilis, and some survivors (of which there were only seventy-four by the time the experiment ended) became blind or otherwise disabled.[58] Most of them never knew that the Tuskegee clinicians had withheld effective antibiotics for decades and hence made their conditions worse. In this betrayal, the Tuskegee clinicians violated their Hippocratic Oath by failing to provide health benefits to their patients and protect them from harm.[59]

The Tuskegee experiment wasn't a secret in the scientific community, producing fifteen publications in the medical literature during its lifetime, but most people only learned about it when a news journalist broke the story in 1972.[60] A national uproar swiftly terminated the experiment, and lawsuits, apologies, and legislation followed in the subsequent decades. In direct response, the National Research Act was enacted by the US Congress, which formalized an institutional review board process to ensure that human subjects research prioritizes human rights and welfare. Nonetheless, the wounds from the experiment haven't yet healed. Nor is it the only reason for distrust by African Americans of medical and public health institutions. None of it began in Tuskegee, just as it didn't end there.

Like the medical distrust that preceded the cholera riots in England, African American fears about exploitation by the medical profession existed for centuries before the Tuskegee experiment.[61] Prior to the passing of anatomy laws, grave robbers regularly plundered African American cemeteries and sold the bodies to medical schools for dissection. Furthermore, dangerous, involuntary, and nontherapeutic experimentation on African Americans has been documented since at least the eighteenth century, as detailed by writer and medical ethicist Harriet Washington in her book *Medical Apartheid*. This kind of inhumane experimentation was so widespread, in fact, that African American stories and folklore warned about kidnappings by doctors who would kill and study Black people in their hospitals.

For instance, during the mid-nineteenth century, physician J. Marion Sims acquired slaves for brutal surgical experiments that were conducted without anesthesia or consent.[62] Famous for his gynecologic research, Sims refused to administer ether to Black women while giving the anesthetic freely to white women, based partly on his belief that Black people didn't feel pain in the same way that white people did.[63] Unfortunately this idea appears to persist in modern medicine today. A 2016 study found that 50 percent of a sample of white US medical students and residents held false beliefs about biological differences between Black and white people, and were less likely to perceive and appropriately treat pain in Black patients.[64]

The Tuskegee experiment seemed to provide only more proof that Black lives weren't valued as more than fodder for the white medical establishment. This deeply entrenched distrust resurfaced during the first decade of the AIDS epidemic as African Americans accounted for more and more new cases. In 1990, a series of polls revealed widespread beliefs among African Americans that the AIDS virus was a tool of genocide created in a laboratory in order to infect and wipe out the African American population.[65] The suspicions extended to AIDS treatments and preventative measures, with notions that the first AIDS drug was the vehicle for a poisoning plot against Black people, condom use was a scheme to reduce the number of Black babies, and clean needle distribution was a means to encourage Black drug addicts.

Although these fears may seem outlandish to many people today, in a historical context they're more understandable. And African Americans aren't alone in having such suspicions or clear reasons for them. Many historically marginalized groups, in the United States and elsewhere, have experiences with institutions and governments that make them feel distrustful and unsafe.[66] This is a major problem when it comes to preventing or controlling a pandemic threat because people everywhere need to be willing participants in the response. And you can't come asking for trust only at the moment you need it. It must be earned over time.

Being Trustworthy

The greatest human achievement in response to a pandemic was watched by the whole world in real time. I didn't truly appreciate this fact until a conversation in June 2020 with Barney Graham, then deputy director of the NIAID's Vaccine Research Center at the National Institutes of Health. He was the first speaker in a public webinar series on COVID-19 vaccines that we produced for the *Outbreak* exhibit, at a time when the Smithsonian was still closed and it was all but impossible to get a test for COVID-19, let alone a shot in the arm. It was common knowledge that scientists were working on vaccines, but few people knew anything about them.

Representing the scientific team developing the Moderna COVID-19 vaccine, Graham spoke plainly to me and our virtual audience about their progress to date. As modest as he was, the work that he described was nothing short of remarkable. The genetic sequence of the novel coronavirus was published on January 10, and within four days Graham's team had designed a mRNA vaccine for testing. They were able to do this, he stressed, because his team had been studying other coronaviruses (the mild endemic ones in humans as well as the highly pathogenic ones that cause SARS and MERS) for the last seven years. If the novel virus hadn't been a coronavirus but rather from any of the other twenty-four viral families, he noted that "we wouldn't have been nearly as well prepared."[67]

Speaking from his home office, Graham explained simply how the vaccine was made, and the process by which his team had collapsed steps and performed studies in parallel so that the product could move forward as quickly as possible without compromising safety. Because the Moderna vaccine used a specific, synthetic subunit of the virus to show to the immune system, he pointed out, it didn't have the same safety risks as a live virus vaccine. He showed us early data from his team's animal experiments, with graphs indicating that the vaccine produced antibodies to neutralize the virus and prevent its replication in mice. Then he took questions from listeners, who asked him about everything from monitoring the long-term effects of the vaccine to expectations about when it would be available. Graham said that he was optimistic about his team's findings to that point, but the vaccine still had to be tested in large-scale trials to see if it worked in humans.

Six months later, the final results were published. In an efficacy trial of 30,000 people, only 11 participants who received two doses of the vaccine had COVID-19 symptoms, and none of them experienced severe disease.[68] In contrast, among the placebo group (which didn't receive the vaccine), there were 185 symptomatic cases, 30 of which were severe, and 1 of which resulted in death. It was, again, absolutely remarkable. With 94 percent efficacy in preventing COVID-19 illness, the Moderna vaccine was authorized for use by the FDA and Health Canada in December 2020. The next year, many other countries approved the use of the vaccine, which was manufactured and distributed in hundreds of thousands of doses, along with numerous other COVID-19 vaccines of various types.

Pandemic solved? Not so fast. Vaccines don't save lives, vaccination does. They can't do their magic unless people take them. And even before the COVID-19 vaccines were ready for the real world, the biggest challenge that lay beyond the laboratory was assuring people that they *wanted* to be vaccinated.

Clearing the trust hurdle was critical for public health, especially in communities with a history of betrayal by institutions that were supposed to protect them. And by no coincidence, these were the communities at greatest risk for infection. In the first few months of the COVID-19 pandemic, federal data showed that Latino, African American, and Native American groups were disproportionately affected by COVID-19 throughout the United States, across urban, suburban, and rural areas.[69] Latino and African American people were three times as likely to become infected as their white neighbors, and nearly twice as likely to die. These disparities were related to factors that increased exposure to COVID-19, such as being front-line workers, relying on public transportation, and living in cramped or multigenerational homes.

Kizzmekia Corbett, the scientific lead of the NIAID team that developed the Moderna vaccine and Graham's supervisee, put these disparities at the forefront of a presentation that she gave for the American Medical Association in March 2021.[70] As a viral immunologist with a background in sociology, Corbett interwove issues of science and society in countless lectures, interviews, and outreach events during the COVID-19 pandemic. She didn't value pipettes over people; she saw both as equally important to her job. Furthermore, as a Black woman who was part of the US medical establishment, employed at a federal health agency, and responsible for a record-setting COVID-19 vaccine, she was uniquely positioned to address issues of distrust in African American communities in particular.

She knew it too. In an interview on the podcast *America Dissected* in January 2021, Corbett spoke about the importance of making institutional distrust widely visible in order to compel more accountability for past failings. "We have no choice but to really show up for people in these moments," she said about scientists and doctors. "It's really all eyes on us, around how we can become more trustworthy."[71] And in her view, they couldn't build trust without first breaking down barriers. With greater accessibility and transparency, and by creating space for questions and answers, scientists could prove their trustworthiness and the public could gain more trust.

Corbett acknowledged the heavy weight on her shoulders, holding a position in which some people had never before seen their mirror image. In matters of trust, it made a difference. But this also reflected another problem, as there were still too few scientists of color representing a huge (non-white) proportion of the US population, often because of a leaky pipeline to success. So while we're redefining what scientists look like, she argued, we may need to redefine what science looks like too.

By committing themselves to public engagement through so many different channels during the pandemic, Graham and Corbett helped forge a new model of a government scientist at a time when one was desperately needed. In so doing, their scientific achievements were even more powerful. In 2021, they were jointly named Federal Employee of the Year in recognition of their public service. (Incidentally, Corbett uses the same term—*public service*—for the act of getting vaccinated.) In addition, the Smithsonian offered another platform to elevate their achievements: in 2021, both Graham and Corbett were honored in the Arts and Industries Building's *FUTURES* exhibit, an exploration of the wealth of possibilities for humanity's next chapter. As "featured futurists," the two scientists were captured in a colorful portrait behind a display of their accomplishments. In it, Corbett wears a T-shirt that reads, "A Black girl will save the world."

Unfortunately, the US government fell short of its goal for 70 percent of the US adult population to have at least one COVID-19 vaccine shot by July 4, 2021. Such widespread vaccination was viewed as a crucial step toward reaching herd (or community) immunity—a situation when enough people in a population have antibodies against a specific disease that vulnerable members of the population are protected.[72] But when the 70 percent milestone was reached a few weeks later, vaccination coverage was still highly uneven across different states and communities throughout the country.

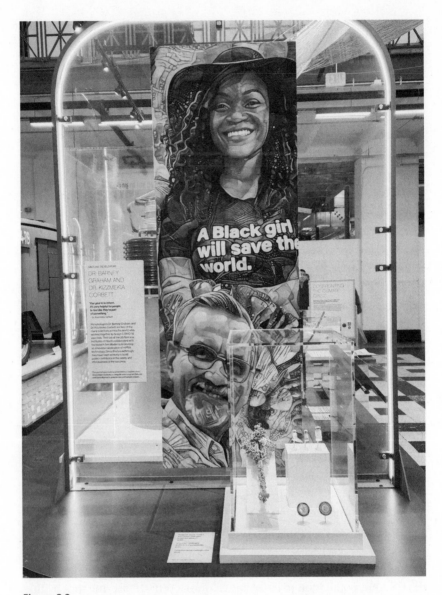

Figure 8.3
Display of Kizzmekia Corbett and Barney Graham, scientific leaders in COVID-19 vaccine development, in the *FUTURES* exhibition at the Smithsonian's Arts + Industries Building in 2021–2022. *Source:* Sabrina Sholts.

The remaining gaps weren't for lack of effort by the NIAID team and many other scientists (including teams at Pfizer and Johnson & Johnson, developers of the other two COVID-19 vaccines used in the United States) to raise awareness and encourage acceptance of the COVID-19 vaccines by the public. The difficulty is that in addition to distrust, there are other reasons that people oppose vaccination and pandemic responses. In the next chapter, we'll focus on the attitude that prizes individual rights over public health. Not everyone wants to be part of the herd.

9 Loss of Liberties

Cooperation is one of the defining characteristics of a society, including and especially ours. In other words, it's a requirement for social living. Across the animal kingdom, in all kinds of ways, groups of individuals of the same species cooperate by organizing and acting in coordination for mutual benefit. Whether they're dividing labor, sharing food, or fending off external threats, in many cases it's all for one and one for all. Of course, the *Three Musketeers* strategy works best when everybody has the same priorities.

Colonial invertebrates, in this sense, make nearly perfect societies. These spineless species, such as corals and sponges, live in colonies composed of members (called zooids) who are physically integrated, wholly interdependent, and genetically identical. Truly, there's no *I* in their tightly knit teams. Zooids are so unified, in fact, that a colony as a whole qualifies as an organism. They may not look like a pinnacle of social evolution, but with their remarkable cohesiveness and cooperative behavior, that's exactly how biologist E. O. Wilson rated these selfless animals.[1]

Social insects, such as ants, termites, and some bees and wasps, occupy another peak in social organization. They also live in colonies, where tasks like foraging or nest construction are doled out between sets of individuals, whose duties can shift with colony demands. All the workers are self-sacrificing in the service of a queen (the only female in the colony who reproduces), but they help one another too. As a case in point, insect foragers are said to have a "social stomach" because they ingest food outside the nest and then regurgitate some of it to share with their nest mates. And even though each colony member is a physically separate entity, none of them can survive for long on their own. Carpenter ants (*Camponotus fellah*), for example, can last for barely a week in social isolation before dying.[2]

Vertebrates, the backboned species like us, are a different story. Cooperation comes in many different forms, along with antisocial behaviors that dial up the drama, such as aggression, competition, and selfishness. Members of vertebrate society can afford to be selfish (that is, act in the interests of their subgroups or themselves at the expense of the collective) because each one is a potentially independent, reproducing unit. That means that sticking with the larger group might increase an individual's chances of survival in some circumstances, but it's not necessary all the time. In any case, vertebrate society can be tense and brutal, remarks Wilson; the sick and injured may be left where they fall, without so much as a pause in the routine business of feeding, resting, and mating, although some members may express concern.[3] In chapter 7, we considered one such episode of indifference in the sad saga of Mr. McGregor, a chimpanzee who was ostracized for illness by all but one of his group members.

Human society is vertebrate in many characteristics, but unique among animals in the manner and means by which we cooperate. Teamwork, as evolutionary biologist David Sloan Wilson writes, is our signature adaptation as a species.[4] Mentally and physically, our teamwork is unmatched in how we cooperate in groups of unrelated individuals, think and communicate in coordination with each other, and transmit learned information across generations. This kind of cooperative sociality is different from how other great apes perceive and do things. And it may have arisen from selective pressures that allowed early humans to begin to think of themselves as a *we* of independent individuals. Whereas chimpanzees act in parallel while chasing a monkey or looking at a banana, our human thinking allows for truly joint activities (for example, we are chasing a monkey together, each with our own role) and joint attention (for instance, we are looking at a banana together, each with our own perspective), argues comparative psychologist Michael Tomasello.[5]

How all of this cooperation developed on a societal level is a heated dispute. Scientists like the Wilsons mentioned above have promoted a theory that natural selection acts on groups rather than only on individual organisms or genes. By favoring some groups over others, group selection supposedly led to the evolution of prosocial traits such as altruism (that is, the opposite of selfishness) among our ancestors. This idea was first raised by Darwin, who introduced the theory of evolution via natural selection with naturalist Alfred Wallace in the 1850s. Darwin suggested that morality doesn't help much in a competition between individuals (such as when one person plays fair and another cheats), but having a high moral standard gives a *group* the upper hand over others (such as when one group is law-abiding and another is chaotic).[6] The Wilsons put it more succinctly in 2007, asserting that "selfishness beats altruism within groups. Altruistic groups beat selfish groups."[7]

I'm not an advocate for group selection as an evolutionary process, but I do see the benefits of group-minded behavior when it comes to infectious diseases. Lots of people do. When rules and restrictions are used to enforce public health measures that limit the transmission of pathogens, however, some people see the hand of tyranny. They see temporary inconveniences to their normal behavior as a violation of their civil liberties by an overreaching authority. And they may refuse to comply, to the disadvantage of us all.

In the last chapter, we examined public distrust as a liability in pandemic prevention. Here we'll look more closely at the pathogen-spreading effects of human individualism, a philosophy that elevates the freedoms of the individual above the welfare of the collective—a complementary social theory to the evolutionary concept of selfishness. After examining some examples of individualism and collectivism during the COVID-19 pandemic, we'll dip into a bit of history of this conflict. Then we'll consider what can and should be done to strengthen our social immune system, the kind of collective response that's essential for ending a pandemic and possibly preventing the next one.

Outside the Norm

My vision of a life altered by COVID-19 began to sharpen during the seismic month of January 2020. For the first few weeks, I had a faint mental sketch of empty streets and crowded hospitals, drawn from reports of the growing emergency in Wuhan. Although COVID-19 cases were starting to pop up in other countries, China was the first place in the world to impose a lockdown because of it. But even in a nation with a recent experience with SARS, it was a fearfully strange turn of events. The quarantine of at least fifty million human beings in Wuhan and other cities in Hubei Province on January 23 was unprecedented in public health history.[8]

One week later, I was watching a presentation on COVID-19 given by my colleague Dan Lucey at the Cannon House Office Building (one of the complexes where members of Congress have offices) in Washington, DC. The new disease didn't even have its official name yet, but everyone was buzzing about it. Speaking in front of colorful, do-it-yourself *Outbreak* panels, Dan addressed a seminar room of mostly congressional staffers, who would presumably pass along the highlights of his presentation to the lawmakers who employed them. Since then, I've often wondered how many other people took away the same flashbulb memory that I did.

It was the last thing that Dan said and did that really stuck with me. After going over the current state of knowledge about the novel coronavirus and reasoning that the extent of its spread was likely underestimated, Dan concluded his talk by pulling a surgical mask out of his pocket. "In case you're wondering how bad this is going to get," he said, scanning rows of faces and holding up the mask for everyone to see. "We should all get used to wearing these." And with that ominous warning, he put the mask on his face and stood silent for a moment, as if posing for a portrait of our pandemic future.

It was January 30, 2020. Not thirty minutes later, the United States reported its first confirmed case of the person-to-person transmission of SARS-CoV-2.

Mask wearing in public was a startling prospect at that time, at least in some parts of the world. Most people in the United States had no cultural preparation for its purpose or practice. Eventually it became common and widely supported across the United States during the COVID-19 pandemic. But not everywhere, not by everyone, and not soon enough. The same could be said of the stay-at-home orders. During the critical early months after the emergence of COVID-19, the United States struggled with an uncoordinated response that created, as journalist Ed Yong wrote in May 2020, a patchwork pandemic: the federal government delegated responsibility to state governments and in effect ceded the country to the virus.[9]

Confusing and contradictory communication by public health authorities was partly to blame for the lack of coordination. After months of actually discouraging healthy people from wearing face masks, the CDC issued a recommendation to wear masks in public places on April 3, 2020, more than two months after Dan tried to sound the alarm on Capitol Hill. But the new guidance was announced by US president Trump, who immediately added that mask wearing was voluntary and he himself wouldn't do it.[10]

The CDC guidance should have come sooner given how much evidence in support of mask wearing was already available. In July 2020, CDC director Robert Redfield acknowledged the mounting data that masking works for preventing SARS-CoV-2 transmission. "I think that if we could get everybody to wear a mask right now," he declared, "I really do think over the next four, six, eight weeks, we could bring this epidemic under control."[11] Two days earlier, Trump wore a mask in public for the first time.

Unfortunately it was too little and far too late. The United States was already leading the world with more than 150,000 COVID-related deaths by then. In August 2020, Redfield and his colleagues made another push for solidarity by publishing an editorial in the *Journal of the American Medical Association* titled "Universal Masking to Prevent SARS-CoV-2 Transmission— The Time Is Now." Citing abundant evidence that face masks can block the transmission of SARS-CoV-2, their article ended with a strong statement that the US public needed "consistent, clear, and appealing messaging that normalizes community masking," which was described as both a small sacrifice and civic duty.[12]

The article would have been more helpful, in my opinion, if it had acknowledged that the United States was a straggling outlier in the world of masking. At least it would have been more honest. The authors didn't mention that more than fifty countries had already imposed mask requirements, some of which had been in place for months.[13] They also failed to acknowledge that Trump and other US leaders had been downplaying the importance of wearing masks since the beginning of the pandemic. Of course, Trump continued to disagree with Redfield on the epidemic-ending potential of universal masking and rejected outright any possibility of a nationwide mask mandate. "I want people to have a certain freedom," he said when asked about it.[14]

Personal freedom was and remains a popular excuse to not wear a mask. For the same reason, many people rallied against lockdown orders that preceded the mask guidance and refused to get vaccinated after COVID-19 vaccines became available. Often buttressed by doubts about the effectiveness of such measures, antimandate mantras framed angry and sometimes violent protests around the country. Protesters launched accusations of socialism, communism, and fascism at local officials, whose health orders were seen as outrageous transgressions of constitutional rights. In mid-April 2020, Trump amplified the antigovernment rhetoric on social media

with Tweets to "LIBERATE MICHIGAN!" and "LIBERATE MINNESOTA!,"
two states whose Democratic governors imposed strict physical distancing
restrictions in response to skyrocketing COVID-19 infections and hospitalizations.[15] As COVID-19 killed more and more people in the United States,
public health actions became increasingly politicized, and more and more
protests became crucibles of antimandate messages.[16]

The freedom argument is a weak defense of selfishness. When a deadly
airborne virus is tearing through vulnerable populations, personal behaviors such as covering your face, avoiding crowds, and getting vaccinated
protect not only yourself but other members of society too. Refusing to
do so violates everyone else's rights to a safe social life along with a return
to school, business, travel, and recreation as soon as possible. Plus there
are plenty of other permanent restrictions that protect public health and
safety, such as smoking bans and speed limits, that antimandate activists
have to follow every day. In fact, since 1980, there have been laws that
require vaccination for school attendance in all fifty US states. Perhaps the
difference with COVID-19 restrictions was their overt packaging as cooperative, community-focused actions. This is an ethos of collectivism that's
absolutely essential to controlling infectious disease, and it's absolutely at
odds with an individual-centered mentality.

*   *   *

The COVID-19 pandemic was experienced differently by every city, region,
and country in the world, not just every US state. And the United States
wasn't the only country with COVID-19 "freedom fighters," although it
was probably the most tolerant of them. Throughout the pandemic, protests against public health measures took place all over the globe, with
huge variation in their scale, motivations, and participants. According to
the 2021 World Global Peace Index, more than 5,000 COVID-related violent incidents in at least 158 countries took place from January 2020 to
April 2021.[17] Some of them were driven by anger about lockdowns and
other restrictions, while others protested lax responses by governments
that didn't acknowledge the severity of the pandemic and its economic
impacts. In the bigger picture, each one of them was an amalgam of numerous causes and accusations.

Outcries for civil liberties arose in a number of western European nations,
where requirements and restrictions were far stricter than in the United

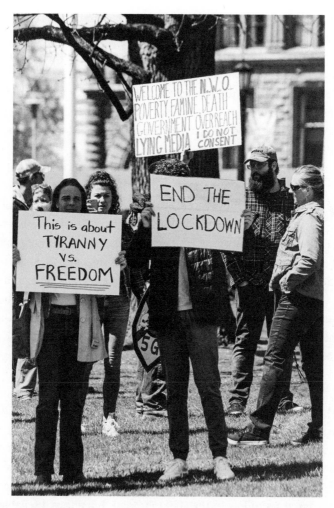

Figure 9.1
COVID-19 protest in Toronto, Canada, in 2020. Protesters in Toronto gathered in Queen's Park with signs that demanded the end of the COVID-19 lockdown and compared the governmental measure to tyranny. *Source:* michael_swan.

States. National mandates and health passes that limited the public activities of unmasked and unvaccinated individuals were compared to slavery, segregation, apartheid, and the Holocaust. Democratic governments were accused of dictatorship, as people in Belgium, France, Germany, Italy, the Netherlands, Spain, and the United Kingdom (plus elsewhere) took to the streets by the thousands. In Austria, the political party Menschen Freiheit Grundrechte was founded largely in opposition to COVID-19 measures, which party members likened to Nazi rule.[18]

But not every country's COVID-19 story is rife with conflict. Although the outbreak started in China, countries in the Asia-Pacific region of the world were on average most successful at containing the spread of SARS-CoV-2 with respect to tests, infections, and deaths.[19] Social cohesion seemed to be an advantage at the outset of the pandemic, along with capable institutions and small populations, although there's no single or simple explanation for each outcome. But some of these nations provide a compelling contrast to the kind of pandemic-prolonging behaviors that contributed to the poor performance of countries like the United States (which ironically, was ranked highest in pandemic preparedness by the Global Health Security Index in 2019).[20]

If we rewind to January 23, 2020, when Wuhan and other cities in Hubei Province began a complete lockdown of untried proportions, the timeline in China follows a different series of events and reactions. Given its well-documented record of censorship and data manipulation during public health crises, including an initial lack of transparency and underreporting about SARS in 2003, the Chinese government was an unreliable narrator of the unfolding disaster.[21] Yet Chinese journalists, doctors, and other brave citizens cracked a window in the Great Firewall that allowed reliable information to reach millions of people on the outside.[22] Chinese author Wang Fang (who uses the pen name Fang Fang) was one of the voices that broke through the seventy-six-day quarantine of Wuhan, writing a diary of her experiences and reflections in daily installments on various Chinese social media platforms and microblogging sites, which were later compiled and translated into English for her book *Wuhan Diary*.

The Chinese public health policy described in Fang's diary is a "zero-COVID" approach that aims to completely stop the community spread of the virus by shutting down normal social and economic activities in an area until the number of new infections drops to and stays at zero. It's the polar opposite of learning to live with the virus, and China's public health restrictions under this policy were the most stringent in the world. It inflicted terrible depression and psychological trauma on Wuhan's residents, who were mostly or entirely confined to their homes for a period of nearly eleven weeks. Despite Fang's unflinching criticism of the Chinese government for its handling of the COVID-19 outbreak, though, she declared that the lockdown was clearly necessary. Her main complaint was not about the collective sacrifice of the people of Wuhan but instead that it should have happened earlier.

As I watched Dan don a face mask on Capitol Hill on January 30, before an audience who probably had never worn one, the residents of Wuhan were utterly desperate for them. Having used face masks as a public health measure for more than a century, Chinese citizens didn't need to be convinced of the effectiveness of these tools. On the contrary, a shortage of masks was their single-greatest worry at the beginning of the lockdown. Against this challenge and others, Fang describes how Wuhan's millions of inhabitants self-organized and worked together in neighborhood groups to make online purchases for their daily necessities. And they cooperated with all the government's requests, according to the diarist, with restraint and patience that made it possible to contain the virus. "Everyone is about at the point where they can no longer take it anymore. . . . [W]e all want to get out," she posted on February 21, adding, "But there is nothing we can do; in order to stay safe, in order to survive, in order to plan for the future, we must just close our doors, stay inside, and wait. If there's one thing we can do to help during this outbreak, this is it."[23] Her sentiments aligned with on-the-ground observations by a Canadian team member of a WHO-China Joint Mission who visited Wuhan and other Chinese cities during the same month. "Everywhere you went, anyone you spoke to, there was a sense of responsibility and collective action," he marveled.[24]

Initially, China suppressed the Wuhan outbreak with greater success than many public health experts thought was possible. When the quarantine was lifted on April 8, after two weeks of no reported new cases, the city's residents were jubilant, and onlookers were amazed. Still, not everyone thought that a zero-COVID policy could or should be attempted elsewhere. Some experts noted that China is rather unique in having an authoritarian political system that assures public compliance with extreme measures as well as an extraordinary ability to complete labor-intensive, large-scale projects with speed. While the mandatory quarantine in Wuhan was a big part of their temporary victory over the virus, Chinese authorities also built two COVID-19 hospitals in just over one week, dispatched more than eighteen hundred contact-tracing teams throughout the city, and used cell phone apps to keep track of people's movements and stop those with confirmed infections from traveling. "Whether it works is not the only measure of whether something is a good public health control measure," argued global health lawyer Alexandra Phelan. "There are plenty of things that would work to stop an outbreak that we would consider abhorrent in a just and free society."[25]

China's zero-COVID measures became more contentious as the pandemic wore on, such as when the residents of Shanghai found themselves in a Wuhan-like situation of mass quarantine and censorship in 2022.[26] In China's commercial capital of 26 million people, the majority of residents were confined to their homes for two months and in some cases denied treatment for serious medical conditions.[27] Similarly grueling lockdowns were enacted in other parts of the country as the Chinese government tried to stamp out every case of COVID-19 wherever the virus was detected. In the far western region of Xinjiang, where some residents of the city of Urumqi spent a hundred days under lockdown, the restrictions were blamed for at least ten deaths that resulted from an apartment fire. In response, across a country in which public dissent is rare, thousands of protesters took to the streets and called for an end to the COVID-19 lockdowns. "Need human rights, need freedom," people chanted.[28]

Before the end of the year, the Chinese government announced a reversal of its pandemic strategy—a dramatic swing from zero-COVID to minimal restrictions. But confusing messaging and guidance about the new rules led to a chaotic national reopening in 2023, with the abrupt abandonment of lockdowns, mass testing, quarantines, and contact tracing.[29] As a consequence, the virus (in particular, the highly transmissible Omicron subvariants) tore through China's population of 1.4 billion people, most of whom lacked protection from previous exposures or high-efficacy vaccines. Without reliable data from Chinese officials, researchers estimated that China's COVID-19 wave may have killed up to 1.5 million people and infected as much as 90 percent of the population in a little more than a month— possibly the fastest spread of a respiratory virus in modern history.[30]

By comparison, some of China's neighboring countries that acted immediately and aggressively in early 2020, but with a less draconian approach, were widely praised for their effective COVID-19 strategies. Even so, public cooperation was vital to containment.

For instance, South Korea announced its first case of COVID-19 on January 20, 2020 (as did the United States) and went from a handful of cases per week to more than nine hundred in a single day by the end of February. Yet the country quickly flattened its epidemic curve without locking down the affected areas. Instead, the South Korean government launched a high-tech system of massive testing, contact tracing, and case isolation, including innovations such as mobile apps and drive-through testing centers. It built innovative, high-capacity screening facilities and worked closely with industry partners to ensure an adequate supply of tests from the onset of the pandemic.

South Korean authorities prioritized communication and transparency about COVID-19 risks after being criticized during a 2015 MERS outbreak in which the names of hospitals treating patients were withheld from the public. Consequently, when someone in South Korea tested positive for COVID-19, people living near them could get a text alert with information about that individual's age, gender, and movements down to the minute—in some cases traced using closed-circuit television and credit card transactions, with the time and names of the businesses they had visited. Numerous websites and mobile apps were created to collect and map the data so that people could avoid places with potential transmission risks. And despite some controversy over privacy concerns, people in South Korea generally supported the disclosures, which placed the public good above individual rights.[31] Having learned from MERS, another coronavirus-caused respiratory disease with an even higher fatality rate than COVID-19, they were also willing to wear masks, cooperate with contract tracers, and otherwise listen to public health officials without excessive complaints.[32]

New Zealand stands out as another example of a successful collective response to the initial spread of COVID-19, helped by its geographic situation as a small island country. Lacking any previous experience with highly pathogenic human coronaviruses (save one probable SARS case in 2003), in February 2020, the New Zealand government began implementing its pandemic influenza plan, which included preparing hospitals for an influx of patients and instituting border-control policies to delay the pandemic's arrival. After confirming its first COVID-19 case at the end of the month, there was clear evidence of community transmission by mid-March, but the country lacked sufficient testing and contact tracing to contain the virus.[33] Switching from a strategy of mitigation to elimination, the government therefore implemented a stringent countrywide lockdown that lasted for seven weeks. On June 8, the pandemic was declared over in New Zealand, 103 days after the first identified case and 20 months before the next surge in 2022.

If there was any single voice that carried the people of New Zealand through quarantine, it belonged to its prime minister, Jacinda Ardern, who spoke to her country as "our team of five million" that could only beat the virus through cooperation. With clear and consistent messaging that kept Kiwis united under the burdens of pandemic restrictions, Ardern's policies garnered high levels of public confidence and compliance; in one poll conducted near the end of the lockdown, more than 90 percent of the respondents said that it was the right decision by the government.[34] By the time the virus did become widespread in New Zealand, the vast majority of adults had been immunized, resulting in fewer than 2,500 COVID-19 fatalities by 2023—the lowest COVID-19-related death rate in the Western world.[35]

Ardern was not without detractors in the end, however, as a small minority of protesters opposed to lockdowns and vaccines compared her to Adolf Hitler and began to follow her around the country. She resigned as New Zealand's prime minister in 2023, leaving behind an admirable legacy of public health protection as well as a new shocking climate of political polarization and extreme rhetoric. In a nod to the far-right movements in the United States and Europe, she called the latter an "imported style of protest that we have not seen in New Zealand before."[36]

*   *   *

From place to place, a multitude of factors contributed to the striking contrasts in experiences during the COVID-19 pandemic. The country-level snapshots above are woefully insufficient to capture the complexity of each situation. But if we zoom out to a panoramic picture of worldwide variation, some of the most glaring failures and successes are unmissable contrasts in individualism and collectivism—a cultural dimension that captures the extent to which people in a society care more about their own needs, goals, and interests than the well-being of the group.[37]

Mask wearing was a deadly lightning rod within individualistic countries like the United States. A survey of in the United States in July 2020 showed that 20 percent of the respondents didn't wear a face mask, despite requirements or recommendations to do so.[38] The number one reason given by 40 percent of them was their right not to wear a mask. (This is ridiculous, by the way, as legal and medical experts have made clear: the US Constitution isn't a suicide pact that guarantees a right to harm others whether refusing masks or vaccines.)[39] About another quarter of them said they didn't wear a mask because it's uncomfortable, making a total of 64 percent of nonmasking people in the United States who refused to cover their faces for reasons of personal inconvenience over protecting themselves and others against COVID-19.

But not all US states are equally individualistic, and mask wearing across the country varied accordingly. Using survey data from July 2020, studies have shown that collectivism and mask usage were linked at the state level, with low mask usage in strongly individualistic states like Montana and North Dakota, and high mask usage in more collectivist states like Hawaii. By no coincidence, Hawaii had the best health outcome from the COVID-19 pandemic in the country.[40]

The same pattern emerged at the country level in a global data set as collectivistic countries like South Korea, Thailand, the United Arab Emirates, and Mexico were high in mask usage, whereas individualistic countries like the United States and United Kingdom were low in mask usage. Unsurprisingly, further research revealed that countries scoring high in individualism generally had more severe COVID-19 situations throughout the trajectory of the pandemic.[41]

Another cultural variable related to individualism is looseness, characterized by weakly defined norms, tolerance for norm-violating behaviors, and a lack of formality and discipline. In culturally loose countries like the United States and Brazil, people therefore faced fewer COVID-19 restrictions and were more likely to violate those put in place. On the other hand, people in culturally tighter countries with strictly defined and enforced norms, such as South Korea and Singapore, were more willing to cooperate with rules that required physical distancing, wearing masks, and avoiding large crowds. By October 2020, looser nations had five times more COVID-19

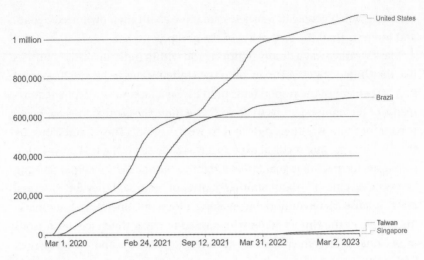

Figure 9.2
Cumulative confirmed COVID-19 deaths across countries. During the COVID-19 pandemic, culturally loose countries with fewer COVID-19 restrictions (such as the United States and Brazil) experienced worse mortality statistics than culturally tighter ones with more restrictions and stronger enforcement of them (such as Taiwan and Singapore). *Source:* Johns Hopkins University CSSE COVID-19 Data.

cases and more than eight times as many COVID-19 deaths than tighter ones. For instance, Singapore and Taiwan reported barely any COVID-19 deaths (5 and 0.3 per 1 million inhabitants, respectively), whereas the United States and Brazil had the highest mortality rates in the world (both around 700 per 1 million inhabitants).[42]

Eighteen months later, the United States and Brazil retained this morbid distinction with more than 3,000 deaths per million people. As of June 2023, the United States reported the most deaths of any country worldwide: more than a million lives lost so far. And this number is almost certainly an undercount.

Ironically, nearly half of the US deaths from COVID-19 occurred after COVID-19 vaccines were made readily available in the United States, a country that produced three of them in record time. This isn't because the vaccines didn't work. On the contrary, they worked extraordinarily well. The problem was that people didn't want them; by the time that the death toll reached the 1 million mark, about one-third of people across the United States still weren't fully vaccinated. Many people declined to be vaccinated out of distrust and misinformation, as we discussed in chapter 8 and will explore further in chapter 10. Others simply didn't see COVID-19 as a real threat, resisting vaccination on the same grounds as they resisted lockdowns and masks as unnecessary and unfair.[43]

Roots of Resistance

Whether they know it or not, people who seek to defend their civil liberties against public health policies are making an unoriginal argument. Public opposition to health mandates started to coalesce in Victorian England after the passage of the Compulsory Vaccination Act of 1853. As the first legislation to require smallpox vaccination for all infants in England and Wales, including a fine or imprisonment for noncompliant parents, the act sparked immediate outrage and resistance.[44] The subsequent Vaccination Act of 1867 extended the compulsory vaccination age requirement to fourteen years old and introduced cumulative penalties for disobedience. Drawing thousands of objectors, the Anti-Compulsory Vaccination League was founded on the premise that the vaccination laws trampled on the civil liberties of parents and that Parliament was failing in its duty to protect them. The organization expanded and evolved over decades as the antivaccination movement spread internationally.

Lest we forget, smallpox was an absolutely horrific disease. Today most of us are fortunate to have never experienced it because of the success of global vaccination. But even as antivaccinationists witnessed endless outbreaks of smallpox during the nineteenth century, they waged a pressure campaign against vaccination laws with a cascade of books, journals, and demonstrations. The protesters reaped success with the Vaccination Act in 1898, which eliminated cumulative penalties and introduced a conscience clause, allowing parents who opposed vaccination to obtain a certificate of exemption. As a result of the new option of conscientious objection, the parents of about two hundred thousand children soon opted out of the procedure. The United Kingdom ultimately repealed vaccination requirements altogether in 1946 because by then nearly half of parents in many areas were claiming conscientious exemptions.[45] As of 2023, there are no mandatory vaccination policies in the United Kingdom for the general public, as the UK government scrapped a plan to require COVID-19 vaccination for workers in certain health and social care roles in 2022.[46]

Interestingly, the United States passed its first vaccination law in 1809 in the state of Massachusetts, which empowered the board of health of a city or town to require as well as enforce smallpox vaccination and revaccination among its inhabitants. And it endured. But almost a century later, the constitutionality of the Massachusetts law was challenged by a Lutheran pastor named Henning Jacobson, who was prosecuted and fined for refusing to be vaccinated during an outbreak of smallpox in the Boston area in 1901.[47] Jacobson had a bad reaction to smallpox vaccination as a child in Sweden and didn't want to risk it again. Thus in a lawsuit that went all the way to the US Supreme Court in 1905, he argued that the law was an "unreasonable, arbitrary, and oppressive" invasion of his liberty, and "hostile to the inherent right of every freeman to care for his own body and health in such way as to him seems best."[48]

The Court disagreed. In a seven-to-two decision, the majority of the justices upheld that US states had the discretion to require smallpox vaccination in order to protect public health. People couldn't be forcibly vaccinated, but they could be arrested, fined, imprisoned, quarantined, isolated, or excluded from school if they refused. And hence the Court wrote, "The liberty secured by the constitution of the United States to every person within its jurisdiction does not import an absolute right in each person to be, at all times and in all circumstances, wholly freed from restraint. There are manifold restraints to which every person is necessarily subject for the common good. On any other basis, organized society could not exist with safety to its members."[49] Furthermore, it pointed out, if each individual had the right to behave without any regard for the potential harm done to others, real liberty for all couldn't exist.

The ruling on *Jacobson v. Massachusetts* mobilized the antivaccination movement in the United States, including the establishment of the Anti-Vaccination League of America several years later. Subsequent generations have carried on this battle for personal freedom against the public health establishment. But US courts have continued to uphold and rely on the case, which provided a 115-year-old legal precedent to justify mask mandates and stay-at-home orders throughout the COVID-19 pandemic as well.

*   *   *

There may be no other country with a deeper history of widespread mask resistance than the United States, starting with the first mask mandate in

San Francisco during the 1918 influenza pandemic. Numerous communities in the US West required mask wearing for a short time, and elsewhere masks were strongly recommended as protection against the fatal flu. Yet like in 2020, masks soon became a symbol of government overreach for some of the public, provoking protests, petitions, defiant bareface gatherings, and conflict.[50] Thousands of San Francisco Bay Area residents even came together as a short-lived organization known as the Anti-Mask League of San Francisco, which opposed the city's second mask ordinance in 1919. Mere weeks into the mandate, the Anti-Mask League submitted a request for a repeal of the ordinance to the city's Board of Supervisors, with one league member calling masks "an infringement on our personal liberty" and "not in keeping with the spirit of a truly democratic people" while urging Mayor James Rolph to end them.[51]

Although Rolph was famous for his affable personality (which earned him the nickname of "Sunny Jim"), he had no smiles for mask slackers. After firmly stating his obligation to respect and enforce the law, he blasted the complaint with a scathing rebuke:

> Do you think I am going to stultify myself here against the wish of 99.5 percent of the doctors; against the officials of the army and navy? The people felt a great relief when the masking ordinance was put in effect. You don't realize the misery and death that has followed this epidemic, nor the forces required to help these people. We should give our minds to serious matters instead of fighting the little inconvenience occasioned by the wearing of a mask for the protection of the general public . . . Why don't you do something for the returning soldiers instead of fighting against the methods employed by the Board of Health to stamp out the influenza epidemic?[52]

Rolph lifted the mask requirement several days later, but only because the Board of Health recommended it. The Anti-Mask League disbanded at the same time, and the pandemic faded into history months later. Both live on in stories and images that provide the closest parallels to the COVID-19 pandemic a century later.

*   *   *

While some zealous San Franciscans were fixating on a piece of cloth, a poor woman with legitimate concerns about personal liberty was imprisoned on the other side of the country. But Mallon, the contagious cook whom we met in chapter 2, wasn't held captive by a temporary or universal

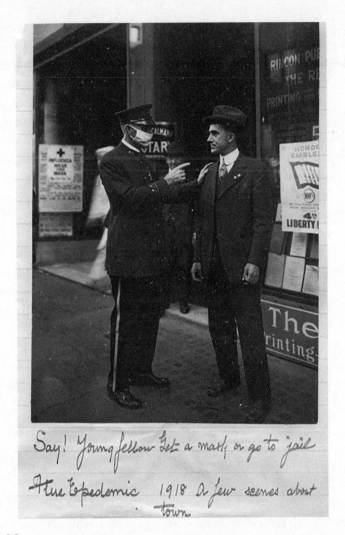

Figure 9.3
Mask resistance in San Francisco in 1918. In this photo, a masked police officer accosts an unmasked man in San Francisco, where city leaders enacted mask requirements during the influenza pandemic. The handwritten caption underneath the photo reads, "Say! Young fellow get a mask or go to jail. Flue [*sic*] Epedemic [*sic*] 1918 A few scenes about town." *Source:* California State Library, photograph by Hamilton Henry Dobbin.

restriction; the sentence was indefinite, and it was hers alone to serve. And her case shows that a demand for personal rights and disdain for public health aren't necessarily the same thing.

Mallon was the first healthy carrier of typhoid fever to be identified in North America, but she wasn't the last.[53] Like hundreds of other New Yorkers who came after her, Mallon was accused of harboring typhoid bacilli in her gallbladder and transmitting the disease through contaminated feces and urine via unwashed hands. Adamantly denying the charge, Mallon was arrested as a health menace under the authority of the New York City Health Department, whose sweeping powers forced her to live in isolation and submit to study (which stopped short of removing her gallbladder, at her refusal) on North Brother Island in the East River of New York City. Health and legal authorities subjugated her freedoms to the safety of society as fiercely as Mallon fought for them.

Following Mallon's incarceration from 1907 to 1910, the New York State Board of Health and health commissioner consented to her release on the conditions that she change her occupation and practice proper hand hygiene. Mallon agreed to the terms, but never accepted that she transmitted typhoid fever to the people for whom she cooked. And when Mallon's cooking was blamed for another typhoid outbreak in 1915, she was cast back into isolation until her death in 1938.

Would it have been possible to protect public health without taking away Mallon's liberty for twenty-six years? In posing this question, historian Judith Leavitt has pointed out that no other healthy carriers identified by health authorities were isolated for life.[54] Not even "Typhoid John," an Adirondack guide who was linked to even more infections and deaths than Mallon in 1909. His case highlighted the absence of a law in the United States for restraining the movements of typhoid carriers, and he consented to experimental therapy for his condition instead.[55] But Mallon didn't benefit from such an arrangement, nor was she offered any financial or reemployment assistance from the state of New York, unlike other healthy typhoid carriers beginning in 1918. Health authorities chose not to exercise their power to create an environment in which Mallon could have become more compliant with their demands, regardless of whether she accepted the theory of healthy carriers.[56]

Mallon's status as an unmarried, Irish-born woman most likely influenced how she was treated by health officials, courts, and the media. Her evocative characterization as Typhoid Mary implied that she purposefully spread the disease, but there's no evidence that she was individualistic or truly understood the risks she posed to others. By many accounts, she was quite caring of the families that she fed. Thus her return to cooking after her first imprisonment may have been a choice of survival rather than an act of malevolence given her limited employment options.

Still, if Mallon did have any disregard for the greater good, maybe that's because she didn't even feel that she had any part in it. Foreign-born people like Mallon were excluded from the collective in merciless ways, not counting her physical removal from US society for disobedience. "If she had confidence in a benevolent system, she would have been more inclined to cooperate with authorities," Leavitt opines. "Instead, she had reason to believe the system would work against her, that who she was—a poor, immigrant, single, middle-aged woman—made her vulnerable to harm by the system rather than protection by it."[57] Mallon's story is a lesson in the importance of equitable and transparent public health policies in the past as well as today.

Embracing Humanity

The various health mandates that come into play during a pandemic are grounded in our interdependence as a species. We evolved with unparalleled success to become highly social, cooperative, and empathetic creatures, most of whom probably couldn't survive isolation for much longer than an errant ant. In this way, as anthropologist Robin Nelson says, we humans have an evolutionary mandate to be generous and take care of one another.[58] But nowadays, our social groups are far bigger and even more interconnected than their foraging-friendly sizes throughout the majority of human history. That means that we have to care about people we don't know and places we haven't even been. We have to understand ourselves and our health in terms of multitude.

Individualism relies on a myth of self-reliance that makes societies sick. Literally. It's the kind of mentality that overlooks the infectious part of an infectious disease. So why do some people buy into it, especially, it seems, during a public health crisis? If eliminating a virus were like chasing a monkey, then maybe more individualists would see the incentives of teamwork. Yet in the case of infectious disease control, the target of the project is invisible, the rewards are intangible, and your partners are often (and sometimes by necessity) nowhere near you. None of it is obvious.

And so education is part of the process. There's formal and family education, which can guide children in thinking and behaving as *we* as well as *me*. But public education, including for adults, is also critical for framing and focusing the challenges at hand. Throughout the COVID-19 pandemic, particularly in the early months, there were subtle and overt pleas for unity and cooperation from leaders and authorities around the world. The top US public health official, Anthony Fauci, emphasized that following public health guidelines was both a personal and societal responsibility, telling the public again and again that "we're all in this together."[59] He nevertheless couldn't do anything about the contradictory messages from the US president and his like-minded allies, who amplified an antithetical ideology of individual independence. Nor were Fauci, CDC officials, and many other scientists perfect in their public communications about the virus and its risks.

Clearly there's a strong cultural component to individualism around the world, meaning that it can be cultivated by our social environment. Some people are much less inclined to sacrifice their personal interests for others because they haven't been raised or reinforced in doing so. This wasn't such an issue when humans lived almost exclusively in small groups. Yet now we're a *we* on a global scale. And to think of a pandemic in terms of *me* is to partake in a lot more suffering than necessary.

As such, many leaders are right to foster a more collectivistic mindset among their constituents regarding promoting safe conduct during the COVID-19 pandemic. But cultural differences in the value of individualism should be considered too. Some researchers have suggested that in cases where the individualistic tendencies are deeply rooted, it might be better to stress the individual benefits of safe conduct and vaccination instead of making the case for collectivistic social responsibility.[60] That is, messages that speak to one's responsibility toward the community might be more effective within collectivistic communities, and within individualistic communities, self-protection messages might work better.

This approach is borne out by evidence. From survey data across the United States, studies have shown that messages about COVID-19 vaccines can be more effective with an individual frame, such as taking care of one's own health, rather than a collective frame that highlights the significance of thinking about community health.[61] People with positive attitudes toward COVID-19 vaccination weren't affected by individual versus collective frames, and so the type of message they read didn't alter their willingness to be vaccinated.[62] Among people who held negative attitudes toward vaccination, however, the individual frame was more persuasive.

Importantly, people exposed to more conservative media were also more impacted by messages with individual framing. One reason for the correlation might be rooted in conservative psychology, which is associated with greater concern for smaller and more well-defined social circles, such as family over friends and the nation versus the world.[63] This interpretation lines up with a global pattern in which people on the ideological Right in most advanced economies favored fewer COVID-19 restrictions.[64] But in the United States at least, another factor is the role of conservative media in shaping misperceptions about COVID-19; research conducted at the outset of the pandemic showed that conservative media users were more likely to believe conspiracy theories and other misinformation promoted by conservative media sources such as Fox News.[65] Two years later, with conservative (Republican) voters accounting for nearly two-thirds of the unvaccinated people in the United States, political partisanship was the single most reliable predictor of vaccination status in the country.[66]

Misinformation is a tragic irony of the world today because communication is a hallmark of humanity. No other species communicates better than we do. But apparently, no other species communicates as harmfully either. In the next chapter, we'll examine this phenomenon as perhaps our most damaging pandemic feature of all.

Human beings are a species defined by knowing a lot. Designating ourselves as *Homo sapiens*, a name invented by Swedish taxonomist Carl Linnaeus in 1758, we're the self-described wise one in the tree of life. And with respect to our mental abilities, it's a fair claim. We have an awesome capacity for producing, sharing, and understanding information. But that doesn't mean that all the information is true.

Broadly speaking, any information that's false is misinformation.[1] We all participate in the spread of misinformation, often with good intentions and frequently by error. "To err is human," as English poet Alexander Pope wrote in 1711. Incidentally, in the same poem, he also wrote that "a little learning is a dangerous thing"—because it can lead someone to believe that they know more than they actually do.[2]

Pope would have appreciated the dangers of misinformation as well as anybody, certainly in matters of health. Suffering from tuberculosis and other debilitating diseases since birth, he was a lifelong subject of eighteenth-century medical knowledge. Much of it was incorrect and possibly harmful, even if it was thought to be effective at the time.[3]

Accurate information about diseases has increased enormously since then, but it's getting harder and harder to separate the facts from the fiction. And false information that's spread deliberately, known as disinformation, has skyrocketed during the so-called information age. According to disinformation expert Renée DiResta, that's because the public is now actively involved in it.[4] Beyond the traditional form of top-down propaganda in which governments, authorities, and institutions shape perceptions of reality, the new propaganda is a bottom-up phenomenon powered by regular people through online amplification. While Roman emperors used messages on coins for mass communication, and Nazis weaponized the printed press, radio, and cinema to promote their ideology, today anyone can disinform (or misinform) millions of people in seconds through the internet and its many social media platforms.[5]

Since the SARS epidemic in 2003, the term *infodemic* has been used to describe this growing problem: an overabundance of information and misinformation that spreads in digital and physical environments during a disease outbreak. During the COVID-19 pandemic, the WHO took this threat seriously, declaring that the concurrent infodemic was as dangerous to human health and security as the virus itself.[6] It was possibly more contagious too. Infodemics can cause confusion and risk-taking behaviors that lead to harm, mistrust in health authorities, and subversion of public health responses, the WHO warned. They also can intensify or lengthen a disease event, making people unsure about what they need to do to protect their health and the health of people around them. Given how the COVID-19 infodemic played out, the WHO's warning was spot-on. A better descriptor, however, might have been *misinfodemic*.

Misinformation is a deadly business. No other species inflicts as much self-damage as humans manage to accomplish with faulty knowledge , thus helping the spread of pathogens that already do quite enough damage without it. By October 2021 of the COVID-19 pandemic, for instance, it was estimated that between two and twelve million people in the United States were not vaccinated against SARS-CoV-2 because of misinformation.[7] Perhaps more than 200,000 of these people died needlessly, according to pediatrician Peter Hotez in his book *The Deadly Rise of Anti-Science: A Scientist's Warning*, considering that every US adult was eligible for COVID-19 vaccines that were over 90 percent protective against severe disease and death by May 2021.[8] The thought is bleak beyond words, especially because COVID-19 is an agonizing way to die. In this chapter, we'll look more closely at how and why humans propagate misinformation, particularly in the guise of conspiracy theories about disease origins and vaccines. Then we'll consider a historical example of how this human habit worsened an epidemic of smallpox in 1885, leading to unnecessary sickness and death. In closing, I'll discuss my own efforts to communicate accurate information and battle misinformation about emerging infectious diseases and pandemic risks, and share some of the lessons that I learned along the way, in addition to highlighting some parallel efforts around the globe.

Mechanisms of Misinformation

People often describe a strong belief as something they feel in their gut or know in their heart. And while that may be true in a sense, our thoughts and emotions are fundamentally the work of our brain. All the activities of the human body, as a matter of fact, are driven by the brain—not just thinking and emotion, but memory, movement, system functions, sensation, and communication. It's like the command center of a cargo ship, with all kinds of technologies that operate simultaneously to ensure smooth sailing. The most critical controls vary with the type of ship, depending on what the ship needs to do and the kind of conditions that it has to navigate.

A lot of things about the human brain, our command center, are nothing special. Nearly every animal has one, although corals and sponges, for instance, are brainless. Furthermore, all vertebrate brains, including ours, follow the same general plan of development. On the other hand, however, they all reflect highly variable adaptations to meet different sensory and behavioral requirements. Thus our large, complex brains evolved from a much simpler and smaller pattern found in the early vertebrates over four million years ago.[9]

With the emergence of early mammals more than two hundred million years ago, a major advance in brain evolution occurred. In contrast to the reptilian brain, mammals developed a thicker, multilayered feature for higher brain functions such as perception and cognition, thereby distinguishing them from other vertebrates today.[10] Called the neocortex, this sheet of neural tissue has widely diversified among mammalian species since the age of the dinosaurs. Ours is distinctive, but not wholly unexpected given our primate status.

Humans have a primate brain that's been supercharged through evolution. We claim the largest brain among living primates, although over a dozen bigger-brained species exist in other realms of the animal kingdom.[11] For example, the brain of a sperm whale (*Physeter macrocephalus*) is six times heavier than ours, and that of an African elephant (*Loxodonta* spp.) weighs three to four times as much. Size doesn't always scale with smarts, despite what you might have heard. But where we outdo all creatures great and small, bar none, is in the cerebral cortex, about 90 percent of which is composed of our neocortex. As it so happens, this wrinkled covering of gray matter around the human brain is responsible for its most complex types of information processing.

Our outsize cerebral cortex contains a mother lode of neurons, the cells that carry nerve signals through the brain and body as electric pulses. And the number of neurons in the cerebral cortex of a human (around sixteen billion on average, out of eighty-six billion in the entire brain) is physically unaffordable for any other species, as neuroscientist Suzana Herculano-Houzel explains in her book *The Human Advantage*. Think of it this way: the human brain accounts for 2 percent of our body mass, but consumes about five hundred kilocalories a day, which is about 25 percent of the energy that the entire human body requires. That's a costly piece of anatomy. By comparison, the brain of a mouse represents about 1 percent of its body mass, but only requires about 8 percent of its total energy it needs.

To feed such an expensive organ as the human brain, Herculano-Houzel reckons that our ancestors would have been forced to forage for more than nine hours a day. But given the rapid increase of brain size in the evolution of *Homo*, particularly over the last 1.5 million years, an equally rapid increase in caloric intake would have been better for business. This happened when early *Homo sapiens* transformed their food through another human singularity, which most of us take for granted nowadays: cooking. From that point on, our species began an ecological transition from a world of scarcity and uncertainty to one of abundance and reliability.

As humans went beyond the basics of raw food to meet their energetic demands, their bulky brains started to pay for themselves. The extraordinary number of neurons packed into our cerebral cortex provided the brainpower for transformative changes in technology, society, and culture that ultimately led us to a human-dominated planet. But this evolutionary success story (from an anthropocentric perspective, at least) also carries the caution of too much, too soon. In the same way that humans have created a world of excess food to which our bodies aren't adapted, we've created a world of ceaseless information that our brains haven't previously encountered. Both have resulted in serious health consequences that we're only beginning to recognize.

*   *   *

If you were born 35,000 years ago, your brain would be more or less identical to the one you have today. For as long as *Homo sapiens* have existed, over a period of at least 300,000 years, human brains have been essentially the same size. Their shapes, however, have changed from an elongated design (sort of like a US football) to a globular one (closer to a basketball) across thousands of generations.[12]

The globular shape of the modern human brain evolved gradually, and finally arrived at its present-day variation between about 100,000 and 35,000 years ago, with bulges in areas of the brain involved in a wide range of functions such as working memory (the ability to remember information for a limited period of time), social cognition (the processes by which people perceive, process, interpret, and respond to social behaviors), and language. At the same time, as some scientists have noted, we see evidence of modern human behavior emerge in the archaeological record: carved bone artifacts, ornaments, pigments, sophisticated stone tools, and material indicators of symbolism and abstract thought.[13]

We also see astonishing artwork. Apparently, with a Stone Age brain, a person could create some of the most spectacular cave paintings ever discovered. Hidden among the limestone gorges of Ardèche in southeastern France, within a wild terrain of honeycombed cliffs, oak forests, river meanders, and scrubland, the Grotte Chauvet-Pont d'Arc preserves breathtaking scenes of a wilder, extinct past. Dated between 37,000 and 28,000 years ago, hundreds of animal paintings and drawings adorn the cave's walls in fine detail and three-dimensional representation, from head-butting woolly rhinoceroses (*Coelodonta antiquitatis*) to snarling cave lions (*Panthera atrox*). With the notable exception of some red ocher handprints, humans are barely visible in the stone tableaux. It was an animal world, in an age when lions ruled France and our brainy forebears lived in small groups separated by miles of wilderness.[14]

Obviously things are different today. Rather than using our brains to hunt mammoths in our midst, we need them to survive in an endless social landscape. Most of us don't have to strategize with anyone in order to acquire food or put much mental energy into doing so, but our cognitive abilities are constantly challenged by nonstop interactions and information in our digital and physical spaces.

Intriguingly, it seems that our brains were already primed for these complexities and demands tens of thousands of years in the past. How and why this happened has perplexed scientists for generations, all the way back to Wallace, an evolutionary theorist who didn't understand how natural selection could endow early humans with an extreme surplus of intellectual capacity—that is, a preadaptation to environments that didn't yet exist.[15] Even if we can reasonably infer how we paid for our brains by inventing cooking, that doesn't explain our need for so much intellect in the first place.

In his book *The Overflowing Brain*, cognitive scientist Torkel Klingberg considers a number of evolutionary psychological theories that attribute the development of our intelligence and possibly our working memory to their benefits for community living, such as by facilitating social interaction and language. But other theories reject the idea of human intelligence as an adaptation, arguing instead that sexual selection (that is, impressing the opposite sex with displays of intelligence) or by-productism (for example, passing along genetic mutations for enhanced cortical areas before they had a useful function) are plausible scenarios.[16]

Another possible solution to "the paradox of how the Stone Age brain handles the twenty-first-century information flood," according to Klingberg, is that our brains adapt to their environments and are shaped by training during life.[17] Called brain plasticity, this ability of the human brain to rewire or restructure itself is well documented. For example, several studies have shown that long periods of musical instrument practice can alter brain morphology, such as enlarging an area activated by sensory impressions in musicians versus nonmusicians.[18]

But such changes can be relatively quick and temporary too. If you start learning to juggle, for instance, neurological evidence shows that a part of the brain that specializes in visual motion perception will grow during a three-month training period and shrink after it ends.[19] Therefore depending on how different parts of the human brain are used or unused, it is ever changing. All types of learning and experience modify the brain, even fleeting and unintentional ones. And so to paraphrase Klingberg, even if your life isn't changed after you finish this book, you'll never again be the person who you were before reading it.[20]

Of course, any single book, article, blog post, or 280-character statement is just a tiny fraction of the amount of information that a human being can consume. Thanks to our 86 billion neurons and the trillions of synaptic connections between them, our brain can store up to 100 terabytes of information over a lifetime. That's more than 50,000 times the text contained in the US Library of Congress.[21] It's a curated collection of memories, though, based on the limits of our brain's ability to receive information. And managing those limits in order to prevent information overload is our attention.

Attention is like a spotlight that illuminates a small piece of information and leaves everything else in the shadows. In cognitive science, it's all the mechanisms by which the brain selects, amplifies, channels, and deepens the processing of information.[22] Our brain needs these mechanisms to filter information from a constant bombardment by sensory stimuli because all of those messages would be impossible to digest in depth. We don't always choose where we direct the spotlight, but we often find the targets that are most important or attractive to us. "My experience is what I agree to attend to," psychologist William James wrote about selective attention in 1890. "Only those items which I notice shape my mind."[23]

*   *   *

As Pope was writing about the dangers of limited information, his friend Jonathan Swift was on a campaign against political lies. "Who first reduced lying into an art, and adapted it to politics, is not so clear from history," wrote the Irish author in 1710, "although I have made some diligent inquiries." The two men had a lot in common, including lifelong illness, and Swift is just as often quoted for his commentary on misinformation. In particular, he called attention to the quick and irreparable damage caused by deception: "Falsehood flies, and truth comes limping after it, so that when men come to be undeceived, it is too late . . . like a physician, who hath found out an infallible medicine, after the patient is dead."[24]

At a time when people transmitted information mostly by word of mouth and the printing press, Swift's metaphor was prescient. Three hundred years later, in a 2018 study about the online spread of true and false claims, researchers found that falsehood diffused significantly farther, faster, deeper, and more broadly than the truth in all categories of information.[25] Their data set consisted of 126,000 fact-checked rumor cascades on Twitter (defined as unbroken retweet chains with a common, singular origin) from 2006 to 2017, involving stories spread by 3 million people more than 4.5 million times. Falsehoods were 70 percent more likely to be retweeted than the truth and reached 1,500 people six times faster. The spread of falsehood was helped by its virality, meaning that the content was shared between individuals rather than simply through a large, single broadcast. And humans were undeniably responsible for it, because robots accelerated the spread of true and false claims at the same rate.

The reasons that falsehoods flew on Twitter—before the COVID-19 pandemic and the platform's rebranding as "X" by entrepreneur Elon Musk, notably—weren't certain. Numerous factors were involved, and novelty (that is, the quality of being new or unusual) may have been one of them. The study's authors found that false rumors were significantly more novel than the truth when compared with tweets to which users were exposed in the sixty days before their retweet. Moreover, false rumors received replies that expressed greater surprise by users than true stories did. This association with novelty and surprise hints at a possible neurological basis for the spread of false tweets.

Novel or unexpected things draw our attention—the kind of attention where the spotlight directs itself. Novel stimuli are also more easily remembered by our brains than predictable or familiar ones, probably because the ability to detect and respond to them is crucial for survival in a rapidly changing environment.[26] Our brain's sensory cortex, for instance, may have evolved to focus on events that are unpredictable or surprising.[27]

When a stimulus is repetitive, our neuronal response to it often decreases rapidly in many parts of the brain. We stop paying so much attention to it because we've seen it many times before. In contrast, we experience an increase in brain activity when the stimulus is novel.[28] Certain neurotransmitters, as chemical substances that carry messages between neurons, may be important for generating this response. Interestingly, the neurotransmitter dopamine has been associated with the human personality trait of novelty seeking—as well as with the addictive nature of online experiences.[29]

Given the apparent surprise elicited by false rumors on Twitter, it's fair to infer that at least some of the users who spread them also believed they might be true. This makes sense, as studies suggest that to the extent that people pay attention to accuracy, they're likely to share things they genuinely believe.[30] (Of course, keep in mind that people are less likely to see posts that contradict their beliefs and biases due to social media algorithms, and tend to favor information and join groups that support them—a phenomenon known as the "echo chamber effect.")[31] If someone doesn't care about whether or not a claim is true, however, they still might intentionally share it. There are numerous possible motivations for this behavior, such as to make others feel better or to trigger their outrage. For instance, in a 2016 poll of over a thousand adults living in the United States, 16 percent of the respondents admitted to knowingly sharing false stories online.[32] Some of them wanted to highlight the stories as fake, whereas others wanted the amusement. More recent research identified additional factors for sharing misinformation in a social media context, such as the desire to attract and please followers and friends, or intention to signal one's group membership, such as political affiliation.[33] Unfortunately, too often the misinformation is actually *disinformation*, created and spread with malicious aims.

Disinformation in the form of organized campaigns of social media manipulation, by which a political party or government uses social media to shape public attitudes, has become "a ubiquitous and pervasive part of the digital information ecosystem," according to researchers at the Oxford Internet Institute in a 2019 report.[34] They identified these campaigns in 70 countries, where the most common communication strategy is the manufacture of misleading content, such as memes, videos, fake news websites, and manipulated media. Generally aiming to increase division and distrust, they sometimes target specific communities or segments of social media users. This strategy has been used by Russian disinformation campaigns, for example, to sow discord in Western societies.[35] During the COVID-19 pandemic, Russian disinformation groups sought to undermine US vaccination efforts by suggesting that COVID-19 vaccines were unsafe and that US President Joe Biden planned to force them on people—including social media posts from Russian state-media accounts that focused in particular on far-right audiences.

One extremely potent form of disinformation and misinformation is the conspiracy theory. Conspiracy theories are commonly defined as beliefs about a group of people that collude in secret to reach malevolent goals.[36] They usually attempt to explain the "real" causes of significant events and circumstances, which can be anything from assassinations to unidentified flying objects to epidemics. But some go much farther than that. Since 2017, the QAnon conspiracy theory has expanded into a vast web of beliefs that the world is run by a cabal of Satan-worshipping pedophiles. That's a strange sentence to write, but millions of people worldwide, especially in the United States, completely buy into it.

Of course, it's important to recognize that conspiracies do exist. Some conspiracy theories, such as the belief that HIV was created by the US government to wipe out Black people, stem from institutional distrust related to the Tuskegee Syphilis Study and other unethical human experiments on African Americans (one of the topics of chapter 8). By all means, questioning institutional power and challenging authority can be a positive act when the abuses being criticized are known or likely to be true. Yet for the most part, conspiracy beliefs have a lot more to do with human psychology and sociology than genuine subterfuge.

Conspiracy theories are a cultural universal across human societies, which has led some researchers to explore evolutionary interpretations of them. Behavioral scientist Jan-Willem van Prooijen and evolutionary psychologist Mark van Vugt have examined the possibility that conspiracy theories are by-products of our unique human brain, resulting from the interaction of psychological mechanisms that evolved for other purposes.[37] They point out, for example, that one key element of any conspiracy theory is pattern perception: an assumption about how people and events are causally connected. Coincidently, pattern recognition is one of the critical cognitive abilities that we acquired through human evolution as the size of our cerebral cortex expanded, thereby providing a neurobiological foundation for intelligence, language, imagination, invention, and the belief in imaginary entities.[38] Another potential predisposition for conspiracy beliefs, the scientists note, is our hyperactive agency detection system, which can ascribe intentionality where none exists (as we discussed in the context of religion in chapter 4).

Alternatively, van Prooijen and van Vugt propose that believing in conspiracy theories isn't a by-product at all but rather an adaptive feature of the human mind. Presuming that humans were frequently confronted with coalitional violence in ancestral environments, they reason that being suspicious of powerful and potentially threatening groups may have been advantageous for survival in earlier times.

Regardless of how conspiracy thinking may or may not reflect our evolutionary past, many people draw benefits from these beliefs today. Conspiracy theories are like rumors in that they act as an ongoing sense-making activity by which inexplicable events become more understandable.[39] By claiming to identify hidden patterns and the culprits behind these events, they can appeal to people who are uncomfortable with uncertainty and randomness.[40] Furthermore, they can make people feel safe, secure, and able to exert control over their environment, such as by allowing them to blame others for their problems or fears about the world. In this way, conspiracy theories can also be a convenient way to reinforce group membership and social exclusion, as they reduce our complex and messy reality to a straight-forward, good-versus-evil story—evidence not required.

To be clear, I'm not saying that conspiracy beliefs are healthy. But I can see why they're attractive. Not all of them are harmful, at least not to society, yet the ones about infectious diseases are dangerous to everyone—those who believe them, those who fight them, those who have nothing to do with them, and certainly those who are targeted by them.

Poisonous Plots

On May 6, 2022, when a person with mpox was identified in the United Kingdom, it wasn't the first time. In previous years, there had been eight cases of mpox related to travel in Nigeria, where the disease is endemic, and this patient was another one. Yet the situation took a dramatic turn as more cases were reported in the United Kingdom over the following days. Two more. Then four more. Two more. Then eleven more. Then thirty-six more. Most of the infected individuals didn't have any links to the first patient, or hadn't traveled to any of the mpox endemic countries in Central and West Africa. Within three weeks, over a hundred cases were confirmed in England, Scotland, Wales, and Northern Ireland.

By the end of the month, the case count had grown to hundreds of people in nearly two dozen countries outside Africa, including Australia, the United Arab Emirates, and much of western Europe and North America. Four months later, the disease had infected more than sixty-seven thousand people in more than a hundred countries. It was an unprecedented level of international spread for mpox. In many patients, the disease appeared to cause a genital or perianal rash, suggesting that close physical contact during sexual contact was helping the spread. And given its sudden appearance simultaneously in numerous nonendemic countries, it seemed likely that the virus had been spreading undetected for some time.[41]

Mpox is a distinct disease from COVID-19. With visible symptoms that include a bumpy rash and pus-filled blisters on the skin, it's caused by a smallpox-like virus that often spreads between people through direct contact with infectious sores, scabs, or body fluids. Nonetheless, the initial reports of mpox in Europe almost immediately provoked the kind of fill-in-the-blanks conspiracy theories that seriously impaired the COVID-19 response over the previous two years.

Social media accounts and news outlets in Ukraine, Russia, China, and the United States pushed stories that the outbreak was the result of a laboratory leak, or the use of mpox as a biological weapon, like COVID-19 was rumored to have been.[42] Many social media users also claimed that COVID-19 vaccines had somehow made people more vulnerable to the mpox virus or infected them with it based on incorrect beliefs about what COVID-19 vaccines contained along with how they worked. Plus there were irrational accusations that the mpox outbreak was a planned pandemic (or a "plandemic") devised by perceived supervillains such as US billionaire Bill Gates. As another cookie-cutter conspiracy in the manner of COVID-19 misinformation, this particular falsehood was shared across Russia media the Chinese social media platform Weibo as well as on Facebook in Romanian, German, English, Arabic, French, Slovenian, Hungarian, and Punjabi languages.

Unsurprisingly, the most nonsensical claims were amplified by far-right public figures in the United States, such as US representative Marjorie Taylor Greene. On Facebook, Greene (who embraced a variety of conspiracy theories, including QAnon, and opposed vaccination and masking during the COVID-19 pandemic) speculated that Gates saw mpox as "something, apparently, he can make a lot of money off of [because] he wants you all to be injected" with a mpox vaccine. She also went on to explain other ways that Gates, a global health philanthropist, wanted to control what people ate and drank, and how an unspecified "they" would frighten the public with images of mpox patients in order to compel mask wearing by the public.[43]

A little learning is a dangerous thing, that's for sure. Conspiracy theories like these ones are spotty misreadings of recent history and warped interpretations of current events. The notion that humans created the mpox virus fails to account for more than half a century of scientific knowledge about its natural occurrence in wildlife and close evolutionary relationships to smallpox and other poxviruses.[44] Even museum specimens of African rodents have shown evidence of mpox infections as early as 1899, as we learned in chapter 1. These conspiracy theories also ignore other recent outbreaks in non-African countries like the United States as well as a long-running outbreak in Nigeria that began in 2017 and may have been the source of its global spread. Climbing to more than 240 confirmed cases from 2017 to 2022, the Nigerian outbreak should have been a warning for the rest of the world.[45] It was only a matter of time until humans carried the virus into communities and continents far and wide.

But many scientists already knew that mpox was a threat. In the 1988 report on the WHO-led smallpox vaccination campaign, which was successfully completed in 1979, there's an entire chapter about mpox and its challenges for the global eradication of smallpox.[46] Human cases of mpox were a concern at the time because they could be confused with smallpox. Surveillance studies in the 1970s and 1980s indicated that mpox cases were scattered widely throughout rainforest areas, mostly in the DRC, and may have only become identifiable after the elimination of smallpox.[47]

Since then, it's been well established that smallpox vaccines are highly protective against mpox. Unlike smallpox, however, as explained in chapter 1, mpox can never be eradicated: it's a zoonotic disease with a number of potential reservoir hosts in nature, from which the virus can spill over to humans and other species at a given moment. After smallpox was stamped out everywhere, and smallpox vaccination ceased around the world, experts suspected that unvaccinated populations would increasingly lose immunity against other poxviruses such as the one that causes mpox. In his 2009 memoir about directing the WHO campaign, *Smallpox: The Death of a Disease*, epidemiologist D. A. Henderson recounted early discussions on this very topic.[48] With the growing spread of mpox in recent decades, it appears those scientific worries were justified.

In a way, conspiratorial worries about mpox aren't new either. At least they're not original. In fact, some of the most colorful claims about mpox have the deepest roots in epidemic history, with rehashed tropes of diseases as pretext, remedies that do harm, doctors out for profit, and elites who want to wipe out or control the masses. Ironically, the same kind of conspiracy theories about smallpox vaccination in the nineteenth century, thereby prolonging the spread of smallpox in some communities, have now been repurposed for mpox (and other diseases) in the twenty-first century. The biggest difference is that the means of communication have changed, and so today's falsehoods fly faster and farther than their forebears.

*   *   *

"VACCINATE! VACCINATE!! VACCINATE!!! THERE'S MONEY IN IT!!! TWENTY THOUSAND VICTIMS!!! will be Vaccinated within the next ten days in this City under the present ALARM!!! That will put $10,000 into the pockets of the Medical Profession." In case all the exclamation points and capitalized letters didn't do the trick, Alexander Milton Ross embellished his poster with a large drawing of a police officer restraining a mother while Death vaccinated her child. It was terrifying, no doubt. For extra emphasis, the police officer held a piece of paper that read "Vaccination for the Jenner-ation of Disease."[49]

In 1885, Canada had no greater adversary of smallpox vaccination than Ross, an Anglo-Canadian physician and naturalist whose medical training was informed by the sanitary movement of the nineteenth century. Opposed to the germ theory emerging in Europe (that same year, Pasteur's rabies vaccine was announced to the world), Ross believed that smallpox was a filth disease and its only antidote was cleanliness.

Vaccination, in his mind, was poisonous. Ross wanted everyone to know it too. Besides papering the city of Montreal with antivaccination posters and pamphlets, writing letters to newspapers and professional journals, and founding a magazine called the *Anti-Vaccinator*, he formed the Canadian Anti-Vaccination League as part of an international antivaccination crusade. "Though Police and the Profession cry Vaccinate! Vaccinate!! Vaccinate!!! and people in thousands follow their blind leaders,—I still say, DON'T," Ross urged in a circular that he distributed throughout the city.[50]

At the time, Montreal was struggling to fight off the largest epidemic of smallpox that it would ever face. For almost a century, smallpox vaccination had been widely used to prevent the disease, but many of the city's inhabitants had refused the procedure.

Some of the holdouts were surely persuaded by Ross and his English-only propaganda. But most of the unvaccinated population and therefore the bulk of the cases consisted of French Canadians. To convince them of the evils of vaccination, French Canadian physician Joseph Emery Coderre formed the first Canadian antivaccination society in Montreal and published numerous antivaccination pamphlets in French in the 1870s. His ardent antivaccination views fed the fervor of protesters who attacked the city council in 1875, halting efforts to enact mandatory smallpox vaccination in Montreal and leaving the city vulnerable to devastating disease ten years later. When compulsory vaccination was attempted again in 1885, the riot was even bigger. Shortly thereafter, Coderre and colleagues created an antivaccination journal, *L'Antivaccinateur canadien-français*, the Francophone counterpart to Ross's magazine.[51]

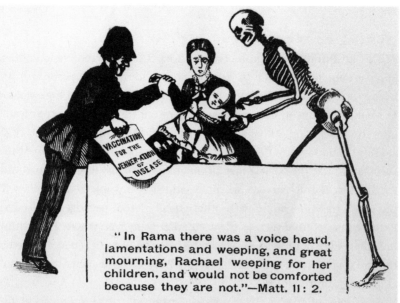

Figure 10.1

Antivaccination poster in 1885. Created by Alexander Milton Ross during the small-pox epidemic in Montreal, the text accuses medical doctors of profiting from small-pox vaccination and urges citizens to refuse it, while the image suggests that the smallpox vaccine is deadly. *Source:* Michael Bliss, *Plague: The Story of Smallpox in Montreal* (Toronto: HarperCollins, 1991).

The misinformation promoted by Ross, Coderre, and their contemporaries should be familiar to anyone with a social media account in the twenty-first century.[52] First off, they downplayed the threat of the epidemic in Montreal. Francophone newspapers wrote little about it, except to dismiss the panic, while Ross stressed in one of his pamphlets, "CAUTION. Do not be alarmed by the smallpox."[53] Simultaneously, they insisted that vaccination was the true danger. In the *Anti-Vaccinator*, Ross explained that vaccination didn't prevent smallpox and actually infected people with the smallpox virus, along with other equally lethal pathogens.[54] Coderre likewise insisted that victims of vaccination were everywhere. His writings included pages of individuals whom he believed were sickened or killed by the vaccine, either from contracting smallpox or some other malady such as gangrene and syphilis.[55]

And then, of course, they spouted conspiracy theories. Provaccination doctors were accused of profiting from the practice, as Ross broadcast in his poster. One French Canadian doctor, in an open letter to Coderre published by the medical journal *L'Union Médicale du Canada* in 1875, laid out the same charge. He also perceived another conspiracy among English physicians in particular, attributing their advocacy of the smallpox vaccine to nationalistic conflicts of interest given that English physician Jenner popularized it.[56] Coderre replied in agreement, affirming that English doctors and public vaccinators practiced vaccination *par intérêt*—purely out of self-interest.[57] These beliefs were consistent with a general distrust of the Anglophone elite, whose vaccines were seen as both poisoning and punishing the French Canadian community, which mostly lived in overcrowded tenements in the poorest quarters of the city.[58]

Their arguments are reminiscent of misinformation during subsequent epidemics and pandemics, all the way up to the present. It's also noteworthy that while Ross thought sanitation was the answer to smallpox, Francophone newspapers printed recipes for at-home remedies, such as buckwheat root or mixtures of zinc sulfate, digitalis, and sugar.[59] (A cure was never found for smallpox before its eradication, and treatments generally consisted of cleaning the wounds and easing the pain of the ill.) These ideas are analogous to the popularization in the United States of non-FDA-approved treatments for COVID-19, such as ivermectin (an antiparasitic agent used to treat patients with certain worm infections and head lice) and hydroxychloroquine (a medication used for malaria and autoimmune conditions such as lupus and rheumatoid arthritis), which many people learned about through the internet, social media, and celebrity testimonials. Despite early hopes, neither of them turned out to be effective for preventing or treating COVID-19.[60] But without any specific treatments for COVID-19 until long into the pandemic, it's not surprising that some patients opted to take risks with these unproven remedies rather than heed public health warnings against them. Some physicians even participated in misinformation about the efficacy of these drugs and continued to prescribe them for COVID-19.[61] And although many studies haven't observed that ivermectin and hydroxychloroquine cause serious adverse effects in COVID-19 patients, they can still be dangerous if the patients forgo evidence-based COVID-19 treatments or vaccination against SARS-CoV-2 as a result of using them, as editors at the *Journal of the American Medical Association* have pointed out.[62]

To be fair, smallpox vaccination was far from perfectly safe in the late nineteenth century. Even Jenner himself couldn't explain how his vaccine worked, and some methods (such as passing infectious material directly from the arm of a vaccinated person to an unvaccinated one) undoubtedly had the potential to introduce other infections. There were also some cases where children may have died as a result of faulty vaccine preparations. Even if the vaccination was successful, it didn't guarantee complete or life-long immunity. Antivaccinationists, though, were incorrect about the risks and effects of the vaccine. And their dishonesty, at least in the case of Ross, raised questions about their own motives.

Ross, the bombastic pamphleteer, was apparently a hypocrite at heart. In October 1885, while the smallpox epidemic was still raging in Montreal, he boarded a train to Toronto. As reported afterward by the *Gazette*, a medical inspector at the Ontario border asked Ross to show proof of recent smallpox vaccination, either in the form of a certificate or scar.[63] It was a standard policy for travelers, but Ross tried his best to get out of it. Then when he couldn't produce a certificate, he reluctantly took off his coat, rolled off his sleeve, and revealed "three perfect vaccination marks" on his arm. One of them was relatively fresh, and the others were from infancy and childhood, according to Ross. The article about the incident offered little by way of commentary, except to note the long history of doctors who believed in the efficacy of vaccination but opposed the practice since they would lose a source of revenue if smallpox declined. (Similarly, during the COVID-19 pandemic, the Fox News channel was a top broadcaster of vaccine skepticism in the United States, even though nearly all of the corporation's employees were vaccinated.)[64]

The news about Ross reached the United States, where it was met with outrage among the public health community. One State Board of Health report called him "a monster in human form who desired that a most terrible disease should decimate his patrons, that he might grow fat on their putrid bodies."[65]

By the end of the smallpox epidemic in Montreal in 1886, more than 3,200 people had died from the disease. The city lost almost 2 percent of its total population in 1885 alone, and more than 3 percent of its French Canadian community. Most of them were children. There were numerous blunders that helped the disease spread, as historian Michael Bliss recounts in his book *Plague: How Smallpox Devastated Montreal*, and the large population of unvaccinated children created by fear and ignorance was a major factor. Every one of the deaths could have been prevented, Bliss emphasizes.[66] Unfortunately, it wasn't until the disease ran out of unvaccinated or otherwise vulnerable hosts that the epidemic finally waned.

Misinformation about diseases is a timeless human challenge. Some opinions offered about the antivaccination riot in Montreal, such as in a *New York Times* editorial in 1875, sound familiar 150 years later. With shock that anyone would harbor such an *absurd* preconception against vaccination, a triumph of modern medicine, the editorial lamented that "in spite of all our boasted progress, curious revelations of popular ignorance and superstition are constantly showing us how little progress has been made." But after laying blame on the fortune tellers in large cities, the quacks in medicine that flourished everywhere, and even the scientific research and scholarly writings that went above the heads of the public, there was still optimism: "When knowledge is more evenly distributed, there will be less of this fantastic and ignorant prejudice."[67]

Evenly distributed knowledge? That sounds a lot like the internet to me.

A Wiser Species

I've read, heard, spoken, written, and thought a lot about public communication about pandemics for over a decade now. It's become part of my job, although it didn't start out that way. As an NMNH curator, my main focus is research in biological anthropology. I'm also responsible for shaping and making decisions about our collections of biological anthropology. But the aspects of my work that involve educating and engaging with the public took center stage when we started discussing ideas for the *Outbreak* exhibit in 2014. Helping people be more informed about emerging infectious diseases and pandemic risks seemed, well, extremely important. I didn't fully appreciate at the time just how crucial it would become.

Serving as the curator of *Outbreak* meant that I was obsessed with the accuracy of information within and related to the exhibit. Nobody wants to see any mistakes on museum walls, but I felt the additional pressure of being someone who had to answer for any errors lurking among the text rails, captions, labels, panels, and screens. My stomach churned at the thought of a single slipup, which might lead a visitor to distrust the rest of the content in the gallery. Or even worse, an inaccuracy—however small or benign—that a visitor might trust, remember, and spread after leaving the building.

In an ideal exhibition, all facts would be bombproof. That is, nothing could challenge or change them, from *Outbreak*'s opening in 2018 until its close in 2022. But obviously this is unrealistic; information changes over time. It's an inherent feature of the scientific method to continually build on and sometimes reassess the best knowledge that's available on a certain topic at a given moment. It doesn't necessarily mean that the previous research was flawed but rather that perhaps new techniques, more evidence, or different questions were brought to bear on a particular problem.

One of the greatest obstacles of public health communication during the COVID-19 pandemic was the dynamic process of explaining and applying information related to the disease as scientists and officials learned more about it. The constant updates were confusing and suspicious to many people, and probably most of all to those who didn't know anything about virology, immunology, or perhaps science as a whole. In these difficult situations, one of the best things that experts can do is to be mindful and honest about the limitations of knowledge as it continues to evolve.

We had to update *Outbreak* numerous times during its lifespan, as we went from looking back on past pandemics to trying to understand a current one. Scientific information is always improving, but anything in the world of emerging diseases can shift before you know it. In 2018, for example, it was a fact that there were two highly human-pathogenic coronaviruses known to exist. Then in 2019, there were three. In addition to this small yet significant change, we had to revise the text about COVID-19's causes, symptoms, and routes of transmission, from when it first emerged to after it spread and mutated globally.

I don't think that the key to combating misinformation, however, is simply providing correct information as though people are simply empty vessels to be filled with facts. And it doesn't make sense to me that lack of exposure to the information is the only barrier to people accepting it. That assumption goes against everything that I know as an anthropologist as well as a lot of we've covered in this chapter.

For starters, there's the matter of human attention. Just because someone sees something doesn't mean that they'll read it. The year that *Outbreak* opened in 2018, the NMNH had around five million visitors, and most of them were looking for the dinosaurs. (Some of them might have been looking for airplanes, not knowing which Smithsonian museum they were in.) Recognizing the limits of their time, energy, and interest, rule number one was to keep the text short, in blocks of no more than fifty to seventy-five words ideally. The fewer the words, the more likely a visitor will read them. If I lobbied to expand or add text to the exhibit script at a late stage of content development, I might get an unblinking response of "nobody's going to read that" or more likely "OK, then tell me what we're going to take out" from my colleague Angela Roberts, *Outbreak*'s exhibit writer.

Angela was also the destroyer of jargon—the technical language that scientists often use and that I struggled to give up as we tried to present information in a simpler way. The more complicated the words, the less likely a visitor will read any further. We wrote all the text at the approximate reading level of a middle school student in the United States, aware that our audience was mostly families and multigenerational groups. Making information understandable to a general audience isn't dumbing it down. It's about meeting people where they are. Knowing your audience is key to effective communication; making them work hard to understand you isn't.

Then there are matters of how people comprehend the information available to them. One of the advantages of an exhibit in a museum is the kind of environment that accommodates many different kinds of learners, such as those who like objects, ideas, or activities. There's also space for conversations and context as visitors interact with the content, which was especially critical for *Outbreak* topics such as vaccination, disease stigma, and the social dimensions of health. My favorite thing to do during public hours was to walk through the gallery and observe how people were discussing the content among themselves, with people whom they know and trust. It's a social learning experience that isn't common outside a formal educational setting. It's an effective way to spark curiosity, raise awareness, and create memories that someone might take home with them too.

Lack of trust in institutions, including the scientific establishment, is a common thread in conspiracy theories and other kinds of misinformation that proliferate during a pandemic. And in the battle for truth, the messengers matter as much as the messages. Knowing this, we trained more than a hundred volunteers to explain content, answer questions, play games, and be ready for challenging conversations with our visitors if needed. We also brought guest scientists into the exhibit in order to discuss their research on *Outbreak*-related topics, including COVID-19 before the novel coronavirus even had a name. We intentionally highlighted and hosted a diversity of individuals ranging in their professions and backgrounds, in whom different people might see a bit of themselves. And with all of our programs, we teamed up with a huge array of speakers to connect with our audiences on a variety of issues and experiences. Those personal connections can make a difference, in any context, when helping people to separate facts from fiction.

* * *

The fight against misinformation is an uphill battle, but many people around the world have joined forces on the side of truth. In 2023, the Duke University Reporters' Lab counted at least 417 fact-checking organizations who were verifying and debunking misinformation in more than 100 countries, 69 languages, and often in collaboration.[68] That's a nearly 40-fold increase since 2008, when there were only eleven organizations. Most of them formed with the rapid rise of social media during the decade prior to the COVID-19 pandemic. Africa Check, for instance, was established as the first independent nonprofit fact-checking organization in 2012, with offices in South Africa, Kenya, Senegal, and Nigeria today. Not by coincidence, it was in Nigeria where the terrible consequences of health misinformation—and the need for organizations like Africa Check—were made clear in 2003, with a year-long boycott of a World Health Organization–sponsored polio vaccination campaign.[69]

Guided by local leaders of several states of northern Nigeria, the boycott grew from rumors that the polio vaccine was contaminated with anti-fertility substances, HIV, and cancer-causing agents intended to wipe out the Muslim population. Sociologist Ayodele Samuel Jegede has teased out a complex interplay of historical, political, and cultural factors in the boycott, including distrust of the federal government (which limited the number of children per woman in the 1980s) and Western health interventions and pharmaceutical companies (especially after Pfizer's controversial clinical trial of an experimental antibiotic during a meningitis epidemic in 1996).[70] But the media magnified the problem of public distrust by reporting the rumors without investigating them, as Africa Check points out, and new polio cases surged—ultimately adding years and hardship to polio elimination efforts in Nigeria and elsewhere.

Similar challenges accompanied a human outbreak of mpox in 2017, thirty-nine years after the last reported case in Nigeria. During the outbreak, there was a rumor that the Nigerian military was injecting school children with the monkeypox virus, causing widespread alarm. In consequence, students were kept at home by their parents and schools closed, which meant that a lot of kids missed out on education as well as on immunizations for other vaccine-preventable diseases. Nigerian public health officials blamed inaccurate, sensationalized, and misleading stories from unauthorized sources for contributing to the panic, with a call for stronger capacity and training for effective factual reporting on science and health issues in Nigeria.[71] Unfortunately, as we've already learned, the outbreak continued for years, and the virus—along with its attendant rumors—went global in 2022.

For some people, trying to stop the spread of misinformation is a full-time job. And even then, it's not easy. For the rest of us, fact-checking isn't possible for every questionable claim that we encounter. Definitely not during an infodemic, when any casual click, swipe, or scroll can lead to a surprising story or attention-grabbing headline. But still, there are simple things that anybody can do to appraise their facts and to determine if, how, and with whom to share newfound knowledge. As a how-to guide for "flattening the infodemic curve," the World Health Organization therefore suggests seven steps that people can take to decide who and what to trust:

1. **Assess the source**. Consider who shared the information with you and where they got it. To verify social media accounts, look at how long they've been active, their number of followers, and their most recent activity. For websites, look for background information and legitimate contact details, such as "About Us" and "Contact Us" pages.

2. **Go beyond headlines**. Read more than just the headline of a story, which may be crafted to get maximum clicks rather than to accurately reflect the content.

3. **Identify the author**. Search the author's name online to see if they are real or credible.

4. **Check the date.** Find the publication date for the story to determine how recent and up-to-date it is.

5. **Examine the supporting evidence**. Verify that experts quoted in a story are reliable and that hyperlinks provided actually support it.

6. **Check your biases**. Ask yourself why you were drawn to a particular headline or story, and whether it challenges or reinforces what you want to hear.

7. **Turn to fact-checkers**. Consult trusted fact checking organizations and global news outlets focused on debunking misinformation, such as the International Fact-Checking Network at the US nonprofit Poynter Institute.[72]

Our human tendency to create and share misinformation is a challenge for all of us. But the same brains that cause it are also highly equipped to fight it. It's not just an issue of knowledge but what we do with it as well. Wisdom counts for nothing if we don't use it.

Conclusion: Being Human

There are a lot of numbers and statistics in this book, and many of them relate to suffering and loss. If you can bear with me, I'll share one more: about 67 million people died from various causes (not just pandemics) in 2022. Probably most of us knew at least one person who passed away. Yet our global species continued to expand, because nearly 134 million babies were born in 2022 too. That means that the human population actually gained about 66 million people that year. My baby was one of them.

Adding a human to the planet makes you think about the future in a different way, especially during the COVID-19 pandemic, when the world was shaken more than anybody could soon forget. You worry about what lies ahead for them and their generation, with the unease of someone who invested their most precious person in a place with a lot of uncertainties. But one thing that I'm certain about, and made the central thesis of this book, is that there are more pandemics ahead of us. I'm certain of this inevitability because pandemics aren't random or uncontrollable like meteorites. We make them happen simply by being human.

Interestingly, a few of the human traits that I've described in this book are already apparent during the first months of life, before a person can walk and talk. They're part of human development, and any new parent or caregiver can watch them in action. For instance, even if they can't articulate words, newborns can definitely vocalize. Oh, do they ever. And the sounds that they produce are emphasized by their urgency to share them, in close-as-possible proximity, with others. When they get sounds in return, such as when I mimic my son's cooing and babbling, it's not really so different from a typical back-and-forth between adults, minus the mundane details.

Touching is, of course, unrelenting during infancy. Human babies learn by touching objects, surfaces, and just about anything else within reach. They touch with their fingers and often their mouths as they explore the environment around them. Yet touching is also a way of soothing and building bonds with other people—something that doesn't change with age. I've found that there's little that a cuddle can't help, and that's not only true for babies.

Infants don't discriminate and distrust as adults do, partly for lack of the kind of experiences that shape these perceptions. But as their brains grow rapidly by cognitive leaps and bounds, they do take note of contrasts, delight in patterns, and start to sort. Plus they're naturally attuned to potential threats, real or imagined. You can tell when babies pick up on social threats, such as angry faces, as well as when they distinguish a stranger from someone they know well. To some extent, these instincts are prepackaged at birth. Other things, like certain behaviors and biases, are influenced by what and how they're taught as they grow up.

My son will never know a pandemic-free life. Then again, neither have I. Like him, I was born at the beginning of a pandemic. AIDS became known to the world around the time that I entered it, when the earliest case reports were published in 1981. It's never been a society-stopping pandemic, largely due to the nature of the virus and its routes of transmission. That is, it's not a crowd disease. But it hasn't been a society-mobilizing pandemic either, and the stigmatization of AIDS patients has a lot to do with it. My mother wasn't aware of AIDS until Rock Hudson died from it in 1985, and neither were a lot of other people at the time. Still, after 40 million deaths and counting, HIV has yet to receive as much attention—or resources—as it deserves.

Some people tried to sound the alarm early. As Laurie Garrett describes in her book *The Coming Plague*, a group of US scientists came together in 1989 in order to raise concerns about emerging microbes as ever-greater threats to humanity.[1] The meeting led to the convening of a special panel by the Institute of Medicine, the health arm of the National Academy of Sciences, which produced the groundbreaking report *Emerging Infections: Microbial Threats to Health in the United States* in 1992. First and foremost, the report's authors pointed to HIV as a harbinger of threats to come, and highlighted the unreadiness of authorities to prevent and control them. The report also identified key elements responsible for the emergence of infectious diseases, including human activities such as land use, air travel, and international commerce, and offered recommendations that would allow the United States to be better prepared to recognize and respond quickly to these public health threats.[2]

More than thirty years later, in the wake of another pandemic, it's fair to wonder if enough people were listening. Maybe it's time for another rallying cry. And so I'd like to conclude this book with some suggestions for what we can all do to manage the pandemic risks that come along with being human. We may not be able to prevent more pandemics entirely, but we have immense power over how frequently they happen and how much damage they do.

1. **Check your anthropocentrism.** We're one species among countless creatures on Earth, and we just got here. By recognizing that we're only as healthy as the other animals and ecosystems with which we share the planet, we can limit the kind of disruptive interactions and activities that create opportunities for the next pandemic pathogen to emerge.

2. **Know your body.** Our unique gifts for talking and touching make us human, but they also make us vulnerable. We don't have to stop using them, yet we can certainly be safer about it. Mask wearing and handwashing are critical actions that people can take to reduce their chances of spreading and catching infectious diseases.

3. **No one is an island.** Humans have become inextricably connected through our rapidly urbanized and globalized society. Understanding the disease risks in the large, dense cities in which half the world lives, and how these risks will shift geographically over the course of this century, will allow us to better focus on and respond to them.

4. **Don't follow the crowd.** Some of our most socially and culturally significant behaviors bring us together—literally. We can avoid some of the infectious disease risks in confined and close-contact gatherings by reducing our exposure to germs, such as by sharing meals outdoors and safely caring for the sick and deceased.

5. **Think like a mountain.** Humans have become an Earth-altering force during our short species span on this planet, and we should make more decisions in consideration of our long-lasting and complex effects on the world. The Anthropocene will go down in Earth history as an age of pandemics unless we think and act with greater concern for

sustainability and environmental responsibility, such as reducing the kind of industrial food production that facilitates the transmission and adaptation of new pathogens.

6. **Fight the virus, not the people.** In viewing some people as others, humans have a tendency to scapegoat them for diseases and epidemics as well. We need to be aware of this predisposition for prejudice when faced with new pathogens so that we don't distract or detract from our efforts to control their spread.

7. **Dismantle stigma.** Humans are exceptionally talented at blaming, shaming, and punishing people for getting sick. Diseases can reach pandemic proportions when people encounter these social barriers for testing and treatment. Eliminating structures and systems that perpetuate stigma can help to end the HIV pandemic and prevent another one like it.

8. **Trust the trustworthy.** Social institutions, such as governments and health care systems, are unique features of human society. So is public distrust of them. These sentiments can lead to vaccine refusal and rejections of other public health measures that are critical for pandemic prevention. Leaders, scientists, and health officials can address these issues by acknowledging past wrongs, explaining the scientific process, and educating the public on how and why guidelines during a health crisis can change.

9. **Love thy neighbors.** Humans evolved to be highly cooperative, but some of us prefer to go it alone. Individualistic countries can do more poorly in pandemics because they prioritize personal freedom over collective well-being. Respecting and following public health measures, such as mask wearing and stay-at-home orders, can mitigate the spread of diseases and potentially lessen the impacts of a pandemic.

10. **Cite your sources.** We're the only species that excels in misinformation and thereby self-harms on a mass scale. Conspiracy theories and falsehoods about infectious diseases can be difficult to discern in an infodemic. Having access to accurate and easy-to-understand information, within a space to discuss and ask questions about it, can serve to differentiate fact from fiction—if people know where to find it. By lending their expertise to science communication, scientists can direct the pubic to credible sources on specific topics and take on misinformation when they see it.

The expression "I'm only human" implies that people are inherently fallible. It's what someone says when they mess up. And it's true. Making errors is part of being human. But so is learning from them, fixing them if you can, and doing better the next time you get a chance. That's the beauty of adaptation. And that's how species survive.

More than anything else, it's my hope that this book will help people understand pandemics through a better understanding of themselves. We have greater potential to influence the trajectory of our pandemic future than many people realize. From our bodies to our beliefs, we need only to look within.

Epilogue: A Museum Changed

In June 2022, when I spotted my colleague Ashley Peery in the Constitution Avenue lobby of the NMNH, we hadn't seen each other for over two years. Not in person at least. Ashley was the *Outbreak* educator in charge of our volunteer training and public programs, so I'd seen her on my computer screen now and then. That was the case for almost all of my much-missed colleagues.

Ashley looked the same, as far as I could tell, behind the mask. We were both wearing them, even though the NMNH lifted its mask requirement two months earlier. That day, over a hundred thousand new COVID-19 cases were reported in the United States.

It was Tuesday.

I still felt strange being there. For weeks, I'd been easing into my prepandemic routine, coming into the office every weekday. Between March 2020, when the Smithsonian closed, and March 2022, when the NMNH ended its capacity restrictions for staff, I'd barely been inside the museum. It was a huge change for someone who until that point had practically lived at the museum. But trying to recover my former lifestyle wasn't easy either.

Funny enough, the first time that I entered the building after March 2020 was in order to get my first dose of COVID-19 vaccine. It was April 2021, and the museum was turned into a vaccination site for federal government employees. A disaster medical assistance team set up stations around the eleven-ton African elephant in the Rotunda, and we filed in one by one. As I pushed up my sleeve, I gestured to the entrance of the *Outbreak* exhibit on the floor above us, visible from the ground floor. I told the uniformed vaccinator that we'd been running an exhibit about pandemics since 2018. He smiled, as far as I could tell, behind the mask.

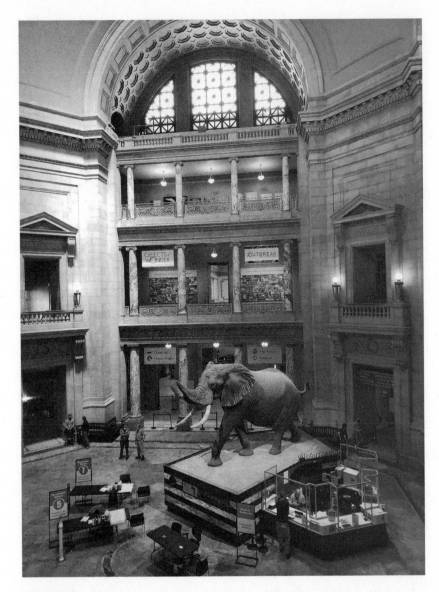

Figure 12.1
The National Museum of Natural History in 2021. While the museum was closed to the public, the Rotunda was used as a space for COVID-19 vaccinations. Ironically, the sign for the entrance to the *Outbreak* exhibit is visible on the floor above. *Source:* Sabrina Sholts.

The next time that I went back to the museum, it was for my second shot. The process seemed smoother, or maybe I was just less disoriented with the added assurance of SARS-CoV-2 antibodies in my system. As I sat there, my mind wandered to the federal clerks and makeshift desks that filled the building during the 1918 influenza pandemic, the most similar event that I knew. I reflected on the surprising ways that history rhymes. *Except that the curators back then could still access their offices*, I thought.

It would be a couple more months before I got into mine. I met a writer who wanted to interview me about some of my work. In her article, she mentioned a plastic skeleton in the corner of my office. She described it as dusty.[1]

When I saw Ashley almost a year later, we were about to meet a group of visitors. There were about twenty of them, all ambassadors from the American Society for Microbiology (ASM) who represented the organization and promoted microbial sciences around the world. Each of them was from a different country, and after spending the week in Washington for a conference, they were all about to fly home to Africa, Asia, and elsewhere. But before heading to the airport, they wanted to visit the *Outbreak* exhibit.

I jumped at the opportunity to accommodate them. The last time that I had taken anyone through the exhibit, it was for an interview with another writer on the day before we closed in March 2020. His article's title was accurate, but depressing: "I Toured This Exhibit on Epidemics before the Coronavirus Pandemic Shut It Down."[2] To me, the ASM ambassadors were a sorely needed counterbalance because many of them had used the Outbreak DIY toolkit in the communities where they lived and worked. ASM ambassadors had helped to keep the exhibit alive in an important way. I hoped that they would leave the tour with motivation to do more of them and thus continue to spread the initiative worldwide.

* * *

Passing through the *Outbreak* exhibit in 2022, my thoughts went back to the 3.5-year-long process of developing it and all of our partners who made it possible. The team of exhibit developers, designers, educators, and fundraisers who made it work. The volunteers who made it accessible. The supporters who made it global.

All of those efforts weren't visible to a visitor who watched a 90-second multiscreen video about One Health, touched a 3D model of a pathogen magnified 2.5 million times, played a 5-minute multiplayer game to stop an outbreak of Virus X, or walked along a wall of objects and stories of HIV survivors. But I saw their impacts in the rapt attention of a family that sat down to watch an ecological explainer, patient expression of a little girl who hugged a plastic Zika virus as her grandmother warned her that the giant *Aedes aegypti* mosquito above her head also transmits dengue fever, high five between young boys who trapped enough virtual bats to identify the source of a mysterious disease, and brief silence between teenagers who regarded a bullhorn used by activist Cleve Jones when he got the inspiration for the AIDS quilt.[3]

I did a lot of people watching over a period of years while the exhibit was open. In anthropological terminology, I guess you would say that I did a lot of observing as I regularly sneaked into the gallery from my office upstairs. Trying to be inconspicuous, I took advantage of the fact that the exhibit was often busy and full, with at least 1.6 million visitors in the first year. Observing how people learned about and understood the causes of epidemics as well as participating (and eavesdropping) in conversations among them was a big part of how I started to develop the ideas that led to this book.

Human-animal-microbe interactions were the primary focus of *Outbreak* and the first factor of disease emergence that people encountered when they stepped through its entrance. This was a logical focus for a natural history museum like ours where visitors saw animals and their human relationships represented in just about every corner of the building. These interactions also make up two-thirds of the One Health triad, our visual theme. It made perfect sense to me to start this book there too.

Human biological factors of pathogen transmission are always and everywhere on display, and the *Outbreak* exhibit was no exception. In pictures and words, we gave visitors tips to reduce their personal risks of disease transmission through the human body, including washing their hands, wearing a mask, and practicing safer sex.[4] But we didn't explain the evolutionary significance and uniqueness of these built-in risks, which as a biological anthropologist are my bread and butter. That's why I thought it was critical to examine these aspects of humanity early and extensively in chapter 2 given that every one of us lives and dies by them.

The major human activities that drive disease emergence, namely land use change, urbanization, and global travel and trade, were the main characters in the show. From Nipah virus outbreaks in Malaysia, to the Ebola virus epidemic in West Africa, to the international spread of SARS from China to dozens of other countries, we wanted our visitors to see how the intensification of these activities over recent human history led to our present epoch of pandemics. In this book, these topics were central to chapters 3 and 5, where I could provide more examples and historical depth than in an exhibit with hundred-word limits allowed.

EVD was the catalyst for the *Outbreak* exhibit owing to Dan Lucey's own experiences on the front lines of the 2014–2016 epidemic. His work alongside so many other doctors and nurses was visualized in a 3D tableau of an emergency treatment unit, accompanied by personal stories from health care workers in West Africa. But the section also highlighted the behavior changes of the public that ended the epidemic, thanks to local leaders and educators in the affected communities. Ebola is discussed throughout this book as a homage to its special role in *Outbreak*'s origin and especially as the dominant story in chapter 4.

Storytelling was an aspect of *Outbreak* that I came to appreciate as an important medium of science communication. It's an approach that shapes the content of all NMNH's exhibits because our visitors respond so well to it. We all do actually; it's a human thing. There were selected stories in the *Outbreak* exhibit, both big and small, but none were bigger than HIV. We dedicated a large, central section of the gallery (and parts of others) to a story that barely scratched the surface of humanity's four-decade battle with this pandemic. For this reason, HIV gets essentially its own chapter near the middle of this book. In recounting its social and physical devastation of marginalized communities, especially through a lens of stigma, I didn't think that I could do justice to the story with anything less.

Apart from stigma, the human sociological factors in epidemics and pandemics were primarily addressed in *Outbreak*'s many public programs. Complicated topics such as xenophobia, distrust, individualism, and misinformation were more conducive to films, seminars, and panel discussions than photos and text. I devoted the second half of this book to them because these phenomena are so specifically and frustratingly human—and thus unavoidable obstacles in reducing pandemic risks. Never more clearly so, I discovered, than when confronted with COVID-19.

Updating the exhibit with COVID-19 information wasn't easy, for a few reasons. First, we didn't have the space or resources to add a lot of additional content to a gallery that was designed and fabricated with millimeter-scale precision. After closing in March 2020, we knew that visitors would need to see *something* about COVID-19 when we reopened, but we had to be economical in our choices. Second, we couldn't very well tell a story about COVID-19 when we were still at the beginning of it and the conclusion was nowhere in sight. The scientific knowledge about the virus and disease was constantly improving, and the ups and downs of the epidemiological curves were like a roller coaster from hell. And lastly, summing up COVID-19 was emotionally excruciating.

The tone of *Outbreak* was supposed to be positive. Sprinkled throughout the exhibit, tidbits of information "on the upside" were clearly marked to encourage visitors to take actions and support changes to promote One Health. But a few months into the COVID-19 pandemic, I struggled to find anything to say about the situation that wasn't, well, angry. I was angry about the avoidable failures of the US government response and furious that many people across the country refused to take the disease seriously. And as time went on, I became heartbroken over all the ways that I'd lost people because of it. Ultimately we opted to create an information rail about what was needed, and in many cases lacking, in order to stop COVID-19 from the beginning: coordination, communication, testing, tracing, and treatment. We paired it with a video that showed how, compared to SARS, the virus might have been more quickly contained on a global scale. *It didn't have to be so bad*, the subtext (and my inner voice) screamed. When we updated the rail a year later, the focus of the content turned to vaccination, ventilation, and variants.

At that point, I had already started to write this book. Still confined to working at home, I needed to channel my knowledge, experiences, and energy into an examination of how and why humans hold responsibility for pandemics, unpacking various novelties of *Homo sapiens* for my own benefit as much as anyone else's. By understanding ourselves a little better, I reasoned, we can better manage our weaknesses and play to our strengths. By seeing pandemics and pathogens from a position of power, we can better see the possible solutions and work to be done.

*   *   *

In the final two weeks before the closing of the exhibit on October 3, 2022, I gave four more tours. The first one was for *Outbreak* stakeholders, a group of donors, advisers, program participants, and supporters whom we invited to the museum for a final discussion of outcomes and insights from the exhibit. In a series of short presentations after the tour, members of the *Outbreak* team shared some highlights of our achievements. Mike Lawrence, the assistant director for exhibits, reported that well over 3.3 million people visited the exhibit, and if prepandemic levels of visitation had remained constant for the entire run, the count would be closer to 5.6 million. Ashley presented on the educational activities associated with the exhibit, which included 45 public programs (28 in-person events and 17 webinars) involving 63 organizations and 108 experts.[5] In addition, we trained a total of 133 volunteers to interact with the public in the *Outbreak* exhibit, resulting in more than 66,000 interactions over the course of 6,700 volunteer hours. DIY Exhibits manager Kerri Dean announced that Outbreak DIY had received more than 300 applications from 60 countries as well as 47 US states and territories to date, mostly from schools and universities, museums, science organizations, and government agencies such as embassies and health departments. She also noted that many applicants were educators who incorporated Outbreak DIY into their curricula, not only teaching their students about the content, but how to engage with the public and communicate science on One Health issues.

The last two tours were for groups with their own interests in One Health. One was for the board of directors of City Wildlife, a nonprofit organization that rescues and rehabilitates sick, injured, and orphaned wildlife in Washington, DC. At the end of it, we had a fascinating conversation about the challenges of avian influenza surveillance among urban ducks. The other tour was for a group of EU delegates and counselors involved in agriculture and food issues within a One Health framework. We discussed the differences between COVID-19 and other epidemics, which I attributed mostly to leadership, coordination, and communication, acknowledging that SARS-CoV-2 posed particular challenges in comparison with other novel viruses. I coaxed some of them into playing the multiplayer game, which provided a lot of amusement as the rest of the group watched—even, ironically, when they failed to contain the outbreak and the game ended with Virus X still spreading.

The exhibit closed in 2022, but *Outbreak* didn't actually end. In addition to the DIY versions around the world, I collaborated with the exhibition team at the Musée des Confluences in Lyon, France, in developing a large-scale interpretation of *Outbreak* to open in April 2024. And at the NMNH, we also installed our own version of Outbreak DIY for a subsequent run in an adjacent gallery that ended in 2023. But our commitment to the One Health message continues. Of all the ways that my museum has changed as a result of COVID-19, including safer infrastructure and more flexible telework options, for me that's the most hopeful one. With a mission to understand the natural world and place of humans with it, we're telling the public that pandemics are part of it. Period. And that's because they're part of being human. The stories that follow will depend on the choices we make—both individually and collectively—to be ready, resilient, and well adapted for changes to come.

Acknowledgments

I had no plans to write any sort of book, let alone one about pandemics, in summer 2020. Like most people, I was literally trying to survive the early months of COVID-19 as the entire world shut its doors. But part of my job was helping the public make sense of it, including by producing free webinars about COVID-19, emerging infectious diseases, and One Health. They were virtual versions of the kind of in-person programs offered by the Smithsonian's NMNH since the opening of the *Outbreak* exhibit in 2018. As the exhibit's curator, I served as the host or moderator for many pandemic-related conversations.

It was through this work that Jill Corcoran at Smithsonian Enterprises got me thinking about catalyzing conversations on a larger scale by putting some of my own knowledge and thoughts about pandemics into a book. And so from 2020 to 2023, I spent a lot of sleepless nights doing just that. I'll always be grateful to Jill for all of her efforts in making this book happen, including introducing me to my agents, Jamie Chambliss and Erin Niumata at Folio Literary Management. Jamie and Erin were a huge support throughout the entire process, and I can't thank them enough for their kindness, encouragement, and professionalism along the way. I also want to thank Paige Towler and Avery Naughton at Smithsonian Enterprises for her contributions to the project.

This book was a journey with my editor at the MIT Press, Bob Prior, who took a big chance on a first-time author when he brought me on board. From the bottom of my heart, I thank Bob and everyone else at the MIT Press who made and promoted the book, including Anne-Marie Bono, Deborah Cantor-Adams, Cindy Milstein, Nicholas DiSabatino, David Olsen, and Jessica Pellien. And I offer my appreciation to the anonymous reviewers who provided excellent comments on the draft manuscript, thereby helping to improve it.

I developed the ideas for this book and cultivated the expertise that I needed to write it from nearly a decade of work on the *Outbreak* exhibit. The NMNH put together a phenomenal team of people to develop and produce the exhibit, which involved countless meetings, emails, and shared docs across a period of four years. We then spent another four years updating the exhibit and expanding on its content with programming, even when the COVID-19 pandemic closed the museum. In so many ways, I appreciate my friends and colleagues on the core team: Robert Costello, Julia Louie, Sally Love, Ashley Peery, Meg Rivers, Angela Roberts, and Shannon Willis. Other NMNH staff members (current or former) who were essential to the *Outbreak* initiative included Kara Blond, Audrey Chang, Junko Chinen, Loretta Cooper, Kerri Dean, Laura Donnelley-Smith, Kristen Hunter, Mike Lawrence, and Kim Moeller. Thank you all.

As I write about in the book, nobody deserves more credit for the *Outbreak* exhibit than Dan Lucey. He not only conceived of the exhibit but then took the steps—and leaps!—to make it a reality. I will forever be grateful to him for his brilliant vision as well as being one of the most dedicated and generous collaborators I've ever had. A lot of what I know about outbreaks I learned from Dan because he never got tired of answering my questions (or never let it show if he did). Much else came from other *Outbreak* advisers, supporters, and stakeholders. Special thanks go to Jon Epstein, the chief science adviser for the exhibit, and the rest of *Outbreak*'s advisory team: Dennis Carroll, David Morens, Larry Madoff, and Suzan Murray. I also want to thank Tony Fauci and many, many others who visited us, spoke with us, guided us, and provided content as we did our best to tell the stories and highlight the heroes of epidemics past and present.

Although I didn't know it at the time, I conducted a lot of research for this book through constant interactions with people from *Outbreak*'s partner organizations: the American Society for Microbiology, District of Columbia Department of Health, EcoHealth Alliance, HealthMap at Boston Children's Hospital, HHMI Tangled Bank Studios, Joint United Nations Programme on HIV/AIDS, ProMED / International Society for Infectious Diseases, Public Health Foundation, Smithsonian Conservation Biology Institute, US Agency for International Development, PREDICT Consortium, US Department of State, World Organisation for Animal Health, and the World Health Organization. I'm grateful for their time and wisdom as well as the resources provided by *Outbreak*'s donors: Ending Pandemics, Johnson and Johnson Innovation, Lyda Hill, Open Philanthropy Project, Rockefeller Foundation, Sanofi Pasteur, CSL Seqirus, Anders Foundation, Biotechnology Innovation Organization, Draper-Hills Family, Infectious Diseases Society of America, National Foundation for Infectious Diseases, National Institute of Allergy and Infectious Diseases, RTI International, and CDC.

Some of the passages in this book draw on my experiences related to the development of an *Outbreak*-inspired exhibit at the Musée des Confluences in Lyon. The *Épidémies* exhibit is an exciting project, thanks to an impressive and extremely kind group of collaborators: Cécilia Fregonara, Mathilde Gallay-Keller, Frédéric Keck, Guillaume Lachenal, Jeanne Matinez, Marianne Rigaud-Roy, Christian Sermet, and Anaïs Vallone. I want to offer special appreciation to Cédric Lesec and Hélène Lafont-Couturier for visiting the *Outbreak* exhibit and bringing me onto the team.

Thank you to all of my colleagues and friends who read and shared comments on sections of the draft manuscript for this book, namely Stephanie Canington, Dennis Carroll, Jon Epstein, Matt Frieman, Logan Kistler, Audrey Lin, Dan Lucey, Dolores Piperno, Briana Pobiner, Torrey Rick, and Angela Roberts. Nick Pyenson offered invaluable advice on the process of book writing as well as feedback on much of the text. Jeff Zhang and William Ristenpart answered some specific questions for me. Nader Khalifa provided some brilliant input.

My family was an incredible source of strength for me as I pushed through years of writing this book. Thank you to my parents, Jill and Jerry Sholts, who let me hole up in my old bedroom when I really needed to focus. Many thanks as well to my sister, Crystal Sholts, and all the Lauridsens for their support: Adam, Pat, Robert, and Helen. I also want to thank the Alexander family—Daniel, Kristi, Sam, Stephanie, Theodore, Eloise, and Rachel—and especially Vernita, who looked after us with immeasurable goodness and grace when David and I began to grow our own little family.

David Alexander, my loving husband, gave me everything that I needed to write this book: a sounding board, a 24-7 morale boost, and the patience of a saint—plus a Nespresso machine. Not only did he read every word of the manuscript, and offered honest and extremely constructive criticism, but his unflappable spirit kept me going through the toughest times. And at the same time, he gave me our son, Issac, the most important reason to write the book in the first place. I love you both more than words can say.

Readers' Guide

The Human Disease was written with the goal of starting conversations about how humans cause pandemics, and what we can do about it. This reading guide is intended to help those conversations take shape. Consisting of a series of open-ended questions, chapter by chapter, the guide can be used for self-reflection or group discussion. By challenging readers to think more deeply about the information and ideas in the book, and encouraging the exchange of different points of view, the answers to each question will vary from person to person, community to community, and place to place. But talking about them is an important first step in recognizing our pandemic risks. The actions that follow are up to us.

Prologue

- Sholts begins the book with her own experience of the COVID-19 pandemic closing down her workplace. What unexpected economic and lifestyle consequences of pandemics have you experienced? How might those consequences change the way we value pandemic prevention measures?

Chapter 1

- At the beginning of the chapter, Sholts writes about the SARS epidemic as a warning that few people recognized. Why do you think that so many people were "unshaken" by SARS in some countries yet the Ebola epidemic caused a panic in other ones?
- In this chapter, there are numerous examples of outbreaks caused by pathogens that are shared between wildlife and people. In your own

community, where do you see the greatest risks for pathogens to spread in this way? How could those risks be reduced—and at what costs?

Chapter 2

• Using stories of outbreaks in a variety of settings, Sholts discusses how we can spread pathogens "simply by being human" through touch and speech. How does this knowledge influence the decisions that you make, such as where and when you choose to wash your hands or wear a face mask?

Chapter 3

• Sholts argues that our pandemic risks are increasing as cities grow in size and connectedness. What are some of the factors that contribute to these concerns?
• More than half the world's population lives in cities and the global urban population is rapidly growing. Should pandemic preparedness be part of urban planning and what would be the trade-offs?

Chapter 4

• In this chapter, Sholts focuses on how cultural behaviors such as funerals can contribute to the spread of pathogens. How would you approach a conversation with someone about how their religious beliefs or practices might be the cause of an outbreak? What would you try to do—or avoid doing—in order to have a productive conversation?
• During the COVID-19 pandemic, which cultural behaviors did you find most difficult to give up or modify? What did you do instead and for how long?

Chapter 5

• This chapter examines some of the ways that human activities have altered Earth's systems, creating potential markers of the Anthropocene such as changes in atmospheric carbon or the appearance of broiler chickens. How have you noticed or experienced the effects of some of these changes during your lifetime?

- Sholts ends this chapter with a quotation about "thinking like a mountain," which means thinking about our impacts on a distant future. How could this kind of perspective be applied to policymaking and what would the changes look like?

Chapter 6

- In chapter 6, what does Sholts mean when she writes that race doesn't exist in biology, but racism has biological consequences?
- Throughout this chapter, Sholts highlights some common xenophobic responses to outbreaks such as naming a disease or pathogen after its suspected source. How can we discuss the geographic origins of a new disease without scapegoating the people associated with it?

Chapter 7

- This chapter focuses on how certain groups of people, such as gay men, were stigmatized and scapegoated at the outset of the AIDS epidemic in the United States. How does scapegoating worsen the spread and effects of pandemics by helping a new disease to become established within a population?
- Despite the widespread availability of effective HIV treatments, stigma often prevents people with HIV from getting the care that they need. In what forms might someone in your community encounter HIV stigma and how could it be eliminated?

Chapter 8

- To what extent do you trust the medical institutions in your country? What kind of experiences, events, or circumstances have shaped your views? And what would it take to change them?
- Fifty years later, the horrors of the Tuskegee experiment have not been forgotten by many people. What more should be done to repair the medical distrust that resulted from it?

Chapter 9

- Who do you think is responsible for the public's health? And how do you think that society should balance individual rights and public health?
- In your opinion, did Mallon deserve a lifelong sentence of imprisonment? If she lived in your country today, how might her experiences have been different?

Chapter 10

- In this chapter, Sholts discusses how "falsehood flies" on social media. How often do you share information online without feeling certain that it's true? What are some ways that you might try to correct misinformation when you see or hear it?
- During the COVID-19 pandemic, where did you get the majority of your information about it? How did you decide who to listen to and what recommendations to follow?

Conclusion

- Does knowing how humans create pandemics make you feel more or less optimistic about our future?
- How will you use the information that you learned in this book? Has it changed any of your behaviors or opinions?

Notes

Prologue

1. *Annual Report of the Director of the Bureau of War Risk Insurance for the Fiscal Year Ended June 30, 1920* (Washington, DC: Government Printing Office, 1920).

2. P. Henson, "How Did the Smithsonian Respond to the 1918 Pandemic?," 2020, https://siarchives.si.edu/blog/how-did-smithsonian-respond-1918-pandemic.

3. Henson, "How Did the Smithsonian Respond to the 1918 Pandemic?"

4. "Influenza Encyclopedia: The American Influenza Epidemic of 1918–1919," University of Michigan Center for the History of Medicine and Michigan Publishing, n.d., https://www.influenzaarchive.org/cities/city-washingtondc.html.

5. "Influenza Epidemic in District Holds Steady Increase," *Washington Herald*, October 7, 1918.

6. L. Saad, "Ebola Ranks among Americans' Top Three Healthcare Concerns," Gallup, November 17, 2014, https://news.gallup.com/poll/179429/ebola-ranks-among -americans-top-three-healthcare-concerns.aspx.

7. G. K. SteelFisher, R. J. Blendon, and N. Lasala-Blanco, "Ebola in the United States—Public Reactions and Implications," *New England Journal of Medicine* 373, no. 9 (2015): 789–791.

8. "Outbreak: Epidemics in a Connected World," video webinar, National Museum of Natural History, n.d., https://naturalhistory.si.edu/education/after-hours/video -webinars-outbreak-epidemics-connected-world.

Chapter 1

1. S. K. Chew, *SARS: How a Global Epidemic Was Stopped* (Manila: WHO Regional Office for the Western Pacific, 2006).

2. R. P. De Vries, W. Peng, O. C. Grant, A. J. Thompson, X. Zhu, K. M. Bouwman, A. T. Torrents de la Pena, et al., "Three Mutations Switch H7N9 Influenza to Human-Type Receptor Specificity," *PLoS Pathogens* 13, no. 6 (2017): e1006390.

3. L. MacPhee, "The History of Life on Earth," 2022, https://jan.ucc.nau.edu/lrm22/lessons/timeline/24_hours.html.

4. M. Madigan, J. M. Martinko, K. S. Bender, D. H. Buckley, and D. A. Stahl, "Microbial Evolution and Systematics," in *Brock Biology of Microorganisms*, 14th ed. (Boston: Pearson, 2015), 347–378.

5. M. H. van Regenmortel and B. W. Mahy, "Emerging Issues in Virus Taxonomy," *Emerging Infectious Diseases* 10, no. 1 (2004): 8–13.

6. S. Payne, *Viruses: From Understanding to Investigation* (London: Academic Press, 2017), 81–86.

7. D. Michieletto, M. Lusic, D. Marenduzzo, and E. Orlandini, "Physical Principles of Retroviral Integration in the Human Genome," *Nature Communications* 10, no. 1 (2019): 1–11.

8. N. Grandi and E. Tramontano, "Human Endogenous Retroviruses Are Ancient Acquired Elements Still Shaping Innate Immune Responses," *Frontiers in Immunology* 9 (2018): 2039.

9. Payne, *Viruses*, 81–86.

10. Payne, *Viruses*.

11. A. van Leeuwenhoek, "An Abstract of a Letter from Mr. Anthony Leevvenhoeck at Delft, Dated Sep. 17. 1683," *Philosophical Transactions of the Royal Society of London* 14, no. 159 (2017): 568–574.

12. Y. M. Bar-On, R. Phillips, and R. Milo, "The Biomass Distribution on Earth," *Proceedings of the National Academy of Sciences* 115, no. 25 (2018): 6506–6511.

13. M. J. Blaser, *Missing Microbes: How the Overuse of Antibiotics Is Fueling Our Modern Plagues* (New York: Macmillan, 2014).

14. A. Casadevall and L. A. Pirofski, "Microbiology: Ditch the Term Pathogen," *Nature* 516, no. 7530 (2014): 165–166.

15. M. Madigan, J. M. Martinko, K. S. Bender, D. H. Buckley, and D. A. Stahl, "Microorganisms and Microbiology," in *Brock Biology of Microorganisms*, 14th ed. (Boston: Pearson, 2015), 1–14.

16. R. Rappuoli, "1885, the First Rabies Vaccination in Humans," *Proceedings of the National Academy of Sciences* 111, no. 34 (2014): 12273–12273.

17. R. J. Dubos, *Louis Pasteur: Free Lance of Science* (Boston: Little, Brown, 1950), 277.

18. Dubos, *Louis Pasteur*, 278.

19. K. E. Jones, N. G. Patel, M. A. Levy, A. Storeygard, D. Balk, J. L. Gittleman, and P. Daszak, "Global Trends in Emerging Infectious Diseases," *Nature* 451, no. 7181 (2008): 990–993.

20. R. A. Fouchier, T. Kuiken, M. Schutten, G. van Amerongen, G. J. van Doornum, B. G. van den Hoogen, M. Peiris, et al., "Koch's Postulates Fulfilled for SARS Virus," *Nature* 423, no. 6937 (2003): 240.

21. L. J. Saif, "Animal Coronaviruses: Lessons for SARS," in *Learning from SARS: Preparing for the Next Disease Outbreak*, ed. S. Knobler, A. Mahmoud, S. Lemon, A. Mack, L. Sivitz, and K. Oberholtzer (Washington, DC: National Academies Press, 2004), 138–149.

22. J. D. Almeida, D. M. Berry, C. H. Cunningham, D. Hamre, M. S. Hofstad, L. Mallucci, K. McIntish, and D. A. J. Tyrell, "Virology: Coronaviruses," *Nature* 220 (1968): 650.

23. J. K. Aronson, "The History of Coronaviruses since 1931," *British Medical Journal* (2020): 369, https://www.bmj.com/content/369/bmj.m1547/rapid-responses.

24. Saif, "Animal Coronaviruses."

25. Y. Guan, B. Zheng, Y. Q. He, X. L. Liu, Z. X. Zhuang, C. L. Cheung, and S. W. Luo, et al., "Isolation and Characterization of Viruses Related to the SARS Coronavirus from Animals in Southern China," *Science* 302, no. 5643 (2003): 276–278.

26. C. Tu, G. Crameri, X. Kong, J. Chen, Y. Sun, M. Yu, H. Xiang, et al., "Antibodies to SARS Coronavirus in Civets," *Emerging Infectious Diseases* 10, no. 12 (2004): 2244.

27. Quoted in J. Parry, "WHO Queries Culling of Civet Cats," *British Medical Journal* 328, no. 7432 (2004): 128.

28. W. Li, Z. Shi, M. Yu, W. Ren, C. Smith, J. H. Epstein, H. Wang, et al., "Bats Are Natural Reservoirs of SARS-Like Coronaviruses," *Science* 310, no. 5748 (2005): 676–679; S. K. Lau, P. C. Woo, K. S. Li, Y. Huang, H. W. Tsoi, B. H. L. Wong, S. S. Y. Wong, et al., "Severe Acute Respiratory Syndrome Coronavirus-Like Virus in Chinese Horseshoe Bats," *Proceedings of the National Academy of Sciences* 102, no. 39 (2005): 14040–14045.

29. L. F. Wang, Z. Shi, S. Zhang, H. Field, P. Daszak, and B. T. Eaton, "Review of Bats and SARS," *Emerging Infectious Diseases* 12, no. 12 (2006): 1834–1840.

30. Lau et al., "Severe Acute Respiratory Syndrome."

31. Lau et al., "Severe Acute Respiratory Syndrome."

32. D. Jebb, Z. Huang, M. Pippel, G. M. Hughes, K. Lavrichenko, P. Devanna, S. Winkler, et al., "Six Reference-Quality Genomes Reveal Evolution of Bat Adaptations," *Nature* 583, no. 7817 (2020): 578–584.

33. World Health Organization, "Prioritizing Diseases for Research and Development in Emergency Contexts," 2022, https://www.who.int/activities/prioritizing-diseases-for-research-and-development-in-emergency-contexts.

34. M. Ruiz-Aravena, C. McKee, A. Gamble, T. Lunn, A. Morris, C. E. Snedden, C. K. Yinda, et al., "Ecology, Evolution and Spillover of Coronaviruses from Bats," *Nature Reviews Microbiology* 20, no. 5 (2022): 299–314.

35. X. Y. Ge, J. L. Li, X. L. Yang, A. A. Chmura, G. Zhu, J. H. Epstein, J. K. Mazet, et al., "Isolation and Characterization of a Bat SARS-Like Coronavirus That Uses the ACE2 Receptor," *Nature* 503, no. 7477 (2013): 535–538.

36. K. N. Durski, A. M. McCollum, Y. Nakazawa, B. W. Petersen, M. G. Reynolds, S. Briand, M. H. Djingarey, et al., "Emergence of Monkeypox—West and Central Africa, 1970–2017," *Morbidity and Mortality Weekly Report* 67, no. 10 (2018): 306.

37. L. V. Patrono, K. Pléh, L. Samuni, M. Ulrich, C. Röthemeier, A. Sachse, S. Muschter, et al., "Monkeypox Virus Emergence in Wild Chimpanzees Reveals Distinct Clinical Outcomes and Viral Diversity," *Nature Microbiology* 5, no. 7 (2020): 955–965.

38. World Health Organization, "Monkeypox," May 19, 2022, https://www.who.int/en/news-room/fact-sheets/detail/monkeypox.

39. M. Kozlov, "How Deadly Is Monkeypox? What Scientists Know," *Nature* 609, no. 7928 (2022): 663.

40. M. G. Reynolds, K. L. Yorita, M. J. Kuehnert, W. B. Davidson, G. D. Huhn, R. C. Holman, and I. K. Damon, "Clinical Manifestations of Human Monkeypox Influenced by Route of Infection," *Journal of Infectious Diseases* 194, no. 6 (2006): 773–780.

41. K. D. Reed, J. W. Melski, M. B. Graham, R. L. Regnery, M. J. Sotir, M. V. Wegner, J. J. Kazmierczak, et al., "The Detection of Monkeypox in Humans in the Western Hemisphere," *New England Journal of Medicine* 350, no. 4 (2004): 342–350.

42. D. R. Croft, M. J. Sotir, C. J. Williams, J. J. Kazmierczak, M. V. Wegner, D. Rausch, M. B. Graham, et al., "Occupational Risks during a Monkeypox Outbreak, Wisconsin, 2003," *Emerging Infectious Diseases* 13, no. 8 (2007): 1150.

43. A. M. Likos, S. A. Sammons, V. A. Olson, A. M. Frace, Y. Li, M. Olsen-Rasmussen, W. Davidson, et al., "A Tale of Two Clades: Monkeypox Viruses," *Journal of General Virology* 86, no. 10 (2005): 2661–2672.

44. C. L. Hutson, K. N. Lee, J. Abel, D. S. Carroll, J. M. Montgomery, V. A. Olson, W. Davidson, et al., "Monkeypox Zoonotic Associations: Insights from Laboratory Evaluation of Animals Associated with the Multi-State US Outbreak," *American Journal of Tropical Medicine and Hygiene* 76, no. 4 (2007): 757–768.

45. Department of Health and Human Services, Food and Drug Administration. 21 CFR Parts 16 and 1240, "Control of Communicable Diseases: Restrictions on African Rodents, Prairie Dogs, and Certain Other Animals," *Federal Register* 73, no. 174 (2008): 51912–51919, https://www.govinfo.gov/content/pkg/FR-2008-09-08/pdf/E8 -20779.pdf.

46. S. Nelson, "Giant 3-Foot-Long Rats Invade Florida Keys," WQAD8 ABC News, June 5, 2014, https://www.wqad.com/article/news/local/drone/8-in-the-air/giant-3 -foot-long-rats-invade-florida-keys/526-2dffbc99-0fb3-4d59-8fde-2530edcaf064; Hutson et al., "Monkeypox Zoonotic Associations."

47. M. F. Antolin, P. Gober, B. Luce, D. E. Biggins, W. E. Van Pelt, D. B. Seery, M. Lockhart, et al., "The Influence of Sylvatic Plague on North American Wildlife at the Landscape Level, with Special Emphasis on Black-Footed Ferret and Prairie Dog Conservation," *Transactions of the 67th North American Wildlife and Natural Resources Conference* 67 (2002): 104–127.

48. W. M. Lotfy, "Current Perspectives on the Spread of Plague in Africa," *Research and Reports in Tropical Medicine* 6 (2015): 21.

49. J. M. Duplantier, J. B. Duchemin, S. Chanteau, and E. Carniel, "From the Recent Lessons of the Malagasy Foci towards a Global Understanding of the Factors Involved in Plague Reemergence," *Veterinary Research* 36, no. 3 (2005): 437–453.

50. J. P. Chippaux and A. Chippaux, "Yellow Fever in Africa and the Americas: A Historical and Epidemiological Perspective," *Journal of Venomous Animals and Toxins Including Tropical Diseases* 24, no. 1 (2018): 20.

51. P. de Oliveira Figueiredo, A. G. Stoffella-Dutra, G. Barbosa Costa, J. Silva de Oliveira, C. Dourado Amaral, J. Duarte Santos, K. L. S. Rocha, et al., "Re-emergence of Yellow Fever in Brazil during 2016–2019: Challenges, Lessons Learned, and Perspectives," *Viruses* 12, no. 11 (2020): 1233.

52. L. Sacchetto, N. I. O. Silva, I. M. D. Rezende, M. S. Arruda, T. A. Costa, E. M. de Mello, G. F. G. Oliveira, et al., "Neighbor Danger: Yellow Fever Virus Epizootics in Urban and Urban-Rural Transition Areas of Minas Gerais State, during 2017–2018 Yellow Fever Outbreaks in Brazil," *PLoS Neglected Tropical Diseases* 14, no. 10 (2020): e0008658.

53. S. Darlington and D. G. McNeil Jr., "Yellow Fever Circles Brazil's Huge Cities," *New York Times*, March 5, 2018, https://www.nytimes.com/2018/03/05/health/brazil -yellow-fever.html.

54. Sacchetto et al., "Neighbor Danger."

55. de Oliveira Figueiredo et al., "Re-emergence of Yellow Fever in Brazil during 2016–2019."

56. Darlington and McNeil, "Yellow Fever Circles Brazil's Huge Cities."

57. S. Romero, "Brazil Yellow Fever Outbreak Spawns Alert: Stop Killing the Monkeys," *New York Times*, May 2, 2017, https://www.nytimes.com/2017/05/02/world/americas/brazil-yellow-fever-monkeys.html.

58. Quoted in Romero, "Brazil Yellow Fever Outbreak Spawns Alert."

59. N. D. Wolfe, C. P. Dunavan, and J. Diamond, "Origins of Major Human Infectious Diseases," *Nature* 447, no. 7142 (2007): 279–283.

60. D. Quammen, *Spillover: Animal Infections and the Next Human Pandemic* (New York: W. W. Norton and Company, 2012); S. Gryseels, T. D. Watts, J. M. K. Mpolesha, B. B. Larsen, P. Lemey, J. J. Muyembe-Tamfum, D. E. Teuwen, et al., "A Near Full-Length HIV-1 Genome from 1966 Recovered from Formalin-Fixed Paraffin-Embedded Tissue," *Proceedings of the National Academy of Sciences* 117, no. 22 (2020): 12222–12229.

61. P. Lemey, O. G. Pybus, B. Wang, N. K. Saksena, M. Salemi, and A. M. Vandamme, "Tracing the Origin and History of the HIV-2 Epidemic," *Proceedings of the National Academy of Sciences* 100, no. 11 (2003): 6588–6592.

62. S. Nyamweya, A. Hegedus, A. Jaye, S. Rowland-Jones, K. L. Flanagan, and D. C. Macallan, "Comparing HIV-1 and HIV-2 Infection: Lessons for Viral Immunopathogenesis," *Reviews in Medical Virology* 23, no. 4 (2013): 221–240.

63. M. Inglis, "Chimps and Gorillas Desperately Need Ebola Vaccine, Too—Virus Has Wiped Out a Third of Them," *Conversation*, January 20, 2015, https://theconversation.com/chimps-and-gorillas-desperately-need-ebola-vaccine-too-virus-has-wiped-out-a-third-of-them-35503.

64. R. Weiss, "Africa's Great Apes Are Imperiled, Researchers Warn," *Washington Post*, April 7, 2003.

65. ProMED, International Society for Infectious Diseases, 2022, https://promedmail.org.

66. L. C. Madoff, "ProMED-Mail: An Early Warning System for Emerging Diseases," *Clinical Infectious Diseases* 39, no. 2 (2004): 227–232.

67. PREDICT, 2022, https://p2.predict.global.

68. M. S. Tiee, R. J. Harrigan, H. A. Thomassen, and T. B. Smith, "Ghosts of Infections Past: Using Archival Samples to Understand a Century of Monkeypox Virus Prevalence among Host Communities across Space and Time," *Royal Society Open Science* 5, no. 1 (2018): 171089.

69. Gryseels et al. "A Near Full-Length HIV-1 Genome from 1966 Recovered."

Chapter 2

1. S. J. Gould and E. S. "Exaptation—A Missing Term in the Science of Form," *Paleobiology* 8, no. 1 (1982): 4–15.

2. J. R. Hurford, *Origins of Language: A Slim Guide* (Oxford: Oxford University Press, 2014).

3. R. J. Eccles, "Dirty Hands," *Dietetic and Hygienic Gazette* 25 (1909): 719.

4. G. A. Soper, "The Work of a Chronic Typhoid Germ Distributor," *Journal of the American Medical Association* 48, no. 24 (1907): 2019–2022.

5. R. Adler and E. Mara, *Typhoid Fever: A History* (Jefferson, NC: McFarland and Company, Inc., 2016).

6. J. W. Leavitt, *Typhoid Mary: Captive to the Public's Health* (Boston: Beacon Press, 1996).

7. Centers for Disease Control and Prevention, "Preventing Norovirus Outbreaks," *CDC Vital Signs*, June 2014.

8. R. R. Yorlets, K. Busa, K. R. Eberlin, M. A. Raisolsadat, D. S. Bae, P. M. Waters, B. I. Labow, et al., "Fingertip Injuries in Children: Epidemiology, Financial Burden, and Implications for Prevention," *Hand* 12, no. 4 (2017): 342–347.

9. S. Almécija, J. B. Smaers, and W. L. Jungers, "The Evolution of Human and Ape Hand Proportions," *Nature Communications* 6, no. 1 (2015): 7717.

10. T. L. Kivell, "Human Evolution: Thumbs Up for Efficiency," *Current Biology* 31, no. 6 (2021): R289–R291.

11. R. Diogo, B. G. Richmond, and B. Wood, "Evolution and Homologies of Primate and Modern Human Hand and Forearm Muscles, with Notes on Thumb Movements and Tool Use," *Journal of Human Evolution* 63, no. 1 (2012): 64–78.

12. M. W. Marzke, "Precision Grips, Hand Morphology, and Tools," *American Journal of Physical Anthropology* 102, no. 1 (1997): 91–110.

13. D. M. Fragaszy, "Preliminary Quantitative Studies of Prehension in Squirrel Monkeys (Saimiri sciureus)," *Brain, Behavior and Evolution* 23, no. 3–4 (1983): 81–92; M. B. Costello and D. M. Fragaszy, "Prehension in Cebus and Saimiri: I. Grip Type and Hand Preference," *American Journal of Primatology* 15, no. 3 (1988): 235–245.

14. G. A. Bortoff and P. L. Strick, "Corticospinal Terminations in Two New-World Primates: Further Evidence That Corticomotoneuronal Connections Provide Part of the Neural Substrate for Manual Dexterity," *Journal of Neuroscience* 13, no. 12 (1993): 5105–5118.

15. R. Arunachalam, V. S. Weerasinghe, and K. R. Mills, "Motor Control of Rapid Sequential Finger Tapping in Humans," *Journal of Neurophysiology* 94, no. 3 (2005): 2162–2170.

16. L. Zhang, L. Lei, Y. Zhao, R. Wang, Y. Zhu, Z. Yu, and X. Zhang, "Finger Tapping Outperforms the Traditional Scale in Patients with Peripheral Nerve Damage," *Frontiers in Physiology* 9 (2018): 1361.

17. A. Mathieu, T. O. Delmont, T. M. Vogel, P. Robe, R. Nalin, and P. Simonet, "Life on Human Surfaces: Skin Metagenomics," *PloS One* 8, no. 6 (2013): e65288.

18. K. R. Feingold and M. Denda, "Regulation of Permeability Barrier Homeostasis," *Clinics in Dermatology* 30, no. 3 (2012): 263–268.

19. H. Yamamoto, M. Hattori, W. Chamulitrat, Y. Ohno, and A. Kihara, "Skin Permeability Barrier Formation by the Ichthyosis-Causative Gene FATP4 through Formation of the Barrier Lipid ω-O-acylceramide," *Proceedings of the National Academy of Sciences* 117, no. 6 (2020): 2914–2922.

20. P. I. Beamer, C. E. Luik, R. A. Canales, and J. O. Leckie, "Quantified Outdoor Micro-Activity Data for Children Aged 7–12 Years Old," *Journal of Exposure Science and Environmental Epidemiology* 22, no. 1 (2012): 82–92.

21. J. L. Spille, M. Grunwald, S. Martin, and S. M. Mueller, "Stop Touching Your Face! A Systematic Review of Triggers, Characteristics, Regulatory Functions and Neuro-Physiology of Facial Self Touch," *Neuroscience and Biobehavioral Reviews* 128 (2021): 102–116.

22. J. A. Hall, N. A. Murphy, and M. S. Mast, "Nonverbal Self-Accuracy in Interpersonal Interaction," *Personality and Social Psychology Bulletin* 33, no. 12 (2007): 1675–1685.

23. A. M. Wilson, M. P. Verhougstraete, P. I. Beamer, M. F. King, K. A. Reynolds, and C. P. Gerba, "Frequency of Hand-to-Head, -Mouth, -Eyes, and -Nose Contacts for Adults and Children during Eating and Non-Eating Macro-Activities," *Journal of Exposure Science and Environmental Epidemiology* 31, no. 1 (2021): 34–44.

24. N. C. Elder, W. Sawyer, H. Pallerla, S. Khaja, and M. Blacker, "Hand Hygiene and Face Touching in Family Medicine Offices: A Cincinnati Area Research and Improvement Group (CARInG) Network Study," *Journal of the American Board of Family Medicine* 27, no. 3 (2014): 339–346.

25. Y. L. A. Kwok, J. Gralton, and M. L. McLaws, "Face Touching: A Frequent Habit That Has Implications for Hand Hygiene," *American Journal of Infection Control* 43, no. 2 (2015): 112–114.

26. S. A. Boone and C. P. Gerba, "Significance of Fomites in the Spread of Respiratory and Enteric Viral Disease," *Applied and Environmental Microbiology* 73, no. 6 (2007): 1687–1696.

27. F. Pancic, D. C. Carpentier, and P. E. Came, "Role of Infectious Secretions in the Transmission of Rhinovirus," *Journal of Clinical Microbiology* 12, no. 4 (1980): 567–571.

28. B. Winther, K. McCue, K. Ashe, J. R. Rubino, and J. O. Hendley, "Environmental Contamination with Rhinovirus and Transfer to Fingers of Healthy Individuals by Daily Life Activity," *Journal of Medical Virology* 79, no. 10 (2007): 1606–1610.

29. M. L. Rotter, "Semmelweis' Sesquicentennial: A Little-Noted Anniversary of Handwashing," *Current Opinion in Infectious Diseases* 11, no. 4 (1998): 457–460.

30. Rotter, "Semmelweis' Sesquicentennial."

31. D. Pittet and B. Allegranzi, "Preventing Sepsis in Healthcare—200 Years after the Birth of Ignaz Semmelweis," *Eurosurveillance* 23, no. 18 (2018): 18–00222.

32. Rotter, "Semmelweis' Sesquicentennial." Semmelweis wasn't the first person to promote hand hygiene for preventing puerperal sepsis, although he was the most effective. Scottish obstetrician Alexander Gordon proved the contagious nature of puerperal sepsis and advocated for handwashing in 1795. Almost fifty years later, in 1843, US physician Oliver Wendell Holmes showed that puerperal fever was frequently carried from patient to patient by physicians, whom he advised to wash themselves and change their clothes following autopsies.

33. Our tendency to reject new knowledge that contradicts established beliefs is a phenomenon sometimes called the Semmelweis effect. That's because Semmelweis's interventions were so unpopular that his contract at the hospital was not renewed in 1849. After continued resistance to his ideas, he ended his days in a mental institution, where he died of sepsis from an infected wound in 1865.

34. M. H. Gordon, *House of Commons (Ventilation): Report and Recommendations* (London: Darling and Son, 1905).

35. C. Flügge, "Die Verbreitung der Phthise durch staubförmiges Sputum und durch beim Husten verspritzte Tröpfchen," *Zeitschrift für Hygiene und Infektionskrankheiten* 30, no. 1 (1899): 107–124.

36. L. P. Garrod, "Mervyn Henry Gordon. 1872–1953," *Obituary Notices of Fellows of the Royal Society* 9, no. 1 (1954): 153–163.

37. B. C. Doust and A. B. Lyon, "Face Masks in Infections of the Respiratory Tract," *Journal of the American Medical Association* 71, no. 15 (1918): 1216–1219.

38. A. Prior, "COVID-19: Why It's So Difficult to Make the Call to Close Parliament," *Conversation*, May 19, 2020, I, https://theconversation.com/COVID-19-why-its-so-difficult-to-make-the-call-to-close-parliament-134082.

39. J. R. Hurford, *Origins of Language: A Slim Guide* (Oxford: Oxford University Press, 2014).

40. A. A. Fernandez, L. S. Burchardt, M. Nagy, and M. Knörnschild, "Babbling in a Vocal Learning Bat Resembles Human Infant Babbling," *Science* 373, no. 6557 (2021): 923–926.

41. S. Asadi, A. S. Wexler, C. D. Cappa, S. Barreda, N. M. Bouvier, and W. D. Ristenpart, "Aerosol Emission and Superemission during Human Speech Increase with Voice Loudness," *Scientific Reports* 9, no. 1 (2019): 1–10.

42. Hurford, *Origins of Language*.

43. M. R. Mehl, S. Vazire, N. Ramírez-Esparza, R. B. Slatcher, and J. W. Pennebaker, "Are Women Really More Talkative Than Men?," *Science* 317, no. 5834 (2007): 82.

44. W. T. Fitch, "The Biology and Evolution of Speech: A Comparative Analysis," *Annual Review of Linguistics* 4 (2018): 255–279.

45. S. Neubauer, J. J. Hublin, and P. Gunz, "The Evolution of Modern Human Brain Shape," *Science Advances* 4, no. 1 (2018): eaao5961.

46. P. Lieberman, "The Evolution of Human Speech: Its Anatomical and Neural Bases," *Current Anthropology* 48, no. 1 (2007): 39–66.

47. W. Tecumseh Fitch and D. Reby, "The Descended Larynx Is Not Uniquely Human," *Proceedings of the Royal Society of London. Series B: Biological Sciences* 268, no. 1477 (2001): 1669–1675.

48. W. T. Fitch, "The Biology and Evolution of Speech: A Comparative Analysis," *Annual Review of Linguistics* 4 (2018): 255–279.

49. D. Lieberman, *The Story of the Human Body: Evolution, Health, and Disease* (New York: Pantheon Press, 2013).

50. A. D. Friederici, N. Chomsky, R. C. Berwick, A. Moro, and J. J. Bolhuis, "Language, Mind and Brain," *Nature Human Behaviour* 1, no. 10 (2017): 713–722.

51. N. Staes, C. C. Sherwood, K. Wright, M. de Manuel, E. E. Guevara, T. Marques-Bonet, M. Krützen, et al., "FOXP2 Variation in Great Ape Populations Offers Insight into the Evolution of Communication Skills," *Scientific Reports* 7, no. 1 (2017): 1–10.

52. C. S. Lai, S. E. Fisher, J. A. Hurst, F. Vargha-Khadem, and A. P. Monaco, "A Forkhead-Domain Gene Is Mutated in a Severe Speech and Language Disorder," *Nature* 413, no. 6855 (2001): 519–523; K. E. Watkins, N. F. Dronkers, and F. Vargha-Khadem, "Behavioural Analysis of an Inherited Speech and Language Disorder: Comparison with Acquired Aphasia," *Brain* 125, no. 3 (2002): 452–464.

53. "Quick Statistics about Voice, Speech, and Language," National Institute on Deafness and Other Communication Disorders, accessed April 23, 2023, https://www.nidcd.nih.gov/health/statistics/quick-statistics-voice-speech-language.

54. A. E. Williams, *Immunology: Mucosal and Body Surface Defences* (Hoboken, NJ: Wiley-Blackwell, 2012).

55. G. Pier, "Molecular Mechanisms of Microbial Pathogenesis," in *Harrison's Infectious Diseases*, ed. D. L. Kasper and A. S. Fauci, 3rd ed. (New York: McGraw-Hill Education Medical, 2017), 11–22.

56. W. W. Busse, "Pathogenesis and Sequelae of Respiratory Infections," *Reviews of Infectious Diseases* 13, supp. 6 (1991): S477–S485.

57. M. Meselson, "Droplets and Aerosols in the Transmission of SARS-CoV-2," *New England Journal of Medicine* 382, no. 21 (2020): 2063.

58. Pier, "Molecular Mechanisms of Microbial Pathogenesis."

59. D. M. Morens, J. K. Taubenberger, and A. S. Fauci, "Predominant Role of Bacterial Pneumonia as a Cause of Death in Pandemic Influenza: Implications for Pandemic Influenza Preparedness," *Journal of Infectious Diseases* 198, no. 7 (2008): 962–970.

60. J. H. K. Chen, C. C. Y. Yip, R. W. S. Poon, K. H. Chan, V. C. C. Cheng, I. F. N. Hung, J. F. W. Chan, et al., "Evaluating the Use of Posterior Oropharyngeal Saliva in a Point-of-Care Assay for the Detection of SARS-CoV-2," *Emerging Microbes and Infections* 9, no. 1 (2020): 1356–1359.

61. V. Stadnytskyi, C. E. Bax, A. Bax, A., and P. Anfinrud, "The Airborne Lifetime of Small Speech Droplets and Their Potential Importance in SARS-CoV-2 Transmission," *Proceedings of the National Academy of Sciences* 117, no. 22 (2020): 11875–11877.

62. S. Asadi, A. S. Wexler, C. D. Cappa, S. Barreda, N. M. Bouvier, and W. D. Ristenpart, "Aerosol Emission and Superemission during Human Speech Increase with Voice Loudness," *Scientific Reports* 9, no. 1 (2019): 1–10."

63. A. Asadi, C. D. Cappa, S. Barreda, A. S. Wexler, N. M. Bouvier, and W. D. Ristenpart, "Efficacy of Masks and Face Coverings in Controlling Outward Aerosol Particle Emission from Expiratory Activities," *Scientific Reports* 10, no. 1 (2020): 1–13.

64. S. Asadi, A. S. Wexler, C. D. Cappa, S. Barreda, N. M. Bouvier, and W. D. Ristenpart, "Effect of Voicing and Articulation Manner on Aerosol Particle Emission during Human Speech," *PloS One* 15, no. 1 (2020): e0227699.

65. Pittet and Allegranzi, "Preventing Sepsis in Healthcare."

66. M. Z. Wahrman, *The Hand Book: Surviving in a Germ-Filled World* (Lebanon, NH: ForeEdge, 2016), 133.

67. World Health Organization, *Hand Hygiene for All*, accessed April 3, 2022, https://www.unicef.org/media/71776/file/Hand-hygiene-for-all-2020.pdf.

68. J. Abaluck, L. H. Kwong, A. Styczynski, A. Haque, A. Kabir, E. Bates-Jefferys, E. Crawford, et al., "Impact of Community Masking on COVID-19: A Cluster-Randomized Trial in Bangladesh," *Science* 375, no. 6577 (2022): eabi9069, https://www.science.org/doi/10.1126/science.abi9069.

69. J. Abaluck, L. H. Kwong, and S. P. Luby. "We Did the Research: Masks Work, and You Should Choose a High Quality Mask if Possible," *New York Times*, September 26, 2021, accessed August 10, 2023, https://www.nytimes.com/2021/09/26/opinion/do-masks-work-for-covid-prevention.html.

70. T. Mitze, R, Kosfeld, J. Rode, and K. Wälde, "Face Masks Considerably Reduce COVID-19 Cases in Germany," *Proceedings of the National Academy of Sciences* 117, no. 51 (2020): 32293–32301.

Chapter 3

1. J. Donne, *Devotions upon Emergent Occasions* (1624; repr., Oxford: Oxford University Press on Demand, 1987), https://www.gutenberg.org/files/23772/23772-h/23772-h.htm.

2. P. Brimblecombe, *The Big Smoke: A History of Air Pollution in London since Medieval Times* (Abingdon, UK: Routledge, 2011).

3. J. Evelyn, *Fumifugium; Or, the Inconvenience of the Aer and Smoake of London* (London: Humphries, 1772).

4. E. Cockayne, *Hubbub: Filth, Noise and Stench in England, 1600–1770* (New Haven, CT: Yale University Press, 2007).

5. E. Vázquez-Espinosa, C. Laganà, and F. Vazquez, "John Donne, Spanish Doctors and the Epidemic Typhus: Fleas or Lice?," *Revista Española de Quimioterapia* 33, no. 2 (2020): 87.

6. Epidemic typhus belongs to a group of typhus fevers associated with different microbes and vectors of transmission. Other notable forms of typhus include scrub (or bush) typhus, which is caused by the bacterium *Orientia tsutsugamushi* and transmitted by some species of chiggers, and flea-borne (or murine or endemic) typhus, which is caused by the bacterium *Rickettsia typhi* and commonly transmitted by the Oriental rat flea (*Xenopsylla cheopis*).

7. When Donne died in 1631, years after he recovered from his illness, he was laid to rest in Saint Paul's Cathedral. Ironically, his burial place is shared with the ashes of Alexander Fleming, the father of antibiotics. Fleming's discovery of penicillin led to a revolution in antibiotic treatments of bacterial diseases, including epidemic typhus.

8. H. Zinsser, *Rats, Lice and History* (Abingdon, UK: Routledge, 1935).

9. S. Badiaga and P. Brouqui, "Human Louse-Transmitted Infectious Diseases," *Clinical Microbiology and Infection* 18, no. 4 (2012): 332–337.

10. P. M. Hohenberg and L. H. Lees, *The Making of Urban Europe, 1000–1994* (Cambridge, MA: Harvard University Press, 1985).

11. G. L. Cowgill, "Origins and Development of Urbanism: Archaeological Perspectives," *Annual Review of Anthropology* 33 (2004): 525–549.

12. Hohenberg and Lees, *The Making of Urban Europe, 1000–1994.*

13. J. Graunt, *Natural and Political Observations Mentioned in a Following Index, and Made upon the Bills of Mortality* (London: Tho. Roycroft, 1662), http://name.umdl .umich.edu/A41827.0001.001.

14. R. Porter, *London, A Social History* (Cambridge, MA: Harvard University Press, 1995).

15. Cockayne, *Hubbub.*

16. S. Ayyadurai, F. Sebbane, D. Raoult, and M. Drancourt, "Body Lice, *Yersinia pestis orientalis*, and Black Death," *Emerging Infectious Diseases* 16, no. 5 (2010): 892; K. R. Dean, F. Krauer, L. Walløe, O. C. Lingjærde, B. Bramanti, N. C. Stenseth, and B. V. Schmid, "Human Ectoparasites and the Spread of Plague in Europe during the Second Pandemic," *Proceedings of the National Academy of Sciences* 115, no. 6 (2018): 1304–1309. In addition to *R. prowazekii* and possibly *Y. pestis*, the body louse is the vector of two other well-known human pathogens: *Bartonella recurrentis*, which causes relapsing fever, and *Bartonella quintana*, which causes trench fever. Several pathogens can infect the same louse at the same time. The other two types of human-adapted lice, the head louse (*Pediculus humanus capitis*) and pubic louse (*Pthirus pubis*), can act as competent vectors under laboratory conditions, and head lice with *Y. pestis* and *B. quintana* infections have been reported.

17. United Nations, "The World's Cities in 2018—Data Booklet" (2018).

18. J.-J. Hublin, A. Ben-Ncer, S. E. Bailey, S. E. Freidline, S. Neubauer, M. M. Skinner, I. Bergmann, et al., "New Fossils from Jebel Irhoud, Morocco and the Pan-African Origin of *Homo sapiens*," *Nature* 546, no. 7657 (2017): 289–292.

19. A. Gibbons, "World's Oldest *Homo sapiens* Fossils Found in Morocco," *Science* (2017).

20. K. Harvati, C. Röding, A. M. Bosman, F. A. Karakostis, R. Grün, C. Stringer, P. Karkanas, et al., "Apidima Cave Fossils Provide Earliest Evidence of *Homo sapiens* in Eurasia," *Nature* 571, no. 7766 (2019): 500–504.

21. M. Stewart, R. Clark-Wilson, P. S. Breeze, M. Janulis, I. Candy, S. J. Armitage, D. B. Ryves, et al., "Human Footprints Provide Snapshot of Last Interglacial Ecology in the Arabian Interior," *Science Advances* 6, no. 38 (2020): eaba8940; D. Bustos, J. Jakeway, T. M. Urban, V. T. Holliday, B. Fenerty, D. A. Raichlen, M. Budka, et al., "Footprints Preserve Terminal Pleistocene Hunt? Human-Sloth Interactions in North America," *Science Advances* 4, no. 4 (2018): eaar7621.

22. A. Brumm, A. A. Oktaviana, B. Burhan, B. Hakim, R. Lebe, J.-X. Zhao, P. H. Sulistyarto, et al., "Oldest Cave Art Found in Sulawesi," *Science Advances* 7, no. 3 (2021): eabd4648.

23. R. Barrett and G. Armelagos, *An Unnatural History of Emerging Infections* (Oxford: Oxford University Press, 2013).

24. D. Richter, R. Grün, R. Joannes-Boyau, T. E. Steele, F. Amani, M. Rué, P. Fernandes, et al., "The Age of the Hominin Fossils from Jebel Irhoud, Morocco, and the Origins of the Middle Stone Age," *Nature* 546, no. 7657 (2017): 293–296.

25. A. G. Henry, A. S. Brooks, and D. R. Piperno, "Plant Foods and the Dietary Ecology of Neanderthals and Early Modern Humans," *Journal of Human Evolution* 69 (2014): 44–54.

26. M. N. Cohen, *Health and the Rise of Civilization* (New Haven, CT: Yale University Press, 1989).

27. K. E. Jones, N. G. Patel, M. A. Levy, A. Storeygard, D. Balk, J. L. Gittleman, and P. Daszak, "Global Trends in Emerging Infectious Diseases," *Nature* 451, no. 7181 (2008): 990–993.

28. K. J. Olival, P. R. Hosseini, C. Zambrana-Torrelio, N. Ross, T. L. Bogich, and P. Daszak, "Host and Viral Traits Predict Zoonotic Spillover from Mammals," *Nature* 546, no. 7660 (2017): 646–650.

29. F. L. Black, "Measles Endemicity in Insular Populations: Critical Community Size and Its Evolutionary Implication," *Journal of Theoretical Biology* 11, no. 2 (1966): 207–211.

30. Barrett and Armelagos, *An Unnatural History of Emerging Infections*.

31. F. W. Marlowe, "Hunter-Gatherers and Human Evolution," *Evolutionary Anthropology* 14, no. 2 (2005): 54–67; R. L. Kelly, *The Lifeways of Hunter-Gatherers: The Foraging Spectrum* (Cambridge: Cambridge University Press, 2013).

32. L. R. Binford, "Mobility, Housing, and Environment: A Comparative Study," *Journal of Anthropological Research* 46, no. 2 (1990): 119–152.

33. E. M. L. Scerri, M. G. Thomas, A. Manica, P. Gunz, J. T. Stock, C. Stringer, M. Grove, et al., "Did Our Species Evolve in Subdivided Populations across Africa, and Why Does It Matter?," *Trends in Ecology and Evolution* 33, no. 8 (2018): 582–594.

34. J. L. A. Webb Jr., "Early Malarial Infections and the First Epidemiological Transition," in *Human Dispersal and Species Movement: From Prehistory to the Present*, ed. N. Boivin, R. Crassard, and M. Petraglia (Cambridge: Cambridge University Press, 2017): 477–493.

35. Why this transition occurred is one of the most debated topics in anthropology, and well beyond the scope of this book. For a comprehensive consideration of this question, see G. Barker, *The Agricultural Revolution in Prehistory: Why Did Foragers Become Farmers?* (Oxford: Oxford University Press, 2009).

36. A. Snir, D. Nadel, I. Groman-Yaroslavski, Y. Melamed, M. Sternberg, O. Bar-Yosef, and E. Weiss, "The Origin of Cultivation and Proto-Weeds, Long before Neolithic Farming," *PLoS One* 10, no. 7 (2015): e0131422; M. A. Zeder, "The Origins of Agriculture in the Near East," *Current Anthropology* 52, no. S4 (2011): S221–S235.

37. Webb, "Early Malarial Infections and the First Epidemiological Transition."

38. C. J. Adler, K. Dobney, L. S. Weyrich, J. Kaidonis, A. W. Walker, W. Haak, C. J. A. Bradshaw, et al., "Sequencing Ancient Calcified Dental Plaque Shows Changes in Oral Microbiota with Dietary Shifts of the Neolithic and Industrial Revolutions," *Nature Genetics* 45, no. 4 (2013): 450. The same research shows a similar shift with the consumption of industrially processed flour and sugar during the Industrial Revolution, beginning in the nineteenth century.

39. L. M. Looi and K. B. Chua, "Lessons from the Nipah Virus Outbreak in Malaysia," *Malaysian Journal of Pathology* 29, no. 2 (2007): 63–67.

40. G. J. D. Smith, D. Vijaykrishna, J. Bahl, S. J. Lycett, M. Worobey, O. G. Pybus, S. K. Ma, et al., "Origins and Evolutionary Genomics of the 2009 Swine-Origin H1N1 Influenza A Epidemic," *Nature* 459, no. 7250 (2009): 1122–1125.

41. A. Düx, S. Lequime, L. V. Patrono, B. Vrancken, S. Boral, J. F. Gogarten, A. Hilbig, et al., "Measles Virus and Rinderpest Virus Divergence Dated to the Sixth Century BCE," *Science* 368, no. 6497 (2020): 1367–1370.

42. S. Rasmussen, M. E. Allentoft, K. Nielsen, L. Orlando, M. Sikora, K.-G. Sjögren, A. G. Pedersen, et al., "Early Divergent Strains of Yersinia Pestis in Eurasia 5,000 Years Ago," *Cell* 163, no. 3 (2015): 571–582; A. Andrades Valtueña, G. U. Neumann, M. A. Spyrou, L. Musralina, F. Aron, A. Beisenov, A. B. Belinskiy, K. I. Bos, et al., "Stone Age *Yersinia pestis* Genomes Shed Light on the Early Evolution, Diversity, and Ecology of Plague," *Proceedings of the National Academy of Sciences* 119, no. 17 (2022): e2116722119, https://www.pnas.org/doi/10.1073/pnas.2116722119.

43. P. Swali, R. Schulting, A. Gilardet, M. Kelly, K. Anastasiadou, I. Glocke, J. McCabe, et al. "*Yersinia pestis* Genomes Reveal Plague in Britain 4000 Years Ago," *Nature Communications* 14, no. 1 (2023): 2930, https://www.nature.com/articles/s41467-023-38393-w.

44. M. A. Spyrou, R. I. Tukhbatova, C.-C. Wang, A. Andrades Valtueña, A. K. Lankapalli, V. V. Kondrashin, V. A. Tsybin, et al. "Analysis of 3800-Year-Old *Yersinia pestis* Genomes Suggests Bronze Age Origin for Bubonic Plague," *Nature Communications* 9, no. 1 (2018): 2234, https://pubmed.ncbi.nlm.nih.gov/29884871.

45. M. Keller, M. A. Spyrou, C. L. Scheib, G. U. Neumann, A. Kröpelin, B. Haas-Gebhard, B. Päffgen, et al., "Ancient Yersinia Pestis Genomes from across Western Europe Reveal Early Diversification during the First Pandemic (541–750)," *Proceedings of the National Academy of Sciences* 116, no. 25 (2019): 12363–12372.

46. M. A. Spyrou, L. Musralina, G. A. Gnecchi Ruscone, A. Kocher, P. G. Borbone, V. I. Khartanovich, A. Buzhilova, et al., "The Source of the Black Death in Fourteenth-Century Central Eurasia," *Nature* 606, no. 7915 (2022): 718–724.

47. R. P. H. Yue, F. L. Lee, and C. Y. H. Wu, "Trade Routes and Plague Transmission in Pre-Industrial Europe," *Scientific Reports* 7, no. 1 (2017): 1–10.

48. B. Bramanti, K. R. Dean, L. Walløe, and N. C. Stenseth, "The Third Plague Pandemic in Europe," *Proceedings of the Royal Society B: Biological Sciences* 286, no. 1901 (2019): 20182429.

49. L. Wade, "From Black Death to Fatal Flu, Past Pandemics Show Why People on the Margins Suffer Most," *Science*, May 14, 2020, https://www.science.org/content /article/black-death-fatal-flu-past-pandemics-show-why-people-margins-suffer-most.

50. F. Roumpani and P. Hudson, "The Evolution of London: The City's Near-2,000-Year History Mapped," *Guardian*, May 15, 2014, https://www.theguardian.com/cities /2014/may/15/the-evolution-of-london-the-citys-near-2000-year-history-mapped.

51. D. Hoornweg and K. Pope, "Socioeconomic Pathways and Regional Distribution of the World's 101 Largest Cities," Global Cities Institute, 2014, http://media.wix .com/ugd/672989_62cfa13ec4ba47788f78ad660489a2fa.pdf.

52. M. Roser and L. Rodés-Guirao, "Future Population Growth," Our World in Data, accessed February 28, 2023, https://ourworldindata.org/future-population-growth.

53. There are four species of Ebola viruses known to cause disease in humans: Ebola virus (Zaire ebolavirus), Sudan virus (Sudan ebolavirus), Taï Forest virus (Taï Forest ebolavirus, formerly Côte d'Ivoire ebolavirus), and Bundibugyo virus (Bundibugyo ebolavirus). Reston virus (Reston ebolavirus) is known to cause disease in nonhuman primates and pigs, but not in people. Bombali virus (Bombali ebolavirus) was recently identified in bats, but its potential to cause disease in other animals is unknown. Zaire ebolavirus is the most fatal Ebola virus and the cause of the largest outbreaks to date.

54. K. Kupferschmidt, "This Bat Species May Be the Source of the Ebola Epidemic That Killed More Than 11,000 People in West Africa," *Science* (2019).

55. World Health Organization, "Origins of the 2014 Ebola Epidemic," January 2015, https://www.who.int/news-room/spotlight/one-year-into-the-ebola-epidemic/ origins-of-the-2014-ebola-epidemic.

56. A. Marí Saéz, S. Weiss, K. Nowak, V. Lapeyre, F. Zimmermann, A. Düx, H. S. Kühl, et al., "Investigating the Zoonotic Origin of the West African Ebola Epidemic," *EMBO Molecular Medecine* 7, no. 1 (2015): 17–23.

57. J. Fairhead, M. Leach, and D. Millimouno, "Spillover or Endemic? Reconsidering the Origins of Ebola Virus Disease Outbreaks by Revisiting Local Accounts in Light of New Evidence from Guinea," *BMJ Global Health* 6 (2021): e005783.

58. B. P. Bell, "Overview, Control Strategies, and the Lessons Learned in the CDC Response to the df2014–2016 Ebola Epidemic," *MMWR Supplements* 65 (2016).

59. K. A. Alexander, C. E. Sanderson, M. Marathe, B. L. Lewis, C. M. Rivers, J. Shaman, J. M. Drake, et al., "What Factors Might Have Led to the Emergence of Ebola in West Africa?," *PLoS Neglected Tropical Diseases* 9, no. 6 (2015): e0003652.

Chapter 4

1. A. Whiten, "The Psychological Reach of Culture in Animals' Lives," *Current Directions in Psychological Science* 30, no. 3 (2021): 211–217.

2. A. Thornton and K. McAuliffe, "Teaching in Wild Meerkats," *Science* 313, no. 5784 (2006): 227–229.

3. P. Marler and M. Tamura, "Song 'Dialects' in Three Populations of White-Crowned Sparrows," *Condor* 64, no. 5 (1962): 368–377.

4. E. J. C. van Leeuwen, K. A. Cronin, and D. B. M. Haun, "A Group-Specific Arbitrary Tradition in Chimpanzees (Pan troglodytes)," *Animal Cognition* 17, no. 6 (2014): 1421–1425.

5. G. Ramsey, "Culture in Humans and Other Animals," *Biology and Philosophy* 28, no. 3 (2013): 457–479.

6. R. M. Sapolsky, *Behave: The Biology of Humans at Our Best and Worst* (New York: Penguin Press, 2017), 271.

7. P. Farmer, *Fevers, Feuds, and Diamonds: Ebola and the Ravages of History* (New York: Farrar, Straus and Giroux, 2020), 47.

8. O. Edwards, "The Skeletons of Shanidar Cave," *Smithsonian Magazine*, March 2010, https://www.smithsonianmag.com/arts-culture/the-skeletons-of-shanidar-cave-7028477.

9. M. C. Stiner, "Love and Death in the Stone Age: What Constitutes First Evidence of Mortuary Treatment of the Human Body?," *Biological Theory* 12, no. 4 (2017): 248–261.

10. M. Martinón-Torres, F. D'errico, E. Santos, A. Álvaro Gallo, N. Amano, W. Archer, S. J. Armitage, et al., "Earliest Known Human Burial in Africa," *Nature* 593, no. 7857 (2021): 95–100.

11. K. N. Swift and J. M. Marzluff, "Occurrence and Variability of Tactile Interactions between Wild American Crows and Dead Conspecifics," *Philosophical Transactions of the Royal Society B: Biological Sciences* 373, no. 1754 (2018): 20170259.

12. K. N. Swift and J. M. "Wild American Crows Gather around Their Dead to Learn about Danger," *Animal Behaviour* 109 (2015): 187–197.

13. M. A. Reggente, F. Alves, C. Nicolau, L. Freitas, D. Cagnazzi, R. W. Baird, and P. Galli, "Nurturant Behavior toward Dead Conspecifics in Free-Ranging Mammals: New Records for Odontocetes and a General Review," *Journal of Mammalogy* 97, no. 5 (2016): 1428–1434.

14. Stiner, "Love and Death in the Stone Age."

15. S. D. Glazier and C. R. Ember, "Religion," Explaining Human Culture, November 28, 2018, https://hraf.yale.edu/ehc/summaries/religion.

16. P. Bloom, "Is God an Accident?," *Atlantic*, December 2005, https://www.the atlantic.com/magazine/archive/2005/12/is-god-an-accident/304425.

17. P. Bloom, "Religion, Morality, Evolution," *Annual Review of Psychology* 63 (2012): 179–199.

18. D. Johnson and J. Bering, "Hand of God, Mind of Man: Punishment and Cognition in the Evolution of Cooperation," *Evolutionary Psychology* 4, no. 1 (2006).

19. J. Schloss, "Introduction: Evolutionary Theories of Religion; Science Unfettered or Naturalism Run Wild?," in *The Believing Primate: Scientific, Philosophical, and Theological Reflections on the Origin of Religion*, ed. M. Murray and J. Schloss (Oxford: Oxford University Press, 2006), 1–25.

20. US Centers for Disease Control and Prevention, "Costs of the Ebola Epidemic," 2019, https://www.cdc.gov/vhf/ebola/history/2014-2016-outbreak/cost-of-ebola.html #N9.

21. C. L. Althaus, "Estimating the Reproduction Number of Ebola Virus (EBOV) during the 2014 Outbreak in West Africa," *PLoS Currents* 6 (2014).

22. Farmer, *Fevers, Feuds, and Diamonds*.

23. World Health Organization, "Ebola Virus Disease," 2021, https://www.who.int /news-room/fact-sheets/detail/ebola-virus-disease.

24. Survival isn't always the end of transmission either. Studies have shown that the Ebola virus can persist in the semen of male survivors for up to a year or longer.

25. P. Vetter, W. A. Fischer, M. Schibler, M. Jacobs, D. G. Bausch, and L. Kaiser, "Ebola Virus Shedding and Transmission: Review of Current Evidence," *Journal of Infectious Diseases* 214, supp. 3 (2016): S177–S184.

26. J. Prescott, T. Bushmaker, R. Fischer, K. Miazgowicz, S. Judson, and V. J. Munster, "Postmortem Stability of Ebola Virus," *Emerging Infectious Diseases* 21, no. 5 (2015): 856.

27. P. Richards and A. Mokuwa, "Village Funerals and the Spread of Ebola Virus Disease," *Cultural Anthropology*, 2014, https://culanth.org/fieldsights/village-funerals -and-the-spread-of-ebola-virus-disease.

28. A. Manguvo and B. Mafuvadze, "The Impact of Traditional and Religious Practices on the Spread of Ebola in West Africa: Time for a Strategic Shift," *Pan African Medical Journal* 22, supp. 1 (2015).

29. World Health Organization, "Sierra Leone: A Traditional Healer and a Funeral, 2015, https://www.who.int/news/item/01-09-2015-sierra-leone-a-traditional-healer-and-a-funeral.

30. Farmer, *Fevers, Feuds, and Diamonds*.

31. K. G. Curran, J. J. Gibson, D. Marke, V. Caulker, J. Bomeh, J. T. Redd, S. Bunga, et al., "Cluster of Ebola Virus Disease Linked to a Single Funeral—Moyamba District, Sierra Leone, 2014," *Morbidity and Mortality Weekly Report* 65, no. 8 (2016): 202–205.

32. K. R. Victory, F. Coronado, S. O. Ifono, T. Soropogui, and B. A. Dahl, "Ebola Transmission Linked to a Single Traditional Funeral Ceremony—Kissidougou, Guinea, December, 2014–January 2015," *Morbidity and Mortality Weekly Report* 64, no. 14 (2015): 386.

33. Curran et al., "Cluster of Ebola Virus Disease Linked to a Single Funeral.".

34. C. F. Nielsen, S. Kidd, A. R. Sillah, E. Davis, J. Mermin, and P. H. Kilmarx, "Improving Burial Practices and Cemetery Management during an Ebola Virus Disease Epidemic—Sierra Leone, 2014," *Morbidity and Mortality Weekly Report* 64, no. 1 (2015): 20.

35. J. B. Blevins, M. F. Jalloh, and D. A. Robinson, "Faith and Global Health Practice in Ebola and HIV Emergencies," *American Journal of Public Health* 109, no. 3 (2019): 379–384.

36. Blevins, Jalloh, and Robinson, "Faith and Global Health Practice in Ebola and HIV Emergencies."

37. W. Williams and M. Mark, "Families Left Haunted by Liberia's Ebola Crematorium," *Guardian*, January 23, 2015, https://www.theguardian.com/world/2015/jan/23/-sp-liberia-ebola-crematorium.

38. D. R. Allen, R. Lacson, M. Patel, and M. Beach, "Understanding Why Ebola Deaths Occur at Home in Urban Montserrado County, Liberia," Centers for Disease Control and Prevention, 2015, http://www.ebola-anthropology.net/wp-content/uploads/2015/07/FINAL-Report-to-Liberia-MoH-Understanding-Why-Ebola-Deaths-Occur-at-Home-Liberia.pdf.

39. A. L. Rogers and R. Dixon, "Ebola's Lingering Pain: Liberians Rue Use of Cremation," *Los Angeles Times*, March 11, 2015, https://www.latimes.com/world/africa/la-fg-ebola-liberia-cremation-20150311-story.html.

40. Rogers and Dixon, "Ebola's Lingering Pain."

41. J. H. Giayhue, "Bones, Ashes at Liberia Crematorium a Reminder of Ebola Trauma," Reuters, January 18, 2015, https://www.reuters.com/article/health-ebola -liberia-idINL3N0UP08J20150118.

42. M. Zhang, "From Respirator to Wu's Mask: The Transition of Personal Protective Equipment in the Manchurian Plague," *Journal of Modern Chinese History* 14, no. 2 (2020): 221–239.

43. L.-T. Wu, *Plague Fighter: The Autobiography of a Modern Chinese Physician* (Cambridge, UK: W. Heffer, 1959).

44. Wu, *Plague Fighter.*

45. R. P. Strong, G. F. Petrie, and A. Stanley, *Report of the International Plague Conference Held at Mukden, April, 1911* (Manila: Bureau of Printing, 1912), 464.

46. Strong, Petrie, and Stanley, *Report of the International Plague Conference*, 262, 464.

47. L.-T. Wu, *A Treatise on Pneumonic Plague* (Geneva: Berger-Levrault, 1926), 428.

48. M. Echenberg, *Plague Ports: The Global Urban Impact of Bubonic Plague, 1894–1901* (New York: NYU Press, 2007), 219.

49. A. V. Jaeggi and M. Gurven, "Reciprocity Explains Food Sharing in Humans and Other Primates Independent of Kin Selection and Tolerated Scrounging: A Phylogenetic Meta-Analysis," *Proceedings of the Royal Society B: Biological Sciences* 280, no. 1768 (2013): 20131615.

50. S. Kerner and C. Chou, introduction to *Commensality: From Everyday Food to Feast*, ed. S. Kerner, C. Chou, and M. Warmind (London: Bloomsbury Publishing, 2015), 2.

51. N. Leite, *Unorthodox Kin: Portuguese Marranos and the Global Search for Belonging* (Berkeley: University of California Press, 2017), 243.

52. C. Fischler, "Commensality, Society and Culture," *Social Science Information* 50, no. 3–4 (2011): 534.

53. K. Woolley and A. Fishbach, "A Recipe for Friendship: Similar Food Consumption Promotes Trust and Cooperation," *Journal of Consumer Psychology* 27, no. 1 (2017): 1–10.

54. K. Woolley and A. Fishbach, "Shared Plates, Shared Minds: Consuming from a Shared Plate Promotes Cooperation," *Psychological Science* 30, no. 4 (2019): 541–552.

55. W. Robertson Smith, *Lectures on the Religion of the Semites* (New York: D. Appleton and Co., 1889), 252.

56. Robertson Smith, *Lectures on the Religion of the Semites*, 253.

57. C.-B. Tan, "Commensality and the Organization of Social Relations," in *Commensality: From Everyday Food to Feast*, ed. S. Kerner, C. Chou, and M. Warmind (London: Bloomsbury Publishing, 2017), 21.

58. Tan, "Commensality and the Organization of Social Relations."

59. L. Yoder, "The Funeral Meal: A Significant Funerary Ritual," *Journal of Religion and Health* 25, no. 2 (1986): 149–160.

60. A. van Gennep, *The Rites of Passage* (Chicago: University of Chicago Press, 1960), 164.

61. Tan, "Commensality and the Organization of Social Relations," 19.

62. World Health Organization," Food Safety," May 19, 2022, https://www.who.int /NEWS-ROOM/FACT-SHEETS/DETAIL/FOOD-SAFETY.

63. L. H. Gould, I. D. A. Rosenblum, D. Nicholas, Q. Phan, and T. F. Jones, "Contributing Factors in Restaurant-Associated Foodborne Disease Outbreaks, FoodNet Sites, 2006 and 2007," *Journal of Food Protection* 76, no. 11 (2013): 1824–1828.

64. A. Collman, "5 Million People Left Wuhan before China Quarantined the City to Contain the Coronavirus Outbreak," *Business Insider*, January 27, 2022, https://www .businessinsider.com/5-million-left-wuhan-before-coronavirus-quarantine-2020-1.

65. J. Lu, J. Gu, K. Li, C. Xu, W. Su, Z. Lai, D. Zhou, et al., "COVID-19 Outbreak Associated with Air Conditioning in Restaurant, Guangzhou, China, 2020," *Emerging Infectious Diseases* 26, no. 7 (2020): 1628.

66. Y. Li, H. Qian, J. Hang, X. Chen, P. Cheng, H. Ling, S. Wang, et al., "Probable Airborne Transmission of SARS-CoV-2 in a Poorly Ventilated Restaurant," *Building and Environment* 196 (2021): 107788.

67. D. Lewis, "Why the WHO Took Two Years to Say COVID Is Airborne," *Nature* 604, no. 7904 (2022): 26–31.

68. K. S. Kwon, J. I. Park, Y. J. Park, D. M. Jung, K. W. Ryu, and J. H. Lee, "Evidence of Long-Distance Droplet Transmission of SARS-CoV-2 by Direct Air Flow in a Restaurant in Korea," *Journal of Korean Medical Science* 35, no. 46 (2020).

69. Lewis, "Why the WHO Took Two Years to Say COVID Is Airborne."

70. G. Hiatt, "In a 4-Month Sample, D.C. Traces 14 Percent of COVID-19 'Outbreaks' to Restaurants," *Eater Washington DC*, December 7, 2020, https://dc.eater .com/2020/12/7/22159468/d-c-releases-COVID-19-outbreak-data-restaurants.

71. K. A. Fisher, M. W. Tenforde, L. R. Feldstein, C. J. Lindsell, N. I. Shapiro, D. C. Files, K. W. Gibbs, et al., "Community and Close Contact Exposures Associated with COVID-19 among Symptomatic Adults ≥ 18 Years in 11 Outpatient Health Care

Facilities—United States, July 2020," *Morbidity and Mortality Weekly Report* 69, no. 36 (2020): 1258.

72. G. P. Guy Jr., F. C. Lee, G. Sunshine, R. McCord, M. Howard-Williams, L. Kompaniyets, C. Dunphy, et al., "Association of State-Issued Mask Mandates and Allowing On-Premises Restaurant Dining with County-Level COVID-19 Case and Death Growth Rates—United States, March 1–December 31, 2020," *Morbidity and Mortality Weekly Report* 70, no. 10 (2021): 350.

73. Tan, "Commensality and the Organization of Social Relations," 20.

74. A. C. B. Tse, S. So, and L. Sin, "Crisis Management and Recovery: How Restaurants in Hong Kong Responded to SARS," *International Journal of Hospitality Management* 25, no. 1 (2006): 3–11.

75. Tan, "Commensality and the Organization of Social Relations," 20.

76. "Partygate: A Timeline of the Lockdown Gatherings," *BBC News*, May 19, 2022, https://www.bbc.com/news/uk-politics-59952395.

77. L. Said-Moorhouse and A. Woodyatt, "This Is Why the Queen Sat on Her Own during Philip's Funeral," CNN, April 18, 2021, https://www.cnn.com/2021/04/17/uk /queen-alone-philip-funeral-gbr-intl-scli/index.html.

78. T. Luna and P. Willon, "Newsom Apologizes for French Laundry Dinner, Says He Will Practice What He Preaches on COVID-19," *Los Angeles Times*, November 16, 2020, https://www.latimes.com/california/story/2020-11-16/gavin-newsom-apology -french-laundry-dinner-COVID-19; K. Willsher, "French Authorities Investigate 'Clandestine' Dinner Parties in Paris," *Guardian*, April 5, 2021, https://www.the guardian.com/world/2021/apr/05/french-authorities-investigate-clandestine-dinner -parties-in-paris.

Chapter 5

1. L. S. Lewis and M. A. Maslin, *The Human Planet: How We Created the Anthropocene* (New Haven, CT: Yale University Press, 2018), 3.

2. P. J. Crutzen and E. F. Stoermer, "The 'Anthropocene,'" *IGSP Global Change Newsletter* 41 (2000): 17–18. While the term *Anthropocene* was coined by Crutzen and Stoermer, similar ideas with different names were offered more than a century ago, such as the *anthropozoic era* suggested by geologist Antonio Stoppani in 1873.

3. Lewis and Maslin, *The Human Planet*, 3.

4. J. Zalasiewicz, C. N. Waters, M. Williams, A. D. Barnosky, A. Cearreta, P. Crutzen, E. Ellis, et al., "When Did the Anthropocene Begin? A Mid-Twentieth Century Boundary Level Is Stratigraphically Optimal," *Quaternary International* 383 (2015): 196–203.

5. T. J. Braje and J. M. Erlandson, "Looking Forward, Looking Back: Humans, Anthropogenic Change, and the Anthropocene," *Anthropocene* 4 (2013): 116–121; B. D. Smith and M. A. Zeder, "The Onset of the Anthropocene," *Anthropocene* 4 (2013): 8–13. The Holocene epoch was proposed by Charles Lyell in 1830. As Lewis and Maslin (*The Human Planet*, 34) discuss, its original meaning was related to the emergence and impacts of humans. When the Holocene was formally ratified by the International Union of Geological Sciences in 2008, the beginning in 11,650 BP was marked by the end of the last glaciation and start of the current warm interglacial conditions, without humans playing a big role in its definition.

6. H. Davis and Z. Todd, "On the Importance of a Date, or Decolonizing the Anthropocene," *ACME: An International Journal for Critical Geographies* 16, no. 4 (2017): 761–780.

7. J. Raff, *Origin: A Genetic History of the Americas* (New York: Twelve, 2022).

8. T. J. Braje, T. D. Dillehay, J. M. Erlandson, R. G. Klein, and T. C. Rick, "Finding the First Americans," *Science* 358, no. 6363 (2017): 592–594.

9. J. J. Halligan, M. R. Waters, A. Perrotti, I. J. Owens, J. M. Feinberg, M. D. Bourne, B. Fenerty, et al., "Pre-Clovis Occupation 14,550 Years Ago at the Page-Ladson Site, Florida, and the Peopling of the Americas," *Science Advances* 2, no. 5 (2016): e1600375; T. D. Dillehay, C. Ocampo, J. Saavedra, A. O. Sawakuchi, R. M. Vega, M. Pino, M. B. Collins, et al., "New Archaeological Evidence for an Early Human Presence at Monte Verde, Chile," *PloS One* 10, no. 11 (2015): e0141923.

10. B. Llamas, L. Fehren-Schmitz, G. Valverde, J. Soubrier, S. Mallick, N. Rohland, S. Nordenfelt, et al., "Ancient Mitochondrial DNA Provides High-Resolution Time Scale of the Peopling of the Americas," *Science Advances* 2, no. 4 (2016): e1501385.

11. Raff, *Origin*, 207.

12. Raff, *Origin*, 210–211.

13. M. Rasmussen, S. L. Anzick, M. R. Waters, P. Skoglund, M. DeGiorgio, T. W. Stafford, S. Rasmussen, et al., "The Genome of a Late Pleistocene Human from a Clovis Burial Site in Western Montana," *Nature* 506, no. 7487 (2014): 225–229; Raff, *Origin*, 211.

14. M. R. Bennett, D. Bustos, J. S. Pigati, K. B. Springer, T. M. Urban, V. T. Holliday, S. C. Reynolds, et al., "Evidence of Humans in North America during the Last Glacial Maximum," *Science* 373, no. 6562 (2021): 1528–1531; D. B. Madsen, L. G. Davis, D. Rhode, and C. G. Oviatt, "Comment on 'Evidence of Humans in North America during the Last Glacial Maximum,'" *Science* 375, no. 6577 (2022): eabm4678; J. S. Pigati, K. B. Springer, M. R. Bennett, D. Bustos, T. M. Urban, V. T. Holliday, S. C. Reynolds, et al., "Response to Comment on 'Evidence of Humans in North America during the Last Glacial Maximum,'" *Science* 375, no. 6577 (2022): eabm6987; C. G. Oviatt, D. B. Madsen, D. Rhode, and L. G. Davis, "A Critical Assessment of Claims

That Human Footprints in the Lake Otero Basin, New Mexico Date to the Last Glacial Maximum," *Quaternary Research* 111 (2022): 1–10; J. S. Pigati, K. S. Springer, J. S. Honke, D. Wahl, M. R. Champagne, S. R. H. Zimmerman, H. J. Gray, et al., "Independent Age Estimates Resolve the Controversy of Ancient Human Footprints at White Sands," *Science* 382, no. 6666 (2023): 73–75.

15. M. M. Bruchac, "Indigenous Knowledge and Traditional Knowledge," in *Encyclopedia of Global Archaeology*, ed. C. Smith (New York: Springer Science and Business Media, 2014), 3814.

16. K. TallBear, "Tell Me a Story: Genomics vs. Indigenous Origin Narratives," *GeneWatch* 26, no. 4 (August–October 2013), 13.

17. C. C. Mann, *1491: New Revelations of the Americas before Columbus* (New York: Alfred A. Knopf, 2005), 16. No writing systems are known among the Native American peoples of North America at the time of European contact, but more than a dozen have been identified in pre-Columbian Mesoamerica as early as about 400 BCE. Maya hieroglyphic writing is among the oldest and most highly developed system found to date (W. A. Saturno, D. Stuart, and B. Beltrán, "Early Maya Writing at San Bartolo, Guatemala," *Science* 311, no. 5765 [2006]: 1281–1283).

18. D. H. Ubelaker, "Population Size, Contact to Nadir," in *Handbook of North American Indians, Volume 3*, ed. D. H. Ubelaker (Washington, DC: Smithsonian Institution, 2006), 694–701.

19. Ubelaker, "Population Size, Contact to Nadir."

20. M. Livi Bacci, *Conquest: The Destruction of the American Indios* (Cambridge, UK: Polity Press, 2008), 158.

21. B. D. Smith, "Plane and Animal Resources: Introduction," in *Handbook of North American Indians, Volume 3*, D. H. Ubelaker (Washington, DC: Smithsonian Institution, 2006), 219.

22. Smith, "Plane and Animal Resources."

23. J. M. Erlandson, "Shell Middens and Other Anthropogenic Soils as Global Stratigraphic Signatures of the Anthropocene," *Anthropocene* 4 (2013): 24–32.

24. T. C. Rick, L. A. Reeder-Myers, C. A., Hofman, D. Breitburg, R. Lockwood, G. Henkes, L. Kellogg, et al., "Millennial-Scale Sustainability of the Chesapeake Bay Native American Oyster Fishery," *Proceedings of the National Academy of Sciences* 113, no. 23 (2016): 6568–6573.

25. Livi Bacci, *Conquest*, 6.

26. T. Inomata, D. Triadan, V. A. Vázquez López, J. C. Fernandez-Diaz, T. Omori, M. B. Méndez Bauer, M. G. Hernández, et al., "Monumental Architecture at Aguada Fénix and the Rise of Maya Civilization," *Nature* 582, no. 7813 (2020): 530–533.

27. C. C. Mann, *1493: Uncovering the New World Columbus Created* (New York: Vintage, 2011).

28. Prior to 1492, the only known and undisputed European presence in the Americas was a fleeting one, evident in the 1,000-year-old Viking settlement of L'Anse aux Meadows on the island of Newfoundland along the Atlantic coast of present-day Canada.

29. K. Deagan and J. M. Cruxent, *Columbus's Outpost among the Taínos* (New Haven, CT: Yale University Press, 2008).

30. F. Guerra, "The Earliest American Epidemic: The Influenza of 1493," *Social Science History* 12, no. 3 (1988): 305–327.

31. V. Tiesler, A. Coppa, P. Zabala, and A. Cucina, "Scurvy-Related Morbidity and Death among Christopher Columbus' Crew at La Isabela, the First European Town in the New World (1494–1498): An Assessment of the Skeletal and Historical Information," *International Journal of Osteoarchaeology* 26, no. 2 (2016): 191–202.

32. Deagan and Cruxent, *Columbus's Outpost among the Taínos*, 138–139.

33. N. D. Cook, "Sickness, Starvation, and Death in Early Hispaniola," *Journal of Interdisciplinary History* (2002): 349–386.

34. A. Crosby, *The Columbian Exchange: Biological and Cultural Consequences of 1492* (Westport, CT: Greenwood Press, 1972).

35. G. J. Smith, D. Vijaykrishna, J. Bahl, S. J. Lycett, M. Worobey, O. G. Pybus, S. K. Ma, "Origins and Evolutionary Genomics of the 2009 Swine-Origin H1N1 Influenza A Epidemic," *Nature* 459, no. 7250 (2009): 1122–1125.

36. B. Pavao-Zuckerman and E. J. Reitz, "Introduction and Adoption of Animals from Europe," in *Handbook of North American Indians, Volume 3*, ed. D. H. Ubelaker (Washington, DC: Smithsonian Institution, 2006), 486.

37. Quoted in Deagan and Cruxent, *Columbus's Outpost among the Taínos*, 280–281.

38. Crosby, *The Columbian Exchange*.

39. Crosby, *The Columbian Exchange*, 96–97.

40. Cook, "Sickness, Starvation, and Death in Early Hispaniola," 361.

41. Deagan and Cruxent, *Columbus's Outpost among the Taínos*, 27.

42. Livi Bacci, *Conquest*.

43. B. Mühlemann, L. Vinner, A. Margaryan, H. Wilhelmson, C. de la Fuente Castro, M. E. Allentoft, P. de Barros Damgaard, et al., "Diverse Variola Virus (Smallpox) Strains Were Widespread in Northern Europe in the Viking Age," *Science* 369, no. 6502 (2020): eaaw8977.

44. S. Duchêne, S. Y. Ho, A. G. Carmichael, E. C. Holmes, and H. Poinar, "The Recovery, Interpretation and Use of Ancient Pathogen Genomes," *Current Biology* 30, no. 19 (2020): R1215–R1231.

45. US Centers for Disease Control and Prevention, "Smallpox: Signs and Symptoms," accessed March 15, 2022, https://www.cdc.gov/smallpox/symptoms/index.html.

46. Quoted in Cook, "Sickness, Starvation, and Death in Early Hispaniola," 364.

47. Cook, "Sickness, Starvation, and Death in Early Hispaniola," 364.

48. Livi Bacci, *Conquest*, 113.

49. Deagan and Cruxent, *Columbus's Outpost among the Taínos*, 173.

50. Livi Bacci, *Conquest*.

51. D. M. Fernandes, K. A. Sirak, H. Ringbauer, J. Sedig, N. Rohland, O. Cheronet, M. Mah, et al., "A Genetic History of the Pre-Contact Caribbean," *Nature* 590, no. 7844 (2021): 103–110.

52. Deagan and Cruxent, *Columbus's Outpost among the Taínos*, 34.

53. C. Zimmer, "Ancient DNA Shows Humans Settled Caribbean in 2 Distinct Waves," *New York Times*, December 23, 2020.

54. J. L. Penn, C. Deutsch, J. L. Payne, and E. A. Sperling, "Temperature-Dependent Hypoxia Explains Biogeography and Severity of End-Permian Marine Mass Extinction," *Science* 362, no. 6419 (2018): eaat1327.

55. L. S. Lewis and M. A. Maslin, "Defining the Anthropocene," *Nature* 519, no. 7542 (2015): 171–180.

56. Lewis and Maslin, *The Human Planet*, 179, 182.

57. Lewis and Maslin, "Defining the Anthropocene."

58. D. R. Piperno, C. H. McMichael, N. C. Pitman, J. E. G. Andino, M. R. Paredes, B. Heijink, and L. A. Torres-Montenegro, "A 5,000-Year Vegetation and Fire History for Tierra Firme Forests in the Medio Putumayo-Algodón Watersheds, Northeastern Peru," *Proceedings of the National Academy of Sciences* 118, no. 40 (2021).

59. V. Peripato, C. Levis, G. A. Moreira, D. Gamerman, H. Ter Steege, N. C. A. Pitman, J. G. de Souza, et al., "More than 10,000 Pre-Columbian Earthworks Are Still Hidden throughout Amazonia," *Science* 382, no. 6666 (2023): 103–109.

60. Lewis and Maslin, *The Human Planet*, 167.

61. E. O. Guerrant, "Genetic and Demographic Considerations in the Sampling and Reintroduction of Rare Plants," in *Conservation Biology*, ed. P. L. Fiedler and S. K. Jain (Boston: Springer, 1992), 321–344.

62. A. Bergström, L. Frantz, R. Schmidt, E. Ersmark, O. Lebrasseur, L. Girdland-Flink, A. T. Lin, et al., "Origins and Genetic Legacy of Prehistoric Dogs," *Science* 370, no. 6516 (2020): 557–564.

63. Deagan and Cruxent, *Columbus's Outpost among the Taínos*, 137.

64. Crosby, *The Columbian Exchange*, 76.

65. M. S. Wang, M. Thakur, M. S. Peng, Y. U. Jiang, L. A. F. Frantz, M. Li, J. J. Zhang, et al., "863 Genomes Reveal the Origin and Domestication of Chicken," *Cell Research* 30, no. 8 (2020): 693–701.

66. J. Peters, O. Lebrasseur, E. K. Irving-Pease, P. D. Paxinos, J. Best, R. Smallman, C. Callou, et al., "The Biocultural Origins and Dispersal of Domestic Chickens," *Proceedings of the National Academy of Sciences* 119, no. 24 (2022): e2121978119.

67. A. A. Storey, J. M. Ramirez, D. Quiroz, D. V. Burley, D. J. Addison, R. Walter, A. J. Anderson, et al., "Radiocarbon and DNA Evidence for a Pre-Columbian Introduction of Polynesian Chickens to Chile," *Proceedings of the National Academy of Sciences* 104, no. 25 (2007): 10335–10339.

68. J. Gongora, N. J. Rawlence, V. A. Mobegi, H. Jianlin, J. A. Alcalde, J. T. Matus, O. Hanotte, et al., "Indo-European and Asian Origins for Chilean and Pacific Chickens Revealed by mtDNA," *Proceedings of the National Academy of Sciences* 105, no. 30 (2008): 10308–10313.

69. M. B. Herrera, S. Kraitsek, J. A. Alcalde, D. Quiroz, H. Revelo, L. A. Alvarez, M. F. Rosario, et al., "European and Asian Contribution to the Genetic Diversity of Mainland South American Chickens," *Royal Society Open Science* 7, no. 2 (2020): 191558.

70. C. E. Bennett, R. Thomas, M. Williams, J. Zalasiewicz, M. Edgeworth, H. Miller, B. Coles, et al., "The Broiler Chicken as a Signal of a Human Reconfigured Biosphere," *Royal Society Open Science* 5, no. 12 (2018): 180325.

71. H. Briggs, "'Planet of the Chickens': How the Bird Took over the World," *.BBC News*, December 12, 2018.

72. Food and Agriculture Organization of the United Nations, "Crops and Livestock Products," accessed March 16, 2022, https://www.fao.org/faostat/en/#data/QCL.

73. H. K. Kim, D. G. Jeong, and S. W. Yoon, "Recent Outbreaks of Highly Pathogenic Avian Influenza Viruses in South Korea," *Clinical and Experimental Vaccine Research* 6, no. 2 (2017): 95–103. Influenza A viruses are divided into many different subtypes based on two proteins on the surface of the virus, hemagglutinin (HA) and neuraminidase (NA). There are eighteen known HA subtypes and eleven known NA subtypes, and in birds, sixteen HA and nine NA subtypes have been identified. Only some H5 and H7 viruses are classified as HPAI viruses, while most that circulate among birds are low pathogenic avian influenza viruses.

74. M. McKenna, "The Looming Threat of Avian Flu," *New York Times*, April 13, 2016.

75. World Health Organization, "Cumulative Number of Confirmed Human Cases for Avian Influenza A(H5N1) Reported to WHO, 2003–2023," March 3, 2023, https:// www.who.int/publications/m/item/cumulative-number-of-confirmed-human-cases -for-avian-influenza-a(h5n1)-reported-to-who-2003-2023-3-march-2023.

76. S. Herfst, E. J. Schrauwen, M. Linster, S. Chutinimitkul, E. de Wit, V. J. Munster, E. M. Sorrell, et al., "Airborne Transmission of Influenza A/H5N1 Virus between Ferrets," *Science* 336, no. 6088 (2012): 1534–1541.

77. K. Kupferschmidt, "'Incredibly Concerning': Bird Flu Outbreak at Spanish Mink Farm Triggers Pandemic Fears," *Science*, January 24, 2023, https://www.science.org /content/article/incredibly-concerning-bird-flu-outbreak-spanish-mink-farm-triggers -pandemic-fears.

78. L. Schnirring, "Researchers Detail H5N1 Avian Flu Outbreak at Mink Farm in Spain," CIDRAP News Brief, University of Minnesota, January 20, 2023, https:// www.cidrap.umn.edu/avian-influenza-bird-flu/researchers-detail-h5n1-avian-flu -outbreak-mink-farm-spain.

79. J. Abbasi, "Bird Flu Has Begun to Spread in Mammals—Here's What's Important to Know," *JAMA*, February 8, 2023, doi:10.1001/jama.2023.1317.

80. E. Anthes, "Bird Flu Sample from Chilean Man Showed Some Signs of Adaptation to Mammals," *New York Times*, April 14, 2023, https://www.nytimes.com /2023/04/14/science/bird-flu-humans.html.

81. J. Vidal, "Factory Farms of Disease: How Industrial Chicken Production Is Breeding the Next Pandemic," *Guardian*, October 18, 2021.

82. Food and Agriculture Organization, *Poultry in the 21st Century: Avian Influenza and Beyond*, ed. O. Thieme and D. Pilling, FAO Animal Production and Health Proceedings, no. 9 (Rome: Food and Agriculture Organization, 2008), 44.

83. M. McKenna, *Plucked: Chicken, Antibiotics, and How Big Business Changed the Way We Eat* (Washington, DC: National Geographic Books, 2019).

84. McKenna, *Plucked*, 169.

85. H. D. Hedman, K. A. Vasco, and L. Zhang, "A Review of Antimicrobial Resistance in Poultry Farming within Low-Resource Settings," *Animals* 10, no. 8 (2020): 1264.

86. McKenna, *Plucked*, 26.

87. Cited in T. Thompson, "The Staggering Death Toll of Drug-Resistant Bacteria," *Nature News*, January 31, 2022.

88. C. J. Murray, K. S. Ikuta, F. Sharara, L. Swetschinski, G. R. Aguilar, A. Gray, C. Han, et al., "Global Burden of Bacterial Antimicrobial Resistance in 2019: A Systematic Analysis," *Lancet* 399, no. 10325 (2022): 629–655.

89. World Health Organization, *Global Action Plan on Antimicrobial Resistance* (Geneva: World Health Organization, 2015), https://ahpsr.who.int/publications/i /item/global-action-plan-on-antimicrobial-resistance.

90. E. C. Ellis, N. Gauthier, K. K. Goldewijk, R. B. Bird, N. Boivin, S. Díaz, D. Q. Fuller, et al., "People Have Shaped Most of Terrestrial Nature for at Least 12,000 Years," *Proceedings of the National Academy of Sciences* 118, no. 17 (2021).

91. S. L. Wing, "Thinking Like a Mountain in the Anthropocene,"in *Living in the Anthropocene Earth in the Age of Humans*, ed. W. J. Kris's and J. K. Stein (Washington, DC: Smithsonian Books, 2017), 22.

Chapter 6

1. R. Bennison, "An Inclusive Re-Engagement with Our Nonhuman Animal Kin: Considerin Human Interrelationships with Nonhuman Animals," *Animals* 1, no. 1 (2011): 40–55.

2. A. Belfer-Cohen and E. Hovers, "Prehistoric Perspectives on 'Others' and 'Strangers,'" *Frontiers in Psychology* 10 (2020): 3063.

3. K. Harper, *Plagues upon the Earth: Disease and the Course of Human History* (Princeton, NJ: Princeton University Press, 2021), 193.

4. Quoted in K. Harper, *The Fate of Rome* (Princeton, NJ: Princeton University Press, 2017), 155.

5. B. Wagemakers, "Incest, Infanticide, and Cannibalism: Anti-Christian Imputations in the Roman Empire," *Greece and Rome* 57, no. 2 (2010): 346, 341.

6. S. K. Cohn Jr., "The Black Death and the Burning of Jews," *Past and Present* 196, no. 1 (2007): 3–36.

7. M. Barber, "Lepers, Jews and Moslems: The Plot to Overthrow Christendom in 1321," *History* 66, no. 216 (1981): 1–17.

8. H. Sidky, *Witchcraft, Lycanthropy, Drugs and Disease: An Anthropological Study of the European Witch-Hunts* (Eugene, OR: Wipf and Stock Publishers, 2010), 256.

9. M. Tampa, I. Sarbu, C. Matei, V. Benea, and S. R. Georgescu, "Brief History of Syphilis," *Journal of Medicine and Life* 7, no. 1 (2014): 4–10.

10. L. Spinney, *Pale Rider: The Spanish Flu of 1918 and How It Changed the World* (New York: PublicAffairs, 2017), 64.

11. "AABA Statement on Race and Racism," American Association of Biological Anthropologists, accessed May 3, 2023, https://physanth.org/about/position -statements/aapa-statement-race-and-racism-2019.

12. D. B. G. Tai, A. Shah, C. A. Doubeni, I. G. Sia, and M. L. Wieland, "The Disproportionate Impact of COVID-19 on Racial and Ethnic Minorities in the United States," *Clinical Infectious Diseases* 72, no. 4 (2021): 703–706; "Hospitalization and Death by Race/Ethnicity," Centers for Disease Control and Prevention, April 24, 2023, https://www.cdc.gov/coronavirus/2019-ncov/covid-data/investigations-discovery /hospitalization-death-by-race-ethnicity.html#print.

13. Y. Hswen, X. Xu, A. Hing, J. B. Hawkins, J. S. Brownstein, and G. C. Gee, "Association of "# covid19" versus "# chinesevirus" with Anti-Asian Sentiments on Twitter: March 9–23, 2020," *American Journal of Public Health* 111, no. 5 (2021): 956–964.

14. Stop AAPI Hate, "National Report (through September 2021)," accessed May 3, 2023, https://stopaapihate.org/national-report-through-september-2021.

15. "UN Chief Appeals for Global Action against Coronavirus-Fueled Hate Speech," UN News, May 8, 2020, https://news.un.org/en/story/2020/05/1063542.

16. "COVID-19 Fueling Anti-Asian Racism and Xenophobia Worldwide," Human Rights Watch, May 12, 2020, https://www.hrw.org/news/2020/05/12/COVID-19 -fueling-anti-asian-racism-and-xenophobia-worldwide.

17. A. Hassan, "'Fight the Virus, Not the People!' SF Chinese-American Leaders Protest Xenophobia Following COVID-19 Outbreak," ABC7, March 1, 2020, https://abc7news .com/coronavirus-china-us-death-age-what-is-xenophobia-definition/5977541.

18. J. 8. Lee and D. E. Murphy, "The SARS Epidemic: Asian-Americans; In U.S., Fear Is Spreading Faster Than SARS," *New York Times*, April 17, 2003, https://www .nytimes.com/2003/04/17/world/the-sars-epidemic-asian-americans-in-us-fear-is -spreading-faster-than-sars.html.

19. N. Shah, *Contagious Divides: Epidemics and Race in San Francisco's Chinatown* (Berkeley: University of California Press, 2001), 7:20.

20. Shah, *Contagious Divides*, 7:20.

21. D. Brekke, "Boomtown, 1870s: 'The Chinese Must Go!,'" KQED, February 12, 2015, https://www.kqed.org/news/10429550/boomtown-history-2b.

22. Shah, *Contagious Divides*, 27. The term *coolie* was a racist stereotype for a Chinese laborer and was used to drive anti-Chinese sentiment.

23. Brekke, "Boomtown, 1870s."

24. Congressional Record, Vol. 2, Part 3. 43rd Congress, 1st Session, March 20, 1874, p. 2300, https://www.congress.gov/bound-congressional-record/1874/03/20.

25. D. K. Randall, *Black Death at the Golden Gate: The Race to Save America from the Bubonic Plague* (New York: W. W. Norton and Company, 2019), 36.

26. Although the act was originally written to last for the duration of ten years, it held strong as a barrier to Chinese immigration far into the twentieth century. It was finally rescinded in 1943, only after China became a US ally in World War II. Still, Chinese immigration did not become on par with that of other countries until the passage of the Immigration Act in 1965. See H. M. Lai, *Island: Poetry and History of Chinese Immigrants on Angel Island, 1910–1940*, 2nd ed. (Seattle: University of Washington Press, 2014).

27. J. Pfaelzer, "Driven Out: Roundups and Resistance of the Chinese in Rural California," *Chinese America: History and Perspectives* (2007): 113–115, 251.

28. M. Szto, "From Exclusion to Exclusivity: Chinese American Property Ownership and Discrimination in Historical Perspective," *Journal of Transnational Law and Policy* 25 (2015): i.

29. R. Ueda, ed., *America's Changing Neighborhoods: An Exploration of Diversity through Places*, 3 vols. (Santa Barbara: ABC-CLIO, 2017), 382.

30. Szto, "From Exclusion to Exclusivity," 66.

31. C. Lynteris, "2. Yellow Peril Epidemics: The Political Ontology of Degeneration and Emergence," in *Yellow Perils: China Narratives in the Contemporary World*, ed. F. Billé and S. Urbansky (Honolulu: University of Hawai'i Press, 2018), 35–59.

32. L. Heinrich, "How China Became the 'Cradle of Smallpox': Transformations in Discourse, 1726–2002," *positions: east asia cultures critique* 15, no. 1 (2007): 7–34.

33. Lynteris, "2. Yellow Peril Epidemics."

34. S. Craddock, "Sewers and Scapegoats: Spatial Metaphors of Smallpox in Nineteenth Century San Francisco," *Social Science and Medicine* 41, no. 7 (1995): 957–968; S. Craddock, Embodying Place: Pathologizing Chinese and Chinatown in Nineteenth-Century San Francisco," *Antipode* 31, no. 4 (1999): 351–371.

35. Craddock, "Embodying Place."

36. Quoted in *Municipal Reports for the Fiscal Year 1887* (San Francisco: Cosmopolitan Printing Company, 1887), 397.

37. Workingmen's Party of California, *Chinatown Declared a Nuisance!* (San Francisco, 1880), 4, http://sfmuseum.org/hist2/nuisance.html.

38. G. B. Risse, *Plague, Fear, and Politics in San Francisco's Chinatown.* (Baltimore: Johns Hopkins University Press, 2012), 9.

39. Workingmen's Party of California, *Chinatown Declared a Nuisance!*, 14.

40. *Municipal Reports for the Fiscal Year 1887*, 397.

41. Craddock, "Sewers and Scapegoats."

42. Lynteris, "2. Yellow Peril Epidemics."

43. Workingmen's Party of California, *Chinatown Declared a Nuisance!*, 16.

44. Szto, "From Exclusion to Exclusivity," 66.

45. Craddock, "Sewers and Scapegoats," 262.

46. Ueda, *America's Changing Neighborhoods*, 378.

47. Craddock, "Sewers and Scapegoats," 262.

48. Randall, *Black Death at the Golden Gate*, 184.

49. C. Lynteris, "A 'Suitable Soil': Plague's Urban Breeding Grounds at the Dawn of the Third Pandemic," *Medical History* 61, no. 3 (2017): 343–357.

50. Lynteris, "A 'Suitable Soil.'"

51. M. Echenberg, *Plague Ports: The Global Urban Impact of Bubonic Plague, 1894–1901* (New York: NYU Press, 2007), 70.

52. A. Yersin, "La peste bubonique à Hong-Kong," *Annales de l'Institut Pasteur* 2 (1894): 664.

53. Echenberg, *Plague Ports*, 7.

54. Echenberg, *Plague Ports*, 236.

55. R. Blue, "Anti-Plague Measures in San Francisco, California, USA," *Epidemiology and Infection* 9, no. 1 (1909): 1–8.

56. "Police Block All Entrance to Chinatown," *San Francisco Examiner*, March 7, 1900.

57. Randall, *Black Death at the Golden Gate*, 45.

58. Risse, *Plague, Fear, and Politics in San Francisco's Chinatown*, 103.

59. "Police Keeping Quarantine Guard over Chinatown," *San Francisco Call*, March 7, 1900.

60. "Chinatown Quarantined," *San Francisco Call*, March 8, 1900.

61. Translated by Prisca Hui in M. Chase, *The Barbary Plague: The Black Death in Victorian San Francisco* (New York: Random House, 2003), 18–19.

62. J. Mohr, *Plague and Fire: Battling Black Death and the 1900 Burning of Honolulu's Chinatown* (New York: Oxford University Press, 2005).

63. Mohr, *Plague and Fire*.

64. "Chinese Consul Protests," *Los Angeles Times*, March 9, 1900.

65. "No Results from Tests of Bacteriologist," *San Francisco Examiner*, March 9, 1900.

66. R. Blue, "Bubonic Plague Control in California in 1903: Origin of Ratproofing as a Control Measure," *California and Western Medicine* 40, no. 5 (1934): 364.

67. Randall, *Black Death at the Golden Gate*, 159–160.

68. Blue, "Bubonic Plague Control in California in 1903," 364.

69. Randall, *Black Death at the Golden Gate*, 160.

70. Randall, *Black Death at the Golden Gate*, 166.

71. F. M. Todd, *Eradicating Plague from San Francisco* (San Francisco: San Francisco Citizen's Health Committee, 1909), 9.

72. W. B. Wherry, "Plague among the Ground Squirrels of California," *Journal of Infectious Diseases* (1908): 485–506.

73. Randall, *Black Death at the Golden Gate*, 167.

74. Wherry, "Plague among the Ground Squirrels of California."

75. Randall, *Black Death at the Golden Gate*, 220.

76. M. Honigsbaum, *The Pandemic Century: One Hundred Years of Panic, Hysteria, and Hubris* (New York: W. W. Norton and Company, 2019), 85.

77. J. Z. Adjemian, P. Foley, K. L. Gage, and J. E. Foley, "Initiation and Spread of Traveling Waves of Plague, Yersinia pestis, in the Western United States," *American Journal of Tropical Medicine and Hygiene* 76, no. 2 (2007): 365–375.

78. J. F. Cully Jr., L. G. Carter, and K. L. Gage, "New Records of Sylvatic Plague in Kansas," *Journal of Wildlife Diseases* 36, no. 2 (2000): 389–392.

79. "Plague in the United States," Centers for Disease Control and Prevention, 2022, https://www.cdc.gov/plague/maps/index.html.

80. Echenberg, *Plague Ports*.

81. Randall, *Black Death at the Golden Gate*, 167.

82. L. Myers, "China Spins Tale That the U.S. Army Started the Coronavirus Epidemic," *New York Times*, March 13, 2020, https://www.nytimes.com/2020/03/13/world/asia/coronavirus-china-conspiracy-theory.html.

83. "Pompeo Ties Coronavirus to China Lab, despite Spy Agencies' Uncertainty," *New York Times*, May 3, 2020, https://www.nytimes.com/2020/05/03/us/politics/coronavirus-pompeo-wuhan-china-lab.html?searchResultPosition=2.

84. L. O. Gostin and G. K. Gronvall, "The Origins of Covid-19—Why It Matters (and Why It Doesn't)," *New England Journal of Medicine* 388 (2023), https://www.nejm.org/doi/full/10.1056/NEJMp2305081.

85. R. F. Garry, "The Evidence Remains Clear: SARS-CoV-2 Emerged via the Wildlife Trade," *Proceedings of the National Academy of Sciences* 119, no. 47 (2022): e2214427119.

86. J. D. Bloom, Y. A. Chan, R. S. Baric, P. J. Bjorkman, S. Cobey, B. E. Deverman, D. N. Fisman, et al., "Investigate the Origins of COVID-19," *Science* 372, no. 6543 (2021): 694–694.

87. S. Mallapaty, "WHO Abandons Plans for Crucial Second Phase of COVID-Origins Investigation," *Nature*, February 14, 2023, https://www.nature.com/articles/d41586-023-00283-y.

88. J. Cohen, "Call of the Wild," *Science* 373, no. 6559 (2023): 951–959.

89. M. Worobey, J. I. Levy, L. Malpica Serrano, A. Crits-Christoph, J. E. Pekar, S. A. Goldstein, A. L. Rasmussen, et al., "The Huanan Seafood Wholesale Market in Wuhan Was the Early Epicenter of the COVID-19 Pandemic," *Science*, September 2, 2021, https://www.science.org/content/article/why-many-scientists-say-unlikely-sars-cov-2-originated-lab-leak.

90. K. J. Wu, "The Strongest Evidence Yet That an Animal Started the Pandemic," *Atlantic*, March 16, 2023, https://www.theatlantic.com/science/archive/2023/03/covid-origins-research-raccoon-dogs-wuhan-market-lab-leak/673390.

91. M. Ruiz-Aravena, C. McKee, A. Gamble, T. Lunn, A. Morris, C. E. Snedden, C. K. Yinda, et al., "Ecology, Evolution and Spillover of Coronaviruses from Bats," *Nature Reviews Microbiology* 20, no. 5 (2022): 299–314.

92. S. Temmam, K. Vongphayloth, E. Baquero, S. Munier, M. Bonomi, B. Regnault, B. Douangboubpha, et al., "Bat Coronaviruses Related to SARS-CoV-2 and Infectious for Human Cells," *Nature* 604, no. 7905 (2022): 330–336.

93. P. Zhou, X. L. Yang, X. G. Wang, B. Hu, L. Zhang, W. Zhang, H. R. Si, et al., "A Pneumonia Outbreak Associated with a New Coronavirus of Probable Bat Origin," *Nature* 579, no. 7798 (2020): 270–273.

94. N. Aizenman, "Why the U.S. Government Stopped Funding a Research Project on Bats and Coronaviruses," NPR, April 29, 2020, https://www.npr.org/sections/goatsandsoda/2020/04/29/847948272/why-the-u-s-government-stopped-funding-a-research-project-on-bats-and-coronaviru.

95. Science News Staff, "Nobel Laureates and Science Groups Demand NIH Review Decision to Kill Coronavirus Grant," *Science*, May 21, 2020, https://www.science.org/content/article/preposterous-77-nobel-laureates-blast-nih-decision-cancel

-coronavirus-grant-demand?adobe_mc=MCMID%3D043845900393746395522628 8
6180388864956%7CMCORGID%3D242B6472541199F70A4C98A6%2540AdobeOrg
%7CTS%3D1677325272.

96. V. L. Hale, P. M. Dennis, D. S. McBride, J. M. Nolting, C. Madden, D. Huey, M. Ehrlich, et al., "SARS-CoV-2 Infection in Free-Ranging White-Tailed Deer," *Nature* 602, no. 7897 (2022): 481–486.

97. M. Kozlov, "NIH to Intensify Scrutiny of Foreign Grant Recipients in Wake of COVID Origins Debate," *Nature News*, June 9, 2023, https://www.nature.com/articles /d41586-023-01930-0.

Chapter 7

1. J. Goodall, *In the Shadow of Man* (Boston: Houghton Mifflin Harcourt, 1971), 213–220.

2. C. Loehle, "Social Barriers to Pathogen Transmission in Wild Animal Populations," *Ecology* 76, no. 2 (1995): 326–335.

3. J. M. Kiesecker, D. K. Skelly, K. H. Beard, and E. Preisser, "Behavioral Reduction of Infection Risk," *Proceedings of the National Academy of Sciences* 96, no. 16 (1999): 9165–9168.

4. D. C. Behringer and M. J. Butler, "Disease Avoidance Influences Shelter Use and Predation in Caribbean Spiny Lobster," *Behavioral Ecology and Sociobiology* 64, no. 5 (2010): 747–755.

5. J. F. Lopes, R. D. S. Camargo, L. C. Forti, and W. O. Hughes, "The Trade-off between the Transmission of Chemical Cues and Parasites: Behavioral Interactions between Leaf-Cutting Ant Workers of Different Age Classes," *Revista Brasileira de Entomologia* 61 (2017): 69–73.

6. J. Goodall, "Social Rejection, Exclusion, and Shunning among the Gombe Chimpanzees," *Ethology and Sociobiology* 7, no. 3–4 (1986): 227–236.

7. D. J. Wilson, "A Crippling Fear: Experiencing Polio in the Era of FDR," *Bulletin of the History of Medicine* 72, no. 3 (1998): 464–495.

8. Wilson, "A Crippling Fear," 466.

9. D. M. Oshinsky, *Polio: An American Story* (Oxford: Oxford University Press, 2005), 31.

10. E. Goffman, *Stigma: Notes on the Management of Spoiled Identity* (New York: Simon and Schuster, 2009).

11. Quoted in *Webinar: End Stigma, End HIV—World AIDS Day 2021*, National Museum of Natural History, December 1, 2021, https://naturalhistory.si.edu

/education/after-hours/video-webinars-outbreak-epidemics-connected-world/end
-stigma-end-hiv.

12. For years before the first *MMWR* publication in 1981, AIDS was apparently spreading among inmates on Riker's Island and unsheltered people on the streets of New York City, although nobody knew at the time what it was. See G. Corea, *The Invisible Epidemic: The Story of Women and AIDS* (New York: HarperCollins, 1992; S. Schulman, *Let the Record Show: A Political History of ACT UP New York, 1987–1993* (New York: Farrar, Straus and Giroux, 2021).

13. US Centers for Disease Control, "Pneumocystis Pneumonia—Los Angeles," *Morbidity and Mortality Weekly Report* 30, no. 21 (1981): 1–3. *Pneumocystis jirovecii*, the fungus that causes PCP, was called *Pneumocystis carinii* until 2002. Rather than change the abbreviation of the disease, which has long been the most common, serious AIDS-defining opportunistic infection in the United States, PCP continues to be used.

14. L. K. Altman, "Rare Cancer Seen in 41 Homosexuals," *New York Times*, July 3, 1981.

15. US Centers for Disease Control, "Kaposi's Sarcoma and Pneumocystis Pneumonia among Homosexual Men—New York City and California," *Morbidity and Mortality Weekly Report* 30, no. 25 (1981): 305–308.

16. Quoted in Altman, "Rare Cancer Seen in 41 Homosexuals."

17. L. K. Altman, "New Homosexual Disorder Worries Health Officials," *New York Times*, May 11, 1982.

18. M. S. Gottlieb, R. Schroff, S. Fligiel, J. L. Fahey, and A. Saxon, "Gay-Related Immunodeficiency (GRID) Syndrome: Clinical and Autopsy Observations," *Clinical Research* 30, no. 2 (1981): 349A; M. C. Flannery, "New Developments in Reproductive Biology," *American Biology Teacher* 44, no. 7 (1982): 434–436, 442.

19. R. O. Brennan and D. T. Durack, "Primary Pneumocystis Carnii and Cytomegalovirus Infections," *Lancet* 318, no. 8259 (1982): 1338–1339; G. A. Oswald, A. Theodossi, and B. G. Gazzard, "Attempted Immune Stimulation in the 'Gay Compromise Syndrome,'" *British Medical Journal* 285 (1982): 1082.

20. Schulman, *Let the Record Show*, 17.

21. ACLU, "Why Sodomy Laws Matter," accessed March 1, 2022, https://www.aclu.org/other/why-sodomy-laws-matter.

22. S. Vider and D. S. Byers, "A Half-Century of Conflict over Attempts to 'Cure' Gay People," *TIME*, February 12, 2015.

23. Quoted in R. D. Lyons, "Psychiatrists, in a Shift, Declare Homosexuality No Mental Illness," *New York Times*, December 16, 1973. See also K. Coleman, "Frank Kameny, Pioneering Gay Rights Activist, Has Died," NPR, October 12, 2011.

24. "Gay Bashings Soar in Portland," *Longview Daily News*, April 18, 1981.

25. S. Sontag, *Illness as Metaphor and AIDS and Its Metaphors* (New York: Macmillan, 2001), 57, 102.

26. R. Shilts, *And the Band Played On* (New York: St. Martin's Press, 1987), 191.

27. US Centers for Disease Control, "Current Trends Update on Acquired Immune Deficiency Syndrome (AIDS)—United States," *Morbidity and Mortality Weekly Report* 31, no. 37 (1981): 507–508, 513–514.

28. M. Cimons and D. McManus, "Student Victims, Terrified Parents: Reagan Sympathizes with Both Sides in AIDS Furor," *Los Angeles Times*, September 18, 1985. Reagan's first-ever public mention of AIDS came in response to questions at a news conference about nationwide protests against children with AIDS in classrooms. Ryan White, a thirteen-year-old who was infected with HIV from a contaminated treatment for hemophilia A, had just been refused entry to his school, even though it was established by then that casual person-to-person contact posed no risk for transmission. Reagan expressed sympathy for both sides, stating that he "well understood" how the protesting parents felt.

29. L. Helmuth, "Hugger-in-Chief," *Slate*, October 26, 2014.

30. In 1983, two separate research groups, US and French, independently proposed that a novel retrovirus was the cause of AIDS. Publishing their findings in the same issue of *Science*, the US group called it the human T-lymphotropic virus type III (HTLV-III), while the French named its lymphadenopathy-associated virus (LAV). In 1986, HTLV-III and LAV were renamed HIV, as both viruses turned out to be the same.

31. T. Kerr, "How Six NYC Activists Changed History with 'Silence = Death.'" *Village Voice*, June 20, 2017.

32. Schulman, *Let the Record Show*, 7. Some people in the United States were eager to take away the civil rights of AIDS patients too. William F. Buckley, in a *New York Times* op-ed in 1986, suggested the forced sterilization and tattooing of people with AIDS in order to protect other members of society from them.

33. P. Staley, *Never Silent: ACT UP and My Life in Activism* (Chicago: Chicago Reviews Press, 2021).

34. "Anthony Fauci on Larry Kramer and Loving Difficult People," *New York Times*, July 4, 2023, https://www.nytimes.com/2023/07/04/opinion/anthony-fauci-larry -kramer.html.

35. Corea, *The Invisible Epidemic*.

36. M. Navarro, "Conversations: Katrina Haslip; An AIDS Activist Who Helped Women Get Help Earlier," *New York Times*, November 15, 1992.

37. T. McGovern, "ACT UP Oral History Project Interview of Terry McGovern," May 25, 2007, https://actuporalhistory.org/numerical-interviews/076-terry-mcgovern.

38. US Centers for Disease Control, "1993 Revised Classification System for HIV Infection and Expanded Surveillance Case Definition for AIDS among Adolescents and Adults," *Morbidity and Mortality Weekly Report* 41 (1993): RR-17; M. Wolfe, "ACT UP Oral History Project Interview of Maxine Wolf," February 19, 2004, https://actuporalhistory.org/numerical-interviews/043-maxine-wolfe.

39. US Centers for Disease Control, "Update: AIDS among Women—United States, 1994," *Morbidity and Mortality Weekly Report* 44, no. 5 (1995): 81–84.

40. McGovern, "ACT UP Oral History Project Interview of Terry McGovern."

41. D. Royles, *To Make the Wounded Whole: The African American Struggle against HIV/AIDS* (Chapel Hill: University of North Carolina NCPress, 2020), 14.

42. E. Ferguson and R. Loftis, "Panic Isn't Warranted, Town Officials Say," *Miami Herald*, August 11, 1985.

43. K. G Castro, S. Lieb, H. W. Jaffe, J. P. Narkunas, C. H. Calisher, T. J. Bush, and J. J. Witte, "Transmission of HIV in Belle Glade, Florida: Lessons for Other Communities in the United States," *Science* 239, no. 4836 (1988): 193–197.

44. L. Villarosa, "America's Hidden HIV Epidemic," *New York Times*, June 6, 2017.

45. US Centers for Disease Control, "Half of Black Gay Men and a Quarter of Latino Gay Men Projected to Be Diagnosed within Their Lifetime," press release, February 24, 2016. *MSM* is a term used to separate behaviors (for example, having sex with men) from social identities (for instance, gay) given that not all MSM self-identify as gay or bisexual.

46. Villarosa, "America's Hidden HIV Epidemic."

47. US Centers for Disease Control, "Opportunistic Infections and Kaposi's Sarcoma among Haitians in the United States," *Morbidity and Mortality Weekly Report* 31, no. 26 (1982): 353–354, 360–361.

48. US Centers for Disease Control, "Current Trends Prevention of Acquired Immune Deficiency Syndrome (AIDS): Report of Inter-Agency Recommendations," *Morbidity and Mortality Weekly Report* 32, no. 8 (1983): 101–103.

49. J. W. Pape, B. Liautaud, F. Thomas, J. R. Mathurin, M. M. A. S. Amand, M. Boncy, V. Pean, et al., "Risk Factors Associated with AIDS in Haiti," *American Journal of the Medical Sciences* 291, no. 1 (1986): 4–7.

50. P. Farmer, *AIDS and Accusation: Haiti and the Geography of Blame* (Berkeley: University of California Press, 2006), 211.

51. M. Simons, "For Haiti's Tourism, the Stigma of AIDS Is Fatal," *New York Times*, November 29, 1983.

52. Farmer, *AIDS and Accusation*, 220, 206.

53. M. T. P. Gilbert, A. Rambaut, G. Wlasiuk, T. J. Spira, A. E. Pitchenik, and M. Worobey, "The Emergence of HIV/AIDS in the Americas and Beyond," *Proceedings of the National Academy of Sciences* 104, no. 47 (2007): 18566–18570; J. W. Pape, P. Farmer, S. Koenig, D. Fitzgerald, P. Wright, and W. Johnson, "The Epidemiology of AIDS in Haiti Refutes the Claims of Gilbert et al.," *Proceedings of the National Academy of Sciences* 105, no. 10 (2008): E13.

54. M. Worobey, A. E. Pitchenik, M. T. P. Gilbert, G. Wlasiuk, and A. Rambaut, "Reply to Pape et al.: The Phylogeography of HIV-1 Group M Subtype B," *Proceedings of the National Academy of Sciences* 105, no. 12 (2008): E16.

55. M. Worobey, T. D. Watts, R. A. McKay, M. A. Suchard, T. Granade, D. E. Teuwen, B. A. Koblin, et al., "1970s and 'Patient 0' HIV-1 Genomes Illuminate Early HIV/AIDS History in North America," *Nature* 539, no. 7627 (2016): 98–101.

56. US Centers for Disease Control, "A Cluster of Kaposi's Sarcoma and Pneumocystis Carinii Pneumonia among Homosexual Male Residents of Los Angeles and Orange Counties, California," *Morbidity and Mortality Weekly Report* 31, no. 23 (1982): 305–307; J. Auerback, W. Darrow, and I. Curran, "Cluster of Cases of AIDS: Patients Linked by Social Contact," *American Journal of Medicine* 76 (1984): 487–492. The process that resulted in the naming of Patient 0 is explained in detail by historian Adam McKay in his book *Patient Zero and the Making of the AIDS Epidemic*. Gaëtan Dugas was identified as the "Out of Town" patient, signified by the letter O by the CDC researchers who conducted the original study. The O was miscopied and/or misread as a zero (0), though, to the extent that he was called "Patient Zero" by the time of the subsequent study—a label that falsely reinforced the notion that he was the original source of the transmission.

57. Shilts, *And the Band Played On*, 439.

58. R. McKay, "Patient Zero: Why It's Such a Toxic Term," *Conversation*, April, 2020.

59. US Centers for Disease Control, "Current Trends Mortality Attributable to HIV Infection/AIDS—United States, 1981–1990," *Morbidity and Mortality Weekly Report* 40, no. 3 (1991): 41–44.

60. D. France, *How to Survive a Plague* (New York: Picador, 2016), 511.

61. D. Brown, "AIDS Death Rate in '97 down 47%," *Washington Post*, October 8, 1998.

62. United Nations Programme on HIV/AIDS, *90-90-90: An Ambitious Treatment Target to Help End the AIDS Epidemic* (Geneva: United Nations Programme on HIV/AIDS, 2014).

63. United Nations Programme on HIV/AIDS, *Global AIDS Strategy 2021–2026: End Inequalities. End AIDS* (Geneva: United Nations Programme on HIV/AIDS, 2021).

64. Centers for Disease Control and Prevention, "Monitoring Selected National HIV Prevention and Care Objectives by Using HIV Surveillance Data—United States and 6 Dependent Areas, 2019," *HIV Surveillance Supplemental Report 2021* 26, no. 2 (May 2021), http://www.cdc.gov/hiv/library/reports/hiv-surveillance.html.

65. T. Straube, "How Did 12 U.S. Cities Do in Reaching Their 90-90-90 HIV Goals?," *POZ*, December 3, 2020.

66. United Nations Programme on HIV/AIDS, *Global AIDS Strategy 2021–2026*.

67. M. C. Sullivan, A. O. Rosen, A. Allen, D. Benbella, G. Camacho, A. C. Cortopassi, R. Driver, et al., "Falling Short of the First 90: HIV Stigma and HIV Testing Research in the 90-90-90 Era," *AIDS and Behavior* 24, no. 2 (2020): 357–362.

68. J. Chikovore, N. Gillespie, N. McGrath, J. Orne-Gliemann, T. Zuma, and ANRS 12249 TasP Study Group, "Men, Masculinity, and Engagement with Treatment as Prevention in KwaZulu-Natal, South Africa," *AIDS Care* 28, supp. 3 (2016): 74–82; P. Mambanga, R. N. Sirwali, and T. Tshitangano, "Factors Contributing to Men's Reluctance to Seek HIV Counselling and Testing at Primary Health Care Facilities in Vhembe District of South Africa," *African Journal of Primary Health Care and Family Medicine* 8, no. 2 (2016): 1–7.

69. M. L. Ekstrand, E. Heylen, A. Mazur, W. T. Steward, C. Carpenter, K. Yadav, S. Sinha, et al., "The Role of HIV Stigma in ART Adherence and Quality of Life among Rural Women Living with HIV in India," *AIDS and Behavior* 22, no. 12 (2018): 3859–3868.

70. S. Kumar, R. Mohanraj, D. Rao, K. R. Murray, and L. E. Manhart, "Positive Coping Strategies and HIV-Related Stigma in South India," *AIDS Patient Care and STDs* 29, no. 3 (2015): 157–163.

71. M. M. Kavanagh, S. C. Agbla, M. Joy, K. Aneja, M. Pillinger, A. Case, N. A. Erondu, et al., "Law, Criminalisation and HIV in the World: Have Countries That Criminalise Achieved More or Less Successful Pandemic Response?," *BMJ Global Health* 6, no. 8 (2021): e006315.

72. United Nations Programme on HIV/AIDS, *Global AIDS Strategy 2021–2026*.

73. Center for HIV Law and Policy, "Map: HIV Criminalization in the United States," 2022, https://www.hivlawandpolicy.org/resources/map-hiv-criminalization-united-states-chlp-2022.

74. United Nations Programme on HIV/AIDS, "UNAIDS Report on the Global AIDS Epidemic Shows That 2020 Targets Will Not Be Met Because of Deeply Unequal Success; COVID-19 Risks Blowing HIV Progress Way Off Course," press release, 2020.

Chapter 8

1. J. M. Engelmann, and E. Herrmann, "Chimpanzees Trust Their Friends," *Current Biology* 26, no. 2 (2016): 252–256.

2. R. Bshary, and A. S. Grutter, "Image Scoring and Cooperation in a Cleaner Fish Mutualism," *Nature* 441, no. 7096 (2006): 975–978.

3. L. A. Bates, K. N. Sayialel, N. W. Njiraini, C. J. Moss, J. H. Poole, and R. W. Byrne, "Elephants Classify Human Ethnic Groups by Odor and Garment Color," *Current Biology* 17, no. 22 (2007): 1938–1942.

4. J. H. Turner, *Human Institutions: A Theory of Societal Evolution* (Lanham, MD: Rowman and Littlefield, 2003), 2.

5. G. Leonetti, M. Signoli, A. L. Pelissier, P. Champsaur, I. Hershkovitz, C. Brunet, and O. Dutour, "Evidence of Pin Implantation as a Means of Verifying Death during the Great Plague of Marseilles (1722)," *Journal of Forensic Science* 42, no. 2 (1997): 744–748.

6. A. Mazque, "In Pictures: A Look Back, One Year after France Went into Lockdown," *France 24*, March 17, 2021, https://www.france24.com/en/france/20210317 -in-pictures-a-look-back-one-year-after-france-went-into-lockdown.

7. P. Peretti-Watel, P. Verger, and O. Launay, "The French General Population's Attitudes toward Lockdown against COVID-19: A Fragile Consensus," *BMC Public Health* 20, no. 1 (2020): 1–8.

8. P. S. Sehdev, "The Origin of Quarantine," *Clinical Infectious Diseases* 35, no. 9 (2002): 1071–1072.

9. Z. Blažina-Tomić and V. Blažina, *Expelling the Plague: The Health Office and the Implementation of Quarantine in Dubrovnik, 1377–1533* (Montreal: McGill-Queen's University Press, 2015).

10. Sehdev, "The Origin of Quarantine."

11. Blažina-Tomić and Blažina, *Expelling the Plague.*

12. P. Slack, "Perceptions of Plague in Eighteenth-Century Europe," *Economic History Review* 75, no. 1 (2022): 138–156.

13. Sehdev, "The Origin of Quarantine."

14. D. G. McNeil Jr., "Using a Tactic Unseen in a Century, Countries Cordon off Ebola-Racked Areas," *New York Times*, August 12, 2014, https://www.nytimes.com /2014/08/13/science/using-a-tactic-unseen-in-a-century-countries-cordon-off-ebola -racked-areas.html.

15. B. Espinoza, C. Castillo-Chavez, and C. Perrings, "Mobility Restrictions for the Control of Epidemics: When Do They Work?," *PLoS One* 15, no. 7 (2020): e0235731.

16. B. Espinoza, V. Moreno, D. Bichara, and C. Castillo-Chavez, "Assessing the Effi-ciency of Movement Restriction as a Control Strategy of Ebola," in *Mathematical and Statistical Modeling for Emerging and Re-emerging Infectious Diseases* (Cham, Switzer-land: Springer, 2016), 123–145.

17. D. Hoffman, "A Crouching Village: Ebola and the Empty Gestures of Quarantine in Monrovia," *City and Society* 28, no. 2 (2016): 246–264.

18. N. Onishi, "As Ebola Grips Liberia's Capital, a Quarantine Sows Social Chaos," *New York Times*, August 28, 2014, https://www.nytimes.com/2014/08/29/world/africa /in-liberias-capital-an-ebola-outbreak-like-no-other.html.

19. Hoffman, "A Crouching Village."

20. "Liberia's West Point Slum Reels from the Nightmare of Ebola," *TIME*, August 22, 2014, https://time.com/3158244/liberia-west-point-slum-ebola-disease-quarantine.

21. S. Fink, "With Aid Doctors Gone, Ebola Fight Grows Harder," *New York Times*, August 16, 2014, https://www.nytimes.com/2014/08/17/world/africa/with-aid-doctors -gone-ebola-fight-grows-harder.html.

22. A. Leaf, "Ebola Spotlights Liberians' Distrust of Their Political Leaders," *Al-Jazeera America*, October 14, 2014, http://america.aljazeera.com/opinions/2014/10 /liberia-ebola-ellenjohnsonsirleafunconstitutionalpowergrab.html.

23. IRIN News, "Disease Rife as More People Squeeze into Fewer Toilets," *New Humanitarian*, November 19, 2014, https://www.thenewhumanitarian.org/news/2009 /11/19/disease-rife-more-people-squeeze-fewer-toilets.

24. Hoffman, "A Crouching Village."

25. Quoted in Onishi, "As Ebola Grips Liberia's Capital, a Quarantine Sows Social Chaos."

26. Hoffman, "A Crouching Village."

27. Leaf, "Ebola Spotlights Liberians' Distrust of Their Political Leaders."

28. S. Towers, O. Patterson-Lomba, and C. Castillo-Chavez, "Temporal Variations in the Effective Reproduction Number of the 2014 West Africa Ebola Outbreak," *PLoS Currents* 6, https://currents.plos.org/outbreaks/article/temporal-variations-in-the -effective-reproduction-number-of-the-2014-west-africa-ebola-outbreak.

29. S. L. Plotkin and S. A. Plotkin, "A Short History of Vaccination," in *Plotkin's Vac-cines*, ed. W. A. Orenstein, P. A. Offit, K. M. Edwards, and S. A. Plotkin (Amsterdam: Elsevier, 2004), 1–16.

30. S. Riedel, "Edward Jenner and the History of Smallpox and Vaccination," in *Baylor University Medical Center Proceedings*, no. 1 (Milton Park, UK: Taylor and Fran-cis, 2005), 18:21–25.

31. E. A. Fenn, *Pox Americana: The Great Smallpox Epidemic of 1775–82* (New York: Macmillan, 2001.

32. Plotkin and Plotkin, "A Short History of Vaccination."

33. Riedel, "Edward Jenner."

34. R. M. Wolfe and L. K. "Anti-Vaccinationists Past and Present," *British Medical Journal* 325, no. 7361 (2002): 430–432.

35. Plotkin and Plotkin, "A Short History of Vaccination."

36. Plotkin and Plotkin, "A Short History of Vaccination."

37. G. L. Geison, *The Private Science of Louis Pasteur* (Princeton, NJ: Princeton University Press, 2014).

38. H. K. Beecher, "Ethics and Clinical Research," in *Biomedical Ethics and the Law*, ed. J. M. Number and R. F. Almeder (Boston: Springer, 1966), 215–227.

39. J. Harkness, S. E. Lederer, and D. Wikler, "Laying Ethical Foundations for Clinical Research," *Bulletin of the World Health Organization* 79 (2001): 365–366.

40. S. Tibi, "Al-Razi and Islamic Medicine in the 9th Century," *Journal of the Royal Society of Medicine* 99, no. 4 (2006): 206–207.

41. M. M. Sajadi, D. Mansouri, and M. R. M. Sajadi, "Ibn Sina and the Clinical Trial," *Annals of Internal Medicine* 150, no. 9 (2009): 640–643.

42. In the 1830s, many people still accepted miasma theory, believing that infectious diseases spread through bad airs and foul smells. It wasn't until 1854 that physician John Snow demonstrated the link between cholera and contaminated drinking water. Snow's groundbreaking contributions to epidemiology are memorialized by a replica of the water pump that he identified as the source of London's 1854 cholera epidemic, located outside a Soho pub renamed as the John Snow on the centenary of his discovery.

43. S. K. Cohn Jr., "Cholera Revolts: A Class Struggle We May Not Like," *Social History* 42, no. 2 (2017): 162–180.

44. S. Burrell and G. Gill, "The Liverpool Cholera Epidemic of 1832 and Anatomical Dissection—Medical Mistrust and Civil Unrest," *Journal of the History of Medicine and Allied Sciences* 60, no. 4 (2005): 478–498.

45. G. Gill, S. Burrell, and J. Brown, "Fear and Frustration—The Liverpool Cholera Riots of 1832," *Lancet* 358, no. 9277 (2001): 233–237; Burrell and Gill, "The Liverpool Cholera Epidemic of 1832 and Anatomical Dissection."

46. Ironically, after Burke was hanged for his crimes in 1829, his body was publicly dissected. His skeleton is currently on display at the Anatomical Museum of the University of Edinburgh.

47. J. Philp, "Bodies and Bureaucracy: The Demise of the Body Snatchers in Nineteenth Century Britain," *Anatomical Record* 305, no. 4 (2022): 827–837.

48. Burrell and Gill, "The Liverpool Cholera Epidemic of 1832 and Anatomical Dissection."

49. Philp, "Bodies and Bureaucracy."

50. Gill, Burrell, and Brown, "Fear and Frustration."

51. "Cholera Subjects," *Morning Chronicle*, March 24, 1832, https://www.newspapers .com/image/393076000.

52. Burrell and Gill, "The Liverpool Cholera Epidemic of 1832 and Anatomical Dissection."

53. S. Boseley, "'Grotesque' Breach of Trust at Alder Hey," *Guardian*, January 29, 2001, https://www.theguardian.com/society/2001/jan/29/health.alderhey.

54. M. Sappol, *A Traffic of Dead Bodies: Anatomy and Embodied Social Identity in Nineteenth-Century America* (Princeton, NJ: Princeton University Press, 2002), 4.

55. C. Stantis, C. de la Cova, D. Lippert, and S. B. Sholts, "Biological Anthropology Must Reassess Museum Collections for a More Ethical Future," *Nature Ecology & Evolution* 7, no. 6 (2023): 786–789.

56. J. Jones, *Bad Blood: The Scandalous Story of the Tuskegee Experiment* (New York: Free Press, 1981), 220.

57. Jones, *Bad Blood*, 93.

58. H. Smith, "Bill Jenkins, Epidemiologist Who Tried to End Tuskegee Syphilis Study, Dies at 73," *Washington Post*, February 27, 2019, https://www.washingtonpost .com/local/obituaries/bill-jenkins-epidemiologist-who-tried-to-end-tuskegee-syphilis -study-dies-at-73/2019/02/27/2319e142-3aa2-11e9-a06c-3ec8ed509d15_story.html.

59. Contrary to popular belief, the participants in the Tuskegee Syphilis Study weren't purposefully infected with syphilis as part of the experiment. The US Public Health Service, however, did *exactly this* in contemporaneous experiments in Guatemala, again without informed consent by the participants. The US STD Research in Guatemala was conducted in partnership with the Pan-American Sanitary Bureau (now the Pan-American Health Organization), with support from a National Institutes of Health grant and cooperation from the Guatemalan government, from 1946 to 1948. Sex workers who already had sexually transmitted diseases (STDs) were paid to have sex with and ideally infect prisoners, mental patients, and soldiers in order to see if penicillin could cure early syphilis and prevent other STDs. At least thirteen hundred subjects were infected with an STD through the experiments, and little more than half of them were treated. The experiments were brought to light

by historian Susan Reverby in 2010, thereby leading—like the Tuskegee Study—to formal investigations, apologies, and lawsuits.

60. J. Heller, "Syphilis Victims in U.S. Study Went Untreated for 40 Years," *New York Times*, July 26, 1972, https://www.nytimes.com/1972/07/26/archives/syphilis-victims-in-us-study-went-untreated-for-40-years-syphilis.html?_r=0.

61. V. N. Gamble, "Under the Shadow of Tuskegee: African Americans and Health Care," *American Journal of Public Health* 87, no. 11 (1997): 1773–1778.

62. H. A. Washington, *Medical Apartheid: The Dark History of Medical Experimentation on Black Americans from Colonial Times to the Present* (New York: Doubleday Books, 2006).

63. C. J. Jones Carney, "The Role of Experimentation and Medical Mistrust in COVID-19 Vaccine Skepticism," *Elm*, January 4, 2021, https://elm.umaryland.edu/voices-and-opinions/Voices--Opinions-Content/The-Role-of-Experimentation-and-Medical-Mistrust-in-COVID-19-Vaccine-Skepticism-.php.

64. K. M. Hoffman, S. Trawalter, J. R. Axt, and M. Norman Oliver, "Racial Bias in Pain Assessment and Treatment Recommendations, and False Beliefs about Biological Differences between Blacks and Whites," *Proceedings of the National Academy of Sciences* 113, no. 116 (2016): 4296–4301.

65. "The AIDS 'Plot' against Blacks," *New York Times*, May 12, 1992, https://www.nytimes.com/1992/05/12/opinion/the-aids-plot-against-blacks.html.

66. Jones Carney, "The Role of Experimentation and Medical Mistrust in COVID-19 Vaccine Skepticism."

67. "The Science of Vaccines," Smithsonian National Museum of Natural History, webinar, June 23, 2020, https://naturalhistory.si.edu/education/after-hours/video-webinars-outbreak-epidemics-connected-world/science-vaccines.

68. L. R. Baden, H. M. El Sahly, B. Essink, K. Kotloff, S. Frey, R. Novak, D. Diemert, et al., "Efficacy and Safety of the mRNA-1273 SARS-CoV-2 Vaccine," *New England Journal of Medicine* 384, no. 5 (2021): 403–416.

69. R. A. Oppel Jr., R. Gebeloff, K. K. R. Lai, W. Wright, and M. Smith, "The Fullest Look Yet at the Racial Inequity of Coronavirus," *New York Times*, July 5, 2020, https://www.nytimes.com/interactive/2020/07/05/us/coronavirus-latinos-african-americans-cdc-data.html.

70. K. S. Corbett, "Everything You Should Know about COVID-19 Vaccines," https://www.youtube.com/watch?v=pL-B30EXBEc.

71. "Black Scientists Matter with Dr. Kizzmekia Corbett," *America Dissected*, podcast, January 5, 2021, https://crooked.com/podcast/black-scientists-matter-with-dr-kizzmekia-corbett.

72. The term *herd immunity* tends to ruffle feathers, so to speak, because of the connotation with herd animals and specifically livestock. It's no coincidence that the concept originated in veterinary medicine as a solution to contagious threats to cattle and sheep, and then was later incorporated into public health language. Many public health professionals avoid the term, however, and favor *community immunity* as more appropriate for human populations.

Chapter 9

1. E. O. Wilson, *Sociobiology: The New Synthesis* (Cambridge, MA: Harvard University Press, 2000), 379.

2. A. Koto, D. Mersch, B. Hollis, and L. Keller, "Social Isolation Causes Mortality by Disrupting Energy Homeostasis in Ants," *Behavioral Ecology and Sociobiology* 69, no. 4 (2015): 583–591.

3. Wilson, *Sociobiology*, 380.

4. D. S. Wilson, *Does Altruism Exist?: Culture, Genes, and the Welfare of Others* (New Haven, CT: Yale University Press, 2015), 72.

5. M. Tomasello, *A Natural History of Human Thinking* (Cambridge, MA: Harvard University Press, 2014), 48.

6. C. Darwin. *The Descent of Man* (London: Penguin Classics, 2004), 157.

7. D. S. Wilson and E. O. Wilson, "Rethinking the Theoretical Foundation of Sociobiology," *Quarterly Review of Biology* 82, no. 4 (2007): 327–348.

8. K. Kupperschmidt and J. Cohen, "China's Aggressive Measures Have Slowed the Coronavirus. They May Not Work in Other Countries," *Science*, March 2, 2020, https://www.science.org/content/article/china-s-aggressive-measures-have-slowed -coronavirus-they-may-not-work-other-countries.

9. E. Yong, "We Live in a Patchwork Pandemic Now," *Atlantic*, May 20, 2020, https://www.theatlantic.com/health/archive/2020/05/patchwork-pandemic-states -reopening-inequalities/611866.

10. L. Sun and J. Dawsey, "New Face Mask Guidance Comes after Battle between White House and CDC," *Washington Post*, April 3, 2020, https://www.washington post.com/health/2020/04/03/white-house-cdc-turf-battle-over-guidance-broad-use -face-masks-fight-coronavirus.

11. "Coronavirus Update with CDC Director, Robert R. Redfield, MD," *JAMA Network*, July 14, 2020, https://www.youtube.com/watch?v=jzHIhSZ_fiA.

12. J. T. Brooks, J. C. Butler, and R. R. Redfield, "Universal Masking to Prevent SARS-CoV-2 Transmission—The Time Is Now," *JAMA* 324, no. 7 (2020): 635–637.

13. "Which Countries Have Made Wearing Face Masks Compulsory?," *Al Jazeera*, August 17, 2020, https://www.aljazeera.com/news/2020/8/17/which-countries-have -made-wearing-face-masks-compulsory.

14. Quoted in N. Robertson, "Trump Doesn't Think US Needs a National Mask Mandate," July 18, 2020, https://www.cnn.com/2020/07/18/politics/trump-us-mask -mandate-coronavirus/index.html.

15. M. D. Shear and S. Mervosh, "Trump Encourages Protest against Governors Who Have Imposed Virus Restrictions," April 17, 2020, https://www.nytimes.com /2020/04/17/us/politics/trump-coronavirus-governors.html.

16. E. Stewart, "Anti-Maskers Explain Themselves," *Vox*, August 7, 2020, https:// www.vox.com/the-goods/2020/8/7/21357400/anti-mask-protest-rallies-donald -trump-COVID-19.

17. *Global Peace Index 2021: Measuring Peace in a Complex World* (Sydney: Institute for Economics and Peace, June 2021), http://visionofhumanity.org/reports.

18. R. Schraer, "COVID: Conspiracy and Untruths Drive Europe's COVID Protests," *BBC News*, November 27, 2021, https://www.bbc.com/news/59390968.

19. Lowry Institute, "COVID Performance Index," March 13, 2021, https://interac tives.lowyinstitute.org/features/covid-performance.

20. E. J. Abbey, B. A. Khalifa, M. O. Oduwole, S. K. Ayeh, R. D. Nudotor, E. L. Salia, O. Lasisi, et al., "The Global Health Security Index Is Not Predictive of Coronavirus Pandemic Responses among Organization for Economic Cooperation and Develop-ment Countries," *PloS One* 15, no. 10 (2020): e0239398.

21. Y. Wang, "Falling for China's Fake COVID-19 News Was Dangerous and Prevent-able," *Quartz*, April 30, 2020, https://qz.com/1847439/trump-blaming-china-for-fake -COVID-19-news-misses-the-point.

22. "China COVID-19: How State Media and Censorship Took on Coronavirus," *BBC News*, December 29, 2020, https://www.bbc.com/news/world-asia-china-55355401.

23. F. Fang and E. W. Zeller, *Wuhan Diary: Dispatches from a Quarantined City*, trans. M. Berry (New York: HarperCollins, 2020), 132.

24. Quoted in Kupperschmidt and Cohen, "China's Aggressive Measures Have Slowed the Coronavirus."

25. Quoted in Kupperschmidt and Cohen, "China's Aggressive Measures Have Slowed the Coronavirus."

26. L. Kuo, "China Shuts Down Talk of COVID Hardship; Users Strike Back," *Wash-ington Post*, May 12, 2022, https://www.washingtonpost.com/world/interactive/2022 /china-coronavirus-voices-of-april-shanghai.

27. J. Liu and P. Mozur, "Shanghai's Lockdown Tests COVID-Zero Policy, and People's Limits," *New York Times*, March 29, 2022, https://www.nytimes.com/2022 /03/29/world/asia/china-shanghai-covid-lockdown.html?searchResultPosition=2.

28. J. Yeung, "China's Lockdown Protests: What You Need to Know," CNN, November 29, 2022, https://www.cnn.com/2022/11/28/china/china-lockdown-protests -covid-explainer-intl-hnk/index.html.

29. L. Kuo, "Why China Dumped Its 'Zero COVID' Policy So Suddenly—and Disastrously," *Washington Post*, January 19, 2023, https://www.washingtonpost.com/world /2023/01/19/why-china-ended-zero-covid.

30. J. Glanz, M. Hvistendahl, and A. Chang, "How Deadly Was China's COVID Wave?," *New York Times*, February 15, 2023, https://www.nytimes.com/interactive /2023/02/15/world/asia/china-covid-death-estimates.html.

31. M. Zastrow, "South Korea Is Reporting Intimate Details of COVID-19 Cases: Has It Helped?," *Nature*, March 18, 2020, https://www.nature.com/articles/d41586 -020-00740-y.

32. J.-H. Kim, J. A.-R. An, S. J. Oh, J. Oh, and J.-K. Lee, "Emerging COVID-19 Success Story: South Korea Learned the Lessons of MERS," Our World in Data, March 5, 2020, https://ourworldindata.org/covid-exemplar-south-korea.

33. M. G. Baker, N. Wilson, and A. Anglemyer, "Successful Elimination of COVID-19 Transmission in New Zealand," *New England Journal of Medicine* 383, no. 8 (2020): e56.

34. J. Lynch, "Newshub-Reid Research Poll: Overwhelming Number of Kiwis Back Government's Lockdown Decision," *Newshub*, May 18, 2020, https://www.newshub .co.nz/home/politics/2020/05/newshub-reid-research-poll-overwhelming-number -of-kiwis-back-government-s-lockdown-decision.html.

35. M. Miller, "Ardern's COVID Policy Was Her 'Greatest Legacy'—but Also Her Undoing," *Washington Post*, January 20, 2023, https://www.washingtonpost.com /world/2023/01/20/jacinda-ardern-new-zealand-covid-resignation.

36. Quoted in Miller, "Ardern's COVID Policy Was Her 'Greatest Legacy.'"

37. J. G. Lu, P. Jin, and A. S. English, "Collectivism Predicts Mask Use during COVID-19," *Proceedings of the National Academy of Sciences* 118, no. 23 (2021).

38. E. D. Vargas and E. R. Sanchez, "American Individualism Is an Obstacle to Wider Mask Wearing in the US," Brookings, August 13, 2020, https://www.brookings.edu /blog/up-front/2020/08/31/american-individualism-is-an-obstacle-to-wider-mask -wearing-in-the-us.

39. M. Hamilton and P. Offit, "You Do Not Have the 'Constitutional Right' to Refuse the COVID-19 Vaccine," CNN August 25, 2021, https://www.cnn.com/2021/08/25

/opinions/unvaccinated-cant-use-constitutional-rights-excuse-hamilton-offit/index
.html.

40. Lu, Jin, and English, "Collectivism Predicts Mask Use during COVID-19."

41. L. Huang, O. Z. Li, B. Wang, and Z. Zhang, "Individualism and the Fight against COVID-19," *Humanities and Social Sciences Communications* 9, no. 1 (2022): 1–20.

42. H. Ritchie, E. Mathieu, L. Rodés-Guirao, C. Appel, C. Giattino, E. Ortiz-Ospina, J. Hasell, et al., "Coronavirus (COVID-19) Deaths." Our World in Data, https://our worldindata.org/covid-deaths.

43. G. Lopez, "The 6 Reasons Americans Aren't Getting Vaccinated," *Vox*, June 2, 2021, https://www.vox.com/2021/6/2/22463223/COVID-19-vaccine-hesitancy-reasons-why.

44. R. M. Wolfe and L. K. Sharp, "Anti-Vaccinationists Past and Present," *British Medical Journal* 325, no. 7361 (2002): 430–432.

45. D. A. Salmon, S. P. Teret, C. R. MacIntyre, D. Salisbury, M. A. Burgess, and N. A. Halsey, "Compulsory Vaccination and Conscientious or Philosophical Exemptions: Past, Present, and Future," *Lancet* 367, no. 9508 (2006): 436–442.

46. G. Iacobucci, "COVID-19: Government Abandons Mandatory Vaccination of NHS Staff," *British Medical Journal* 376 (2022): o269.

47. "Henning Jacobson Loses His Fight with the Board of Public Health over Vaccination," New England Historical Society, accessed May 18, 2022, https://www .newenglandhistoricalsociety.com/henning-jacobson-loses-his-freedom-to-the -board-of-public-health.

48. Quoted in Jacobson v. Massachusetts, 197 U.S. 11 (1905), accessed May 18, 2022, https://supreme.justia.com/cases/federal/us/197/11/#tab-opinion-1921099.

49. Jacobson v. Massachusetts.

50. C. Hauser, "The Mask Slackers of 1918," *New York Times*, August 3, 2020, https:// www.nytimes.com/2020/08/03/us/mask-protests-1918.html.

51. Quoted in *Journal of Proceedings Board of Supervisors*, City and County of San Francisco, January 6, 1919, 50.

52. Quoted in *Journal of Proceedings Board of Supervisors*, 50.

53. J. W. Leavitt, *Typhoid Mary: Captive to the Public's Health* (Boston: Beacon Press, 1997).

54. Leavitt, *Typhoid Mary*.

55. "Guide a Walking Typhoid Factory," *New York Times*, December 2, 1910, https://timesmachine.nytimes.com/timesmachine/1910/12/02/105101972.html ?pageNumber=6.

56. Leavitt, *Typhoid Mary*, 50.

57. Leavitt, *Typhoid Mary*, 245.

58. R. Nelson, "A Microbe Proved That Individualism is a Myth," *Scientific American* 326, no. 3 (2022): 32–33.

59. Quoted in A. D. Sorkin, "Anthony Fauci Issues a New Coronavirus Plea," *New Yorker*, July 1, 2020, https://www.newyorker.com/news/daily-comment/as-trumps-hostility-to-masks-fuels-a-public-health-nihilism-fauci-issues-a-new-plea.

60. Y. Maaravi, A. Levy, T. Gur, D. Confino, and S. Segal, "'The Tragedy of the Commons': How Individualism and Collectivism Affected the Spread of the COVID-19 Pandemic," *Frontiers in Public Health* 9, no. 37 (2021).

61. P. Borah, J. Hwang, and Y. C. Hsu, "COVID-19 Vaccination Attitudes and Intention: Message Framing and the Moderating Role of Perceived Vaccine Benefits," *Journal of Health Communication* 26, no. 8 (2021): 523–533.

62. P. Borah, "Message Framing and COVID-19 Vaccination Intention: Moderating Roles of Partisan Media Use and Pre-Attitudes about Vaccination," *Current Psychology* (2022): 1–10.

63. A. Waytz, R. Iyer, L. Young, J. Haidt, and J. Graham, "Ideological Differences in the Expanse of the Moral Circle," *Nature Communications* 10, no. 1 (2019): 1–12.

64. A. Connaughton, "Those on Ideological Right Favor Fewer COVID-19 Restrictions in Most Advanced Economies," Pew Research Center, July 30, 2021, https://www.pewresearch.org/fact-tank/2021/07/30/those-on-ideological-right-favor-fewer-COVID-19-restrictions-in-most-advanced-economies.

65. K. H. Jamieson, and D. Albarracin, "The Relation between Media Consumption and Misinformation at the Outset of the SARS-CoV-2 Pandemic in the US," *Harvard Kennedy School Misinformation Review*, April 20, 2020, https://misinforeview.hks.harvard.edu/article/the-relation-between-media-consumption-and-misinformation-at-the-outset-of-the-sars-cov-2-pandemic-in-the-us.

66. J. Kates, J. Tolbert, and K. Orgera, "The Red/Blue Divide in COVID-19 Vaccination Rates," Kaiser Family Foundation, January 19, 2022, https://www.kff.org/policy-watch/the-red-blue-divide-in-COVID-19-vaccination-rates-continues-an-update.

Chapter 10

1. U. K. Ecker, S. Lewandowsky, J. Cook, P. Schmid, L. K. Fazio, N. Brashier, P. Kendeou, et al., "The Psychological Drivers of Misinformation Belief and Its Resistance to Correction," *Nature Reviews Psychology* 1, no. 1 (2022): 13–29.

2. A. Pope, *An Essay on Criticism* (1711), Project Gutenberg, February 8, 2015, e-book #7409, https://www.gutenberg.org/files/7409/7409-h/7409-h.htm.

3. E. M. Papper, "The Influence of Chronic Illness upon the Writings of Alexander Pope," *Journal of the Royal Society of Medicine* 82, no. 6 (1989): 359–361.

4. R. DiResta, "It's Not Misinformation. It's Amplified Propaganda," *Atlantic*, October 9, 2021, https://www.theatlantic.com/ideas/archive/2021/10/disinformation-propaganda-amplification-ampliganda/620334.

5. Ecker et al., "The Psychological Drivers of Misinformation Belief and Its Resistance to Correction."

6. World Health Organization, "Health Topics: Infodemic," 2022, https://www.who.int/health-topics/infodemic#tab=tab_1.

7. R. Bruns, D. Hosangadi, M. Trotochaud, and T. Kirk Sell, "COVID-19 Vaccine Misinformation and Disinformation Costs an Estimated $50 to $300 Million Each Day," Johns Hopkins Center for Health Security, 2021, https://www.centerforhealthsecurity.org/sites/default/files/2023-02/20211020-misinformation-disinformation-cost.pdf.

8. P. J. Hotez, *The Deadly Rise of Anti-Science: A Scientist's Warning* (Baltimore: Johns Hopkins University Press, 2023).

9. H. Kaas, "From Mice to Men: The Evolution of the Large, Complex Human Brain," *Journal of Biosciences* 30, no. 2 (2005): 155–165.

10. Kaas, "From Mice to Men."

11. S. Herculano-Houzel, *The Human Advantage: A New Understanding of How Our Brain Became Remarkable* (Cambridge, MA: MIT Press, 2016), 24.

12. S. Neubauer, J. J. Hublin, and P. Gunz, "The Evolution of Modern Human Brain Shape," *Science Advances* 4, no. 1 (2018): eaao5961.

13. Neubauer, Hublin, and Gunz, "The Evolution of Modern Human Brain Shape."

14. C. Packer and J. Clottes, "When Lions Ruled France," *Natural History* 109, no. 9 (2000): 52–57.

15. T. Klingberg, *The Overflowing Brain: Information Overload and the Limits of Working Memory* (Oxford: Oxford University Press, 2009), 84.

16. Whereas adaptations are features that evolved through natural selection to increase survival and reproduction (that is, fitness) in specific environments and ecosystems, evolutionary by-products are carried along with these features without providing any fitness benefits of their own. For instance, the umbilical cord evolved to provide nutrients from a mother to her in utero offspring, while the functionless belly button is a by-product of this adaptation. See J. W. van Prooijen and M. van Vugt, "Conspiracy Theories: Evolved Functions and Psychological Mechanisms," *Perspectives on Psychological Science* 13, no. 6 (2018): 770–788.

17. Klingberg, *The Overflowing Brain*, 100.

18. T. Elbert, C. Pantev, C. Wienbruch, B. Rockstroh, and E. Taub, "Increased Cortical Representation of the Fingers of the Left Hand in String Players," *Science* 270, no. 5234 (1995): 305–307.

19. D. Bogdan, G. Christian, B. Volker, S. Gerhard, B. Ulrich, and M. Arne, "Neuroplasticity: Changes in Grey Matter Induced by Training," *Nature* 427, no. 6972 (2004): 311–312.

20. Klingberg, *The Overflowing Brain*, 11.

21. R. Marois and J. Ivanoff, "Capacity Limits of Information Processing in the Brain," *Trends in Cognitive Sciences* 9, no. 6 (2005): 296–305.

22. S. Dehaene, *How We Learn: The New Science of Education and the Brain* (London: Penguin, 2020).

23. W. James, *The Principles of Psychology, Volume 1* (1890), Project Gutenberg, August 2, 2018, e-book #57628, 403, https://www.gutenberg.org/files/57628/57628-h/57628 -h.htm.

24. J. Swift, "Number XIV," *Examiner*, November 9, 1710, https://en.wikisource.org /wiki/The_Works_of_the_Rev._Jonathan_Swift/Volume_3/The_Examiner.

25. S. Vosoughi, D. Roy, and S. Aral, "The Spread of True and False News Online," *Science* 359, no. 6380 (2018): 1146–1151.

26. C. Ranganath and G. Rainer, "Neural Mechanisms for Detecting and Remembering Novel Events," *Nature Reviews Neuroscience* 4, no. 3 (2003): 193–202.

27. L. Itti and P. Baldi, "Bayesian Surprise Attracts Human Attention," *Vision Research* 49, no. 10 (2009): 1295–1306.

28. Ranganath and Rainer, "Neural Mechanisms for Detecting and Remembering Novel Events."

29. R. P. Ebstein, O. Novick, R. Umansky, B. Priel, Y. Osher, D. Blaine, E. R. Bennett, et al., "Dopamine D4 Receptor (D4DR) Exon III Polymorphism Associated with the Human Personality Trait of Novelty Seeking," *Nature Genetics* 12, no. 1 (1996): 78–80; A. Lembke, *Dopamine Nation: Finding Balance in the Age of Indulgence* (New York: Penguin, 2021).

30. Ecker et al., "The Psychological Drivers of Misinformation Belief and Its Resistance to Correction."

31. M. Cinelli, G. De Francisci Morales, A. Galeazzi, W. Quattrociocchi, and M. Starnini, "The Echo Chamber Effect on Social Media," *Proceedings of the National Academy of Sciences* 118, no. 9 (2021): e2023301118, https://www.pnas.org/doi/epdf /10.1073/pnas.2023301118.

32. Pew Research Center, "Many Americans Believe Fake News Is Sowing Confusion," 2016, https://assets.pewresearch.org/wp-content/uploads/sites/13/2016/12/14154753/PJ_2016.12.15_fake-news_FINAL.pdf.

33. G. Pennycook, Z. Epstein, M. Mosleh, A. A. Arechar, D. Eckles, and D. G. Rand, "Shifting Attention to Accuracy Can Reduce Misinformation Online," *Nature* 592, no. 7855 (2021): 590–595.

34. S. Bradshaw and P. N. Howard, "The Global Disinformation Disorder: 2019 Global Inventory of Organised Social Media Manipulation," Working Paper 2019.2, Project on Computational Propaganda, Oxford, UK.

35. J. B. Barnes, "Russian Disinformation Targets Vaccines and the Biden Administration," *New York Times*, August 5, 2021, https://www.nytimes.com/2021/08/05/us/politics/covid-vaccines-russian-disinformation.html.

36. J. W. van Prooijen and K. M. Douglas, "Belief in Conspiracy Theories: Basic Principles of an Emerging Research Domain," *European Journal of Social Psychology* 48, no. 7 (2018): 897–908.

37. Van Prooijen and van Vugt, "Conspiracy Theories."

38. M. P. Mattson, "Superior Pattern Processing Is the Essence of the Evolved Human Brain," *Frontiers in Neuroscience* 8 (2014): 1–17.

39. M. J. Wood, "Propagating and Debunking Conspiracy Theories on Twitter during the 2015–2016 Zika Virus Outbreak," *Cyberpsychology, Behavior, and Social Networking* 21, no. 8 (2018): 485–490.

40. Y. Y. Hong, H. W. Chan, and K. M. Douglas, "Conspiracy Theories about Infectious Diseases: An Introduction," *Journal of Pacific Rim Psychology* 15 (2021): 18344909211057657.

41. World Health Organization, "Multi-Country Monkeypox Outbreak in Non-Endemic Countries: Update," accessed June 1, 2022, https://www.who.int/emergencies/disease-outbreak-news/item/2022-DON388.

42. R. Schraer, "Monkeypox Wasn't Created in a Lab—and Other Claims Debunked," *BBC News*, May 29, 2022, https://www.bbc.com/news/health-61580089.

43. Quoted in A. Slisco, "Marjorie Taylor Greene Pushes Bill Gates Monkeypox Conspiracy," *Newsweek*, May 20, 2022, https://www.newsweek.com/marjorie-taylor-greene-pushes-bill-gates-monkeypox-conspiracy-1708789.

44. There are currently eighty-three species of poxviruses in the *Poxviridae* viral family. And for centuries there was a tradition of naming poxvirus diseases after the animals in which they were first observed, but not necessarily the animals who serve as their principal reservoir hosts. Thus some of the names are misleading. Cowpox virus, for example, is primarily a disease of rodents, but has a wide host range, and

occasionally infects cows, cats, zoo animals, and humans. Likewise, monkeypox (mpox) virus was first identified in monkeys, but rodents are thought to be its main reservoirs in the wild. See F. Fenner, D. A. Henderson, I. Arita, Z. Jezek, and I. D. Ladnyi, *Smallpox and Its Eradication* (Geneva: World Health Organization, 1988), 6:1–1421.

45. H. Branswell, "Warning Signs Ahead of Monkeypox Outbreak Went Unheeded, Experts Say," *STAT*, May 26, 2022, https://www.statnews.com/2022/05/26/warning-signs-ahead-of-monkeypox-outbreak-went-unheeded-experts-say.

46. Fenner et al., *Smallpox and Its Eradication*.

47. D. A. Henderson, *Smallpox: The Death of a Disease: The Inside Story of Eradicating a Worldwide Killer* (Amherst, NY: Prometheus Books, 2009), 254.

48. Henderson, *Smallpox*, 254.

49. M. Bliss, *Plague: A Story of Smallpox in Montreal* (Toronto: HarperCollins, 1991).

50. Bliss, *Plague*, 262.

51. H. MacDougall and L. Monnais, "Not without Risk: The Complex History of Vaccine Resistance in Central Canada, 1885–1960," *Public Health in the Age of Anxiety: Religious and Cultural Roots of Vaccine Hesitancy in Canada*, ed. P. Bramadat, M. Guay, J. A. Bettinger, and R. Roy (Toronto: University of Toronto Press, 2017), 129–161.

52. P. Larsson, "COVID-19 Anti-Vaxxers Use the Same Arguments from 135 Years Ago," *Conversation*, October 4, 2020, https://theconversation.com/COVID-19-anti-vaxxers-use-the-same-arguments-from-135-years-ago-145592.

53. A. M. Ross, *Stop!! A Pitiable Sight! People Driven Like Dumb Animals to the Shambles!! Tyranny of Doctorcraft!!!* (1885), HathiTrust, accessed June 1, 2022, https://catalog.hathitrust.org/Record/100314945.

54. A. M. Ross, *The Anti-Vaccinator, and Advocate of Cleanliness* (October 1885), National Library of Medicine Digital Collections, accessed June 1, 2022, https://collections.nlm.nih.gov/bookviewer?PID=nlm:nlmuid-101235983-bk.

55. J. E. Coderre, *Vaccination: Etude Lue à la Société Médicale de Montréal, les 31 janvier, 14 & 28 février, 1872* (1872), Des presses à vapeur de La Minerve, accessed June 1, 2022, https://babel.hathitrust.org/cgi/pt?id=aeu.ark:/13960/t78s5b18g&view=1up&seq=6&skin=2021.

56. A. Dagenais, "Vaccination: Letter au Docteur Coderre," *L'Union Medicale du Canada* 6, no. 2 (1875): 55–62.

57. J. Emery-Coderre, *Vaccination: Etude Sur les Effets de la Vaccination* (1875), Des presses à vapeur de La Minerve, 15, accessed June 1, 2022, :https://babel.hathitrust.org/cgi/pt?id=aeu.ark:/13960/t05x2pd8x&view=1up&seq=4&skin=2021.

58. J. Marsh, "The 1885 Montreal Smallpox Epidemic, *Canadian Encyclopedia*, 2021, https://www.thecanadianencyclopedia.ca/en/article/plague-the-red-death-strikes-montreal-feature.

59. M. Côté-Gendreau, "Witnessing History through Parish Registers: The 1885 Smallpox Epidemic," *Généalogie et Histoire du Québec: Le Blog l'Institut Drouin*, 2020, https://www.genealogiequebec.com/blog/en/2020/08/03/witnessing-history-through-parish-registers-the-1885-smallpox-epidemic.

60. Both ivermectin and hydroxychloroquine were studied as potential candidates for drug repurposing (that is, identifying novel uses for existing drugs) at the beginning of the COVID-19 pandemic. Although in vitro studies showed that these drugs could block SARS-CoV-2 in cell cultures derived from monkey kidneys, subsequent studies and trials failed to demonstrate that they were beneficial for the prevention or treatment of COVID-19.

61. R. Rubin, "When Physicians Spread Unscientifi Information about COVID-19," *JAMA* 327, no. 10 (2022): 904–906.

62. K. Bibbins-Domingo and P. N. Malani, "At a Higher Dose and Longer Duration, Ivermectin Still Not Effective against COVID-19," *JAMA* (2023), doi:10.1001/jama.2023.1922.

63. "Three Times Vaccinated, Dr. A. M. Ross, of This City, in a New Light," *Gazette*, October 14, 1885, https://www.newspapers.com/image/419312936/?terms=Three%20times%20vaccinated&match=1.

64. S. Sadeque, "Nearly All Fox Staffers Vaccinated for Covid Even as Hosts Cast Doubt on Vaccine," *Guardian*, September 15, 2021, https://www.theguardian.com/media/2021/sep/15/fox-news-vaccines-testing-tucker-carlson.

65. "Smallpox and Its Prophylaxis," *First Annual Report of the State Board of Health of the State of Kansas* (Topeka: Kansas Publishing House, 1886), 126–144, https://babel.hathitrust.org/cgi/pt?id=mdp.39015062312114&view=1up&seq=7&skin=2021.

66. Bliss, *Plague*.

67. "An Absurd Prejudice," *New York Times*, August 17, 1875, https://www.nytimes.com/1875/08/17/archives/an-absurd-prejudice.html.

68. M. Stencel, E. Ryan, and J. Luther, "Misinformation Spreads, but Fact-Checking Has Leveled Off," Duke University Reporters' Lab, June 21, 2023, https://reporterslab.org/misinformation-spreads-but-fact-checking-has-leveled-off.

69. Africa Check, "Africa's First Independent Fact-Checking Organisation," n.d., https://africacheck.org/who-we-are.

70. A. S. Jegede, "What Led to the Nigerian Boycott of the Polio Vaccination Campaign?," *PLoS Medicine* 4, no. 3 (2007): e73, https://www.ncbi.nlm.nih.gov/pmc

/articles/PMC1831725/#:~:text=The%20fear%20of%20vaccines%3A%20Fear
,the%20disease%20from%20West%20Africa.

71. O. Oyebanji, U. Ofonagoro, O. Akande, I. Nsofor, C. Ukenedo, T. B. Mohammed, C. Anueyiagu, et al. "Lay Media Reporting of Monkeypox in Nigeria," *BMJ
Global Health* 4, no. 6 (2019): e002019.

72. World Health Organization, "Let's Flatten the Infodemic Curve," n.d., https://
www.who.int/news-room/spotlight/let-s-flatten-the-infodemic-curve.

Conclusion

1. L. Garrett, *The Coming Plague: Newly Emerging Diseases in a World Out of Balance*
(New York: Farrar, Straus and Giroux, 1994), 6.

2. S. C. Oaks Jr., R. E. Shope, and J. Lederberg, eds., *Emerging Infections: Microbial
Threats to Health in the United States* (Washington, DC: National Academies Press,
1992).

Epilogue

1. J. Lepore, "When Black History Is Unearthed, Who Gets to Speak for the Dead?,"
New Yorker, September 27, 2021, https://www.newyorker.com/magazine/2021/10/04
/when-black-history-is-unearthed-who-gets-to-speak-for-the-dead.

2. J. Barajas, "I Toured This Exhibit on Epidemics before the Coronavirus Pandemic
Shut It Down," *PBS NewsHour*, March 18, 2020, https://www.pbs.org/newshour/arts
/i-toured-this-exhibit-on-epidemics-before-the-coronavirus-pandemic-shut-it-down.

3. Without question, the bullhorn was my favorite object in the show. It originally
belonged to Harvey Milk, the assassinated human rights leader, and symbolized
decades of struggles for social justice. When Jones offered to loan it to us for the
Outbreak exhibit, I cried.

4. When I showed the ASM ambassadors some examples of how the *Outbreak* team
created tactile experiences to attract and hold visitors' attention, such as the colorful
3D models of viruses affixed to text rails, they nodded approvingly. When I admitted to deep concerns about fomite transmission, they nodded knowingly. Keeping
hand sanitizer dispensers filled was a constant and critical challenge, especially
during the COVID-19 pandemic.

5. Nineteen of these programs were recorded and made available on the NMNH's
website, where they continue to live on and educate the public. See "Video Webinars—Outbreak: Epidemics in a Connected World," National Museum of Natural
History, accessed May 14, 2023, https://naturalhistory.si.edu/education/after-hours
/video-webinars-outbreak-epidemics-connected-world.

Index